Essential Values-Based Practice

Clinical Stories linking Science with People

Essential Values-Based Practice

Clinical Stories linking Science with People

K. W. M. (Bill) Fulford
Emeritus Professor of Philosophy and Mental Health, University of Warwick Medical School, UK

Ed Peile
Emeritus Professor of Medical Education, University of Warwick Medical School, UK

Heidi Carroll
General Practitioner, Aberdeenshire, UK

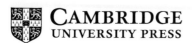

CAMBRIDGE
UNIVERSITY PRESS

CAMBRIDGE UNIVERSITY PRESS
Cambridge, New York, Melbourne, Madrid, Cape Town,
Singapore, São Paulo, Delhi, Mexico City

Cambridge University Press
The Edinburgh Building, Cambridge CB2 8RU, UK

Published in the United States of America by Cambridge University Press, New York

www.cambridge.org
Information on this title: www.cambridge.org/9780521530255

© Cambridge University Press 2012

First published 2012

Printed in the United Kingdom at the University Press, Cambridge

A catalogue record for this publication is available from the British Library

ISBN 978-0-521-53025-5 Paperback

Review quotes

As a primary care physician who has spent over 25 years in the USA caring for patients, teaching, and developing curricula, I am continually searching for strategies to help patients, medical students, and physicians get "unstuck" and get on with the business of healing and health. *Essential Values-based Practice: Linking Science with People* provides coherent tools and frameworks that I am eager to use as a provider, a teacher, and a carer. The values-based practice framework outlined in the premise, the process, and the point offers information that can be used to support self-awareness, reflective practice, and exploration of values – the provider's and the patient's. Alicia D. H. Monroe, MD Vice Dean Educational Affairs, University of South Florida College of Medicine.

"*Essentials* is an outstanding example of clear writing, essential references and useful clinical reasoning." Professor Giovanni Stanghellini, Co-Chair of the World Psychiatric Association (WPA) Section on the Humanities and Chair of the Association of European Psychiatrists (AEP) Section on Philosophy and Psychiatry.

"Constantly reinforce(s) the reality of value issues in everyday practice." Dr Roger Neighbour, Past President Royal College of General Practitioners and author of *The Inner Consultation* and *The Inner Apprentice*.

Contents

Part 5. Bringing it all together

Foreword

Julia Samuel
Founder Patron and Trustee of the Child Bereavement Charity

This is truly brilliant book. In the twenty-first-century medical environment, driven by the dual pulls of high costs and cost effectiveness. Patients can get submerged in technology, protocols, and paperwork, to the extent they lose their humanity and experience themselves as a case number, not a person. This book highlights the challenge medical teams, having a plethora of scientific knowledge, encounter every day when faced with the uniquely human problems of each individual patient. Its guidance puts the heart back into medicine.

My experience with families whose children have died has taught me that, even when medicine fails as tragically as when a child dies, how the family is responded to at the time has a life-long impact on that family, for good or ill. Every conversation, every decision, every gesture is burned in their memory for life. Often the unforgiveable errors are more to do with the lack of attuned care than with medicine: not enough proper reflection on the needs of this family, careless assumptions made, insensitive communication, which might be appropriate for another family, but is received with fury by this particular family, too much haste to get "it over with." Any medical professional reading this book is given both a map and a way of thinking which protects against these all too frequent irrevocable mistakes, and ensures the family receives the best possible care at such a difficult time.

The coherence with which the authors unpick complex and usually intangible, as well as explicit, situations is extraordinary. They keep the same themes running throughout the text, linking and reinforcing them with each case study, giving their arguments a lot of weight. I was fascinated by the different scenarios, which echoed some of my own experiences with patients and made the text come alive and easy to read. They intentionally didn't describe the "nightmare" examples where bad practice, bad stories, and bad outcomes come together, recognizing that it is the more subtle everyday situation that is the key learning in this book, because it is from them that individual patients receive genuine person-centered care.

This book is a hugely welcome clarion call back to the essential values in medicine, that keys into the natural motivation of most doctors, to reach out to the individual patient and make a difference. It is a very impressive book, and I couldn't be more delighted to endorse the importance and value of its messages.

Acknowledgments

The development of values-based practice has been a strongly collaborative enterprise involving a wide range of stakeholders, including patients, carers, clinicians, managers and policy-makers, in the UK and internationally. We are grateful to all these and to the many individual colleagues whose particular contributions are acknowledged in the body of this book or in the website supporting the series (see Prologue).

Early work on developing values-based practice in mental healthcare was generously supported by a number of institutions including the Mental Health Foundation, the Sainsbury Centre for Mental Health, Turning Point, the UK's Department of Health and the World Psychiatric Association. Much of the thinking behind this book was developed through two Warwick-Wellcome conferences, and we gratefully acknowledge the support of both the Wellcome Trust and the Laces Trust in assembling experts from the UK and around the world interested in developing values-based practice in all areas of clinical practice and policy.

The stories at the heart of this book have taken us into areas of practice beyond our respective areas of personal experience and clinical expertise. While the responsibility for any errors remains our own, we are very grateful to the many colleagues from other specialty areas at Warwick Medical School and elsewhere who have given generously of their time and expertise in reviewing either individual chapters or the book as a whole: Gillian Bendelow, Kamaldeep Bhui, Mark Bratton, Matthew Broome, Amanda Burls, Iain Chalmers, Graham Clarke, Janet Cooper, Annabelle Crauford, Jeremy Dale, Peter Gilbert, Christopher Heginbotham, Jeremy Howick, Sally Johnson, Jane Kidd, Malcolm King, Sudhesh Kumar, John Launer, Judith Lees, Alicia Monroe, Daniel Munday, Roger Neighbour, Alec O'Rourke, Vimmi Passi, Mila Petrova, Hanna Pickard, Christopher Poole, John Sadler, Julia Samuel, Ajit Shah, Suzanne Shale, Janet Smith, Anne-Marie Slowther, Lanre Sorinola, Giovanni Stanghellini, Jill Thistlethwaite, Philip Thomas, Jan Trott, Werdie van Staden, Tom Viggiano, Malcolm Walker, Veronica Wilkie and Sue Ziebland

Finally, we want to acknowledge the late Yvonne Carter, who, as the first Dean of Warwick Medical School, worked with and supported us in extending values-based practice from mental health into other areas of health and social care.

A bold claim to start this book

The aim of most patient–clinician consultations is to improve health outcomes. Most often they succeed, and patients are to a greater or lesser extent satisfied and empowered. However, some consultations are unsatisfactory and result in failure to improve health outcomes; dissatisfaction on the part of patients, carers or clinicians; complaints and litigation; and even unnecessary morbidity or mortality.

In our experience, when consultations fail to achieve the desired results, the cause is not usually a failure of evidence-based practice. Today's clinicians are trained in evidence-based medicine, educated, updated and appraised to a point where they can find most of the accurate scientific information they need to assist patients in decision-making. *The most likely reason why things go wrong is a failure of values-based practice* – not ascertaining the relevant values perspectives and acting on them in a coherent and purposeful manner, evolving individual patient-centered decisions that are informed by values as well as evidence.

This book aims to help clinicians acquire and develop the processes of values-based practice that support evidence-based practice in the particular situations facing individual patients.

Prologue: linking science with people

A young woman with schizophrenia finds a turning point towards recovery when a new member of the mental health team recognizes and acknowledges her aspirations.

A middle-aged car sales manager finally engages positively with evidence-based management of his hypertension when a cardiologist appointed through his firm's occupational health scheme links the need for treatment to his ambitions as an amateur racing car enthusiast.

A young couple at risk of being torn apart by conflicting views over IVF are reconciled when their parish priest helps them to understand the real rather than fancied implications of the techniques being proposed by the local infertility clinic.

These are some of the stories – based on those of real people, although biographically disguised – that are at the heart of this book. Each story presents a familiar clinical problem; for each problem, there are a variety of possible evidence-based solutions, but in each case matching solution to problem depends critically on engaging with the *values* of those concerned.

Values, evidence and complexity

There is nothing new as such about values in medicine. The Hippocratic Oath, on which modern codes of practice still draw, goes back over 2000 years. There is similarly nothing new as such about evidence in medicine. David Sackett and his colleagues, in their early and still influential *Evidence-Based Medicine: How to Practice and Teach EBM*, to which we will be returning at several points in this book, locate what is possibly the earliest recorded use of evidence-based methods in ancient Chinese medicine.

What *is* new is the ever-growing complexity of modern health care, and it is this complexity that drives the need equally for values-based and for evidence-based decision-making. We need evidence-based practice as a process for factoring *complex evidence* into individual clinical decision-making; and we need values-based practice as a process for factoring *complex values* into individual clinical decision-making. The actual processes involved are different of course. Values-based practice is different from evidence-based practice in that it relies primarily on learnable clinical skills working within a person-centered and multidisciplinary model of practice. But the essential reliance on good process to support clinical decision-making in the growing complexity of current practice is the same.

Linking science with people

Even before the processes for values-based practice were defined, there were several tools in medicine's toolbox for working with values, including ethics, decision analysis and health economics. We will be returning to these and other tools and to how they fit together with values-based practice at various points in the book.

One of the skills needed by the workman with a plethora of tools is to know *how* to use *which* tool in which sequence to achieve the optimal result. To work the toolbox analogy, the problem facing the carpenter when the door is sticking is *how* to best reduce the size. He has at his disposal saws, chisels, planes and sanders, and the good carpenter will put his hand on the right tool for the job in the right sequence. Values-based practice adds a number of specific tools to the toolbox: for example, not many clinicians carry "dissensus" in their toolbox until they have learnt a bit about values-based practice. But what values-based practice adds above all is an approach or process that focuses on *the unique values of the particular individuals* involved (clinicians, patients and carers) in a given clinical situation.

This is why values-based practice links science with people. The power of science is that it produces knowledge that is generalizable across all relevant cases. But people are unique. Values-based practice thus links the generalizable evidence that we get from science with the unique values – the needs, wishes, preferences, expectations and so forth – of the individual people involved in the particular clinical decisions we make in everyday practice.

What this book covers

This book provides an introduction to values-based practice as a new skills-based approach to working with complex and sometimes conflicting values in health care.

It is not a textbook of values. There is already much that has been written from both theoretical and practical perspectives about values in medicine. We cover much of this in Part 1. This book is about the values of particular individuals – individual patients and their family members, and individual clinicians – and the skills and other resources needed to support balanced decision-making where their (often very different) values come into conflict.

Story lines of the book

In line with the person-centered focus of the book, our core chapters, in Parts 2, 3, 4 and 5, are all built around the stories of individual patients and clinicians. Each story illustrates how a given element of the process of values-based practice sits alongside and complements evidence-based practice in the clinical encounter.

We cover a range of different clinical contexts in both hospital and the community settings, with some of our case histories being overtly value-laden (for example, cross-cultural presentations of abdominal pain, and child protection and multidisciplinary team working) and others less so (for example, compliance in the management of hypertension, and avoiding chronicity with low back pain). But in each case, it is the values (whether overt and/or hidden, and of patient and/or clinician) that are vital to effective evidence-based management of the situation in question.

The five parts of the book

In Part 1, we give an overview of values and values-based practice in medicine, drawing in this instance on the story of a primary care physician or general practitioner (GP), Dr. Gulati, and how she works with a patient, Roy Walker, who is demanding a clinically inappropriate off-work certificate for low back pain. Parts 2–4 then pick up on the details of values-based practice with further stories illustrating each of the key process elements of values-based practice considered individually. Finally, in the two chapters in Part 5, we draw the elements of values-based practice together, first through a story of partnership in decision-making

in end-of-life care, and then by returning to Dr. Gulati from Part 1 and following how she and her colleagues work in partnership with their local Patients' Forum to develop a shared framework of values for their practice.

The book and the series

This book is the launch volume for a new series from Cambridge University Press on values and values-based practice in medicine. The series will be edited by Bill Fulford and Ed Peile with the support of an international advisory board representing each of the main stakeholder groups in values-based practice including patients and carers, clinicians, policy-makers and managers.

Although the stories in this book are mainly UK focused, we believe the issues they raise are important across healthcare in all parts of the world. Through the series as a whole, we will be exploring some of these issues further as they arise in other cultures and systems of healthcare and as they are perceived from the perspectives of patients, carers, managers and policy-makers, as well as from those of clinicians.

Ways of using this book

One way in which the book can be read is by working through sequentially from Chapter 1 and developing your understanding of values-based practice as you go.

As a collection of stories, on the other hand, another way to read the book is by starting from whichever case study is closest to your own clinical or personal experience. Having explored that case in detail, you can then broaden your knowledge of values-based practice by going back to the introductory chapters and working through some of the other case stories in the book.

Although not a textbook as such, the case studies and supporting materials can be used for Continuing Professional Development (CPD) and other teaching and learning activities. To this end, we have included in each of the case histories a number of brief reflection points at which the reader is invited to think about a key issue for themselves before reading on. Each chapter starts with a topic box setting out the main points covered in that chapter. The final chapter, Chapter 14, includes an example of a workshop in values-based practice. Appendix B gives a teaching framework with detailed learning outcomes for each element of values-based practice together with possible methods of assessment. A diagrammatic "map" showing how the elements of values-based practice fit together, which first appears as Fig. 3.4 in the initial overview of values-based practice, is repeated at the start of each subsequent chapter to help you to orientate yourself within the overall approach. You may also want to turn to the end of the book for additional features that you may find helpful in navigating your way around the book:

- Appendix A gives a summary of values-based practice with brief definitions of its key 'terms of art'
- These key terms are highlighted in blue for ease of reference in the index.

The index is backed up by a spreadsheet (the VBP Index Spreadsheet) on the VBP website (see below) showing how each element of values-based practice is introduced, explained and illustrated across the book as a whole.

The book is further supported by the series website jointly hosted by Cambridge University Press and Warwick Medical School at http://www.go.warwick. ac.uk/values-basedpractice/. This includes full-text versions of many of the key sources and resources noted in the individual chapters.

Our characters

In linking the theoretical points to clinical practice, some of our characters may at times seem overly conscientious and self-aware. Dr. Gulati, for example, the GP in our opening Chapters 1 and 2, takes time out to review what she knows about some of the resources from ethics, decision analysis and evidence-based practice that might help her in deciding what she should do about a patient who is demanding a clinically inappropriate off-work certificate.

We could have presented the theoretical points here discursively and, while taking time out might be good "reflective practice," Dr. Gulati's investment in this one case clearly goes beyond what would be possible on a day-to-day basis in a busy inner city general practice. But we hope nonetheless that our narrative presentation of the theoretical points will help to underline the reality of value issues in everyday practice and the strongly practical nature of values-based practice as a resource for responding to them.

It is important to add finally that our characters, although fictional, are all based on experience. As such, we hope you will find them realistic in the range and diversity of perspectives that between them they represent. It is by engaging with the diversity of real people that values-based practice aims to link science with people.

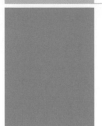

Introduction to Part 1

In this Part 1, we set out by way of introduction a number of key ideas respectively about values, individuals and values-based practice and the tools we have for working with them in medicine and healthcare.

- Chapter 1 is about values in clinical decision-making. It sets the scene with three key points about values as these emerge from the opening scenario in a consultation for chronic low back pain between a GP, Dr. Gulati, and her patient, Roy Walker.
- Chapter 2 is about individuals. It takes us to the starting point for values-based practice in the complex values that bear on individual clinical judgment in clinical decision-making. Again, we get to these complex values not in a theoretical way but by following a further stage in Dr. Gulati's story as she works through some of the tools in medicine's values toolbox (professional codes, ethics, decision analysis and evidence-based practice).
- Chapter 3 gives an overview of values-based practice setting out briefly its point (it is about balanced decision-making), its premise (in mutual respect) and ten elements of the process by which it supports clinical decision-making in practice. The chapter also includes examples of how values-based approaches have been developed and applied in various areas of mental health.

Part 1 as a whole thus paves the way for the more detailed description of values-based practice that follows in the rest of the book. The chapters in Parts 2–4 illustrate a number of key elements of values-based practice considered separately, while Part 5 shows how these elements come together in practice.

"It's my back, Doctor!" (episode 1): values and clinical decision-making

Topics covered in this chapter

Three key points about values in medicine are outlined as illustrated by a GP consultation for chronic low back pain between Dr. Gulati and her patient, Roy Walker.
Other topics include:

- Ethical and other values
- Clinician and patient values
- Foreground and background values
- The network of values
- Values, decisions and actions
- NICE guidelines for low back pain.

Take-away message for practice

*Values in medicine (i) include but are **wider than ethics**, (ii) are **everywhere** and (iii) are **action-guiding**.*

Values-based practice, as we indicated in our introduction, is a new skills-based approach to working more effectively with complex and sometimes conflicting values in medicine. As such, values-based practice is like evidence-based practice: both are responses to the growing complexity of clinical decision-making. Evidence-based practice supports clinical decision-making where complex and sometimes conflicting *evidence* is in play. Values-based practice supports clinical decision-making where complex and sometimes conflicting *values* are in play.

In this chapter, we illustrate the complexities of values in medicine not with a high-profile "ethics case" but rather as they emerge from the everyday scenario of a GP consultation for chronic low back pain. Three key points will emerge from this scenario, namely that values in medicine:

- are *wider than just ethics*, which nonetheless are an important aspect of our values;

- are *everywhere in medicine*, although not always recognized for what they are;
- are important because they stand alongside evidence in *guiding decisions and actions*.

In Chapter 2, these three key points about values in medicine will take us (still with the story of Dr. Gulati and Roy Walker) to the starting point for values-based practice in individual clinical decision-making.

The clinical context

Roy Walker, a 36-year-old laborer with a poor work record and a history of alcohol abuse, walked into Dr. Rushi Gulati's consulting room as the first patient in a busy Monday morning clinic saying, "I've come for my sick note." Roy Walker was normally seen by a different partner in the practice, Dr. Austin, who had a relatively relaxed attitude to off-work certification. However, Dr. Austin was on 2 months' study leave.

Dr. Gulati saw from Roy Walker's notes that he had been receiving increasingly strong analgesics for low back pain for some months following a strain at work. Repeated investigations had, however, been negative, and Dr. Gulati's examination on this occasion showed no significant clinical signs. When she tried to explain this to Roy Walker and to suggest ways of starting to get himself back to work, he became agitated and refused to leave "until I've got my usual."

The variety of values in the clinical encounter

The complexity of the values base of decision-making in current practice is clearly evident in this opening clinical scenario between Roy Walker and Dr. Gulati. The standoff that is developing between them is not the stuff of high-profile ethical debates. Yet into this familiar, perhaps all too familiar, situation of everyday clinical experience are packed many of the different kinds of values we encounter in health care.

Values, individuals and an overview of values based practice

Reflection point

Before reading on, you may want to think for a moment for yourself about the variety of different kinds of values that are important in health care. Some of these are mentioned in our introduction but you may find you think of others as well.

Which of these different kinds of values are in play in the opening scenario between Roy Walker and Dr. Gulati?

Faith	How we treat people
Internalization	Attitudes
Acting in best interests	Principles
Integrity	Autonomy
Conscience	Love
Best interests	Relationships
Autonomy	
Respect	Non-violence
Personal to me	Compassion
Difference . . . diversity	Dialogue
Beliefs	Responsibility
Right/wrong to me	Accountability
What I am	Best interests
Belief	What I *believe*
Principles	What makes me tick
Things held dear	What I won't compromise
Subjective merits	Objective "core"
Meanings	Confidentiality
Person-centered care	Autonomy
A *standard* for the way	Significant
I conduct *myself*	Standards
Belief about how things should be	Truth
Things you would not want to	
change	

Fig. 1.1. What are values?

Dr. Gulati's values

First, there are clearly ethical issues for Dr. Gulati. Some of these are general ethical issues, around honesty and fair-dealing for instance. There are also specifically medical ethical issues: Roy Walker was demanding "his usual" and autonomy of patient choice is an important principle of patient-centered practice to which Dr. Gulati was committed. But she was also equally committed to the principle of acting in her patient's best interests, which, in this instance, given the clear evidence of poor outcomes from chronicity (see below), seemed to be pushing her towards refusing his demands.

However, there are also values of many other kinds bearing on Dr. Gulati. Thus, the evidence of poor outcomes with low back pain just noted is relevant also to quality-of-life issues, and to the quality of life not just of the patient but of the patient's family. In the present case, Dr. Gulati was well aware of the implications (positive and negative) for Roy Walker's wife and children of how she responded to his demands.

Then again, Dr. Gulati was conscious of the fact that she and other partners in the practice had worked hard to establish a rigorous approach to clinical governance, and that in a recent practice audit, Dr. Austin's willingness to issue off-work certificates on apparently tenuous grounds had stood out like a sore thumb. There was also "value for money" to think about – the practice had recently been celebrated in the local media for providing a first-class clinical service within tight budgetary controls based on evidence-based prescribing.

The variety of values in general

We should not be surprised by the variety of values bearing on Dr. Gulati in this opening scenario from her consultation with Roy Walker. The Scandinavian philosopher Georg Henrik von Wright devoted a whole book to exploring the varieties of values (von Wright, 1963). This indeed is an important aspect of the complexity of values that, as we noted in the introduction to this part of the book, lies behind the need for values-based alongside evidence-based approaches in medicine.

Fig. 1.1 illustrates a further aspect of the complexity of values in medicine. It shows the wide variety of different meanings associated with the very word "values" by a group of trainee doctors.

The triplets of words in this table were produced as part of an exercise during a training workshop on values-based practice. Everyone was asked to write down "three words or short phrases that mean 'values' to you." As an exercise in word association, the task aimed to be personal and individual. Thus, the triplets of words show what each of the trainees individually associated with the word "values" rather than trying to come up with anything in the way of a consensus.

As you can see, although there were some shared meanings, everyone came up with a different set of words. The variety of meanings associated with the word "values" by just this one small group of trainees included as you might expect ethical values – "principles," "right/wrong to me," "standards," etc. as in Fig. 1.1; but they also included needs ("things held dear"), preferences ("personal to me", "what makes me tick"), hopes and ideals ("belief about how things should be") and a wide selection of specific values ("compassion", "loyalty", "faith", etc.). There are still further kinds of values that are not even represented in the table, such as cultural and aesthetic values and prudential values (wise, foolish).

Key point 1: values are wider than ethics

Fig. 1.1 thus takes us straight to the first key point about values that we need to be aware of clinically, namely that *values are wider than just ethical values*. Health-related values *include* ethical values, of course, and we will be seeing later how ethical and other values come together in clinical decision-making. But health-related values include much else besides.

Values are everywhere in the clinical encounter

Besides the sheer variety of health-related values, it is important to be aware of where and how and (crucially) *whose* values are involved in the clinical encounter. Again, this is well illustrated by the opening scenario between Dr. Gulati and Roy Walker.

> **Reflection point**
>
> You may want to go back to the opening clinical scenario between Roy Walker and Dr. Gulati at this point.
>
> We have noted the *variety* of values in play. But exactly *whose* values are important here? And where and how do they come into the clinical encounter?

Meet Roy Walker

One way to think about these questions is in terms of the individuals most directly involved. In the last section, we focused on the values bearing on Dr. Gulati. But the clinical encounter is, of course, a *two*-way encounter. So it is the *interaction* between Dr. Gulati's values and Roy Walker's values that will determine how the consultation goes.

Roy Walker has thus far come across to Dr. Gulati as an obstreperous and bullying man who is at best a hypochondriac and at worst simply work shy. Certainly, he is potentially aggressive. But behind the bluster, as we will see when we return to their story in Chapter 14, is a man who had always lacked confidence and whose self-esteem had suffered a further severe blow with his back injury and (as he saw it) his inability to work. As a younger man, Roy Walker had been athletically built, and much of his fragile sense of self-worth was invested in his well-muscled physique. Now, with a developing "middle-aged spread" since he had stopped working, even this seemed to be slipping away.

Correspondingly, Roy Walker, whose only successes in life had been achieved by rather aggressively asserting himself, reacted in the only way he knew how when he found himself in front of Dr. Gulati instead of Dr. Austin. He was in fact very much aware that he needed help (we look at why this was so in Chapter 14) but, in his culturally influenced perception, "maleness" did not go with talking about your problems. Notwithstanding this, he had been plucking up courage to ask for help from Dr. Austin and had thus been completely taken aback to find himself seeing not only a different doctor but a female doctor. A more self-confident man might have managed this set-back better. But for Roy it felt as though he could never win.

Added to that, his appearance was against him. Demoralized and unhappy man that he was, he had clung on to his self-image as a strong man by wearing vest-style T-shirts to show off his bull-like shoulders. Dr. Gulati was wrong-footed by this. Partly she was concerned about physical violence, although she prided herself about taking no nonsense from bullying men. Partly also her deep-rooted aesthetic and cultural values contributed to her finding his appearance rather distasteful. As she became aware of this, she was able to mediate this "personal taste" value by reminding herself how her experience as an Asian woman had taught her just how damaging it could be to be judged by appearances. Professional objectivity was thus also an important value for Dr. Gulati.

Clinician *and* patient

In the clinical encounter, then, the values of both clinician and patient are important. This might seem obvious. But it is a point worth emphasizing in the context of current policy and service development priorities that increasingly emphasize "patient power."

These priorities reflect a perceived need to shift away from a traditional emphasis on professional power, sometimes characterized as "the doctor as God." However, the shift risks taking us to the opposite extreme of "the patient as God," a consumerist model in which the patient, like a customer, is always right.

Values-based practice, as we will see in Chapter 3, seeks to avoid these extremes with an approach that starts from a premise of mutual respect and relies on a robust process to support balanced decision-making in the particular circumstances of the particular individuals involved in a given clinical decision.

Foreground and background values

Digging a little deeper into our opening scenario also makes a further point about the ubiquity of values in medicine, namely that they are not all equally self-evident – there are, as it were, background values as well as more obvious foreground values in the clinical encounter.

In the present case, Dr. Gulati's commitment to evidence-based prescribing and Roy Walker's wish for an off-work certificate are both foreground values, being relatively transparent and up front. This is what the consultation is all about. Dr. Gulati was also aware of the way in which she was affected by appearances and, as a doctor, was able to counteract this. But in the background to their encounter, there is a wide range of other values, to a greater or lesser extent deeply hidden, and yet no less important to how the consultation goes.

Among background values we have already noted are, for example, the influences on Dr. Gulati and Roy Walker of their respective social groups, the strong commitment among a majority of Dr. Gulati's colleagues to the cost-effective use of resources, and the very different but equally powerful peer pressures on Roy Walker arising from local cultural models of maleness.

There are many other background values in play. Dr. Gulati's professional values, for example, gave her a strong sense of loyalty to her colleagues, including Dr. Austin who, although now causing problems by being rather too ready to issue off-work certificates, had originally encouraged Dr. Gulati to join the practice and had supported her strongly in her early years as a GP. Then again, there were also the interests of Roy Walker's family to consider. Dr. Gulati, as we noted, was concerned that Roy Walker might take out his frustration on his wife and children if she refused to give him "his usual."

The network of values

Background values, furthermore, are very far from being confined to the values of those directly concerned in a given clinical encounter. Indeed, once you start thinking along these lines, it becomes clear that there is a whole web of people and institutions whose values, foreground and background, will critically influence how the consultation between Dr. Gulati and Roy Walker goes. Relevant values include:

- The values (needs, wishes, expectations, etc.) of the wider community, including in this instance Dr. Gulati's cultural group.
- The commercial imperatives of Roy Walker's employers and the job center's targets.
- The policy priorities of each of the many UK National Health Service (NHS) organizations within which general practice is embedded and those of central government.
- The standards embedded in the codes and guidelines of the General Medical Council (GMC; the regulatory authority for doctors in the UK) and other professional organizations.
- The targets set by the Care Quality Commission and the many other groups with responsibility for monitoring standards in the NHS.

Still other important components of the network of values are all the policy priorities and other values that go into shaping both the primary research and the derived evidence-based guidelines that underpin clinical practice and on which, therefore, Dr. Gulati is directly or indirectly relying.

Key point 2: values everywhere

Values then, to come to our second key point, *are everywhere in medicine.* Like the air we breathe, they are not always noticed for what they are (many are in the background rather than the foreground). But also like the air we breathe, whether they are noticed or not, values are always important.

Values-based practice is in part about making explicit the range and variety of values bearing on the clinical consultation and managing them more effectively. We will be exploring the values network within which the consultation between Dr. Gulati and Roy Walker was embedded further at several points in this and the next chapter and also when we return to their story in Chapter 14. But first it will be worth stepping back for a moment to think about what exactly all these different kinds of values have in common. This will take us to our third key point, namely that values in all their range and variety of forms are all action-guiding.

Values are action-guiding

Thus far, and drawing only on a brief snapshot of the initial encounter between Dr. Gulati and Roy Walker, we have seen that values are:

- *wider than just ethics*, extending to needs, wishes, preferences and so forth;
- *everywhere*, including the values of *clinician as well as patient*, extending to *background as well as more obvious foreground values*, and all set within an extensive *network of values*.

But if values cover such a remarkably wide terrain, what exactly *are* values? What is the common factor? What is it that makes all these very different things *values*? And exactly how does such a diversity of values *bear on clinical decision-making*?

What then *are* values?

"Values" is one of those words that everyone uses assuming they know what it means but which turns out on reflection to be remarkably difficult to define. The word "values" is not alone in this. In evidence-based medicine, for example, there is much discussion of "best evidence" but what exactly the word "evidence" means is left largely unquestioned.

Nonetheless, various definitions of "values" have been suggested by, among others, some of the pathfinders for *evidence*-based medicine. David Sackett and his colleagues, for example, in their foundational book on evidence-based medicine (to which we referred earlier) put it this way:

> By patient values we mean the unique preferences, concerns and expectations each patient brings to the clinical encounter and which must be integrated [with best research evidence and clinical experience] into clinical decisions if they are to serve the patient.
>
> Sackett *et al.* (2000, p. 1)

This is a helpful definition in many ways. True, Sackett's definition focuses only on patients' values, and, as we have already seen, Dr. Gulati's values are as material as those of Roy Walker to values-based decision-making, while the relevant network of values extends well beyond those of the clinician and patient directly involved. Nonetheless, Sackett's definition:

- reminds us that values in medicine are wider than ethics: values in Sackett's definition include "preferences, concerns and expectations";
- explicitly links values, both positive ("preferences") and negative ("concerns"), with evidence in clinical decision-making: values, he says, have to be *integrated* with evidence and clinical experience in clinical decision-making;
- makes clear the importance of values in, as we put it in the subtitle to this book, linking science (represented by generalizable evidence) with people (as unique individuals each with what might be called their own "values fingerprint"). In Sackett's words values are "the *unique* preferences, concerns and expectations *each patient* brings to the clinical encounter."

Helpful as it is, however, Sackett's explanation of the meaning attached to values in their book falls short of actually nailing what exactly values *are* and hence exactly *why* values (in all their remarkable range and diversity) are relevant to clinical decision-making.

Values, decisions and actions

For a deeper understanding of values and their relevance to clinical decision-making, we turn to the work of an Oxford philosopher, R. M. Hare. As a former White's Professor of Moral Philosophy in Oxford, Hare worked in what is sometimes called "ordinary language" philosophy. This mid-twentieth-century school of analytic philosophy explored the meanings of complex concepts like "values" by looking carefully at how the concepts in question are actually *used* in everyday (i.e. ordinary) contexts.

With its down-to-earth and somewhat empirical approach, ordinary language philosophy has many resonances with medicine – one of its practitioners called it "philosophical field work" (Austin, 1956–1957, p. 25). Values-based practice is essentially a practical spin-off from the work of the Oxford School (see Fulford, 1989 and the series website) and remains an area of ongoing study. Hare's work, however, takes us straight to the bottom line for clinical decision-making, for what Hare showed was that the many and diverse varieties of values are all *action-guiding* – "prescriptive" is the term he used (Hare, 1952).

Key point 3: values are action-guiding

That values are all action-guiding is the third of our three key points about values in medicine. The implications for clinical decision-making are clear – actions

7

in a clinical context are guided not only by evidence *but also by values*. Clinical decisions thus stand on two feet. They are guided by evidence and by values. The evidence footing is broadly construed as including both research evidence and the evidence of clinical experience. The elements of the values footing will become clearer as we move on.

It will be worth considering this point about the two feet of decision-making (the need for a values foot as well as an evidence foot) in a little more detail as it plays out in different kinds of clinical situation.

Clinical decision-making

Values guide clinical decision-making

In this book, we use the term "values," following Hare, to include anything positively or negatively weighted as a guide to healthcare decision-making. This action-guiding sense of the term is clearly evident in the scenario between Dr. Gulati and Roy Walker. Her dilemma was the product of a tension between different values that were "guiding" her in different directions about what to do. The values of patient autonomy and of best interests, for example, were in tension in this respect. There was a similar if more deeply hidden tension arising from Roy Walker's appearance between Dr. Gulati's professional values of objectivity and her cultural and personal aesthetic values.

Roy Walker, too, was "values-guided" – by his fears about his back, his concerns for the future, his self-image as a well-muscled man and so forth. So his values have to be factored into the weightings that will guide the clinical decisions Dr. Gulati has to make. The doctor and the patient, although the central protagonists in this clinical situation, are but part of a wider network of people and institutions whose values – positive and negative – are in different ways critical to how things work out between them.

Evidence also guides clinical decision-making

In her clinical decision-making, Dr. Gulati was also guided by the evidence represented by her clinical experience and relevant research. She was accustomed to using the terms "red flags" and "yellow flags" in her assessment of back disorders. The former alerted her to look out for potentially serious disease like cauda equina compression, while the latter term was based on work by Kendall and Burton in 1997 on the psycho-social factors predicting chronicity and poor outcomes with low back pain (Kendall *et al.*, 2009). These yellow flags are summarized in Table 1.1. As you can see, Roy Walker had a full house. Was his back pain already chronic, or was there a last window of opportunity to affect this?

Evidence that Dr. Gulati relied on quite heavily in her practice was that emanating from the influential UK National Institute for Health and Clinical Excellence, commonly known as NICE guidance. Although reducing work-loss is not part of the NICE brief, yellow flags (as further developed by others, e.g. Corbett *et al.*, 2009) are mentioned in NICE guidance (NICE, 2009). The therapeutic guidance at this point would be that Roy should be referred for an intensive rehabilitation program.

Values as well as evidence in *all* clinical decisions

We chose to present the scenario between Roy Walker and Dr. Gulati as our opening narrative precisely because it is on the one hand so richly values-laden and on the other so strongly evidence-based. But Hare's point was that *all* decisions, clinical or otherwise, and whether overtly value-laden or not, are values- as well as evidence-driven.

Table 1.1. Psycho-social yellow flags for chronic low back pain

A negative attitude that back pain is harmful or potentially severely disabling

Fear avoidance behavior and reduced activity levels

An expectation that passive, rather than active, treatment will be beneficial

A tendency to depression, low morale and social withdrawal

Social or financial problems

From Samanta *et al.* (2003).

Generally speaking, we do not have to reflect too hard on why we take the decisions we do in everyday practice. Just "getting on with the job" working mostly on automatic is integral to what it means to be a skilled professional.

It can often be quite difficult to reconstruct our decisions. When we *do* reflect on any particular decision we have taken, we can generally come up with the evidence base on which we acted – not necessarily the detailed research evidence but at least the broad area of medical knowledge that, together with our individual clinical experience, informs the decision in question. This was the case with Dr. Gulati.

What is perhaps not always so self-evident, even on reflection, is the *values* base of our decisions. In Dr. Gulati's situation, the importance of the weightings provided by values is clear. Her knowledge of the factors associated with poor outcomes with low back pain was, on its own, not sufficient to drive her clinical decisions. Her view that she ought not to issue an off-work certificate was the result of *combining* (or "integrating" as Sackett *et al.*, 2000, put it) this evidence-based knowledge with her values-based commitment to acting in her patient's best interests. And her *dilemma* about what to do in this instance consisted, as we noted a moment ago, precisely in the fact that *other* values (such as patient autonomy) ran directly counter to the importance she placed on "best interests."

Values and prescribing an antibiotic

Hare's point is that *all* decisions, even those that are not overtly value-laden like Dr. Gulati's, depend not only on evidence but also on the positive and negative weightings provided by values. If you tried reflecting on your own last decision, as in the reflection point above, you may well have found this for yourself.

Suppose, for example, that your decision was about prescribing an antibiotic for, say, pneumococcal pneumonia. Your choice of antibiotic will clearly have been evidence-based. It is likely to have been guided by your local formulary, which combines evidence on local resistance patterns, for instance, with the cost of the different options.

The role of values, on the other hand, is initially less obvious in a case like this. When you think about your antibiotic-prescribing decision further, however, it becomes clear that a whole series of background values have to be connected up with the relevant evidence base – the balance of benefits (antimicrobial efficacy) and harms (side effects), the cost-effectiveness of the antibiotic in question ("cost" and "effectiveness" both being value-laden concepts), wider economic issues around health budgets, and so on. Indeed, a decision as apparently un-value-laden as prescribing an antibiotic turns out, on reflection, to be embedded in much the same network of values as Dr. Gulati's overtly value-laden dilemma about issuing an off-work certificate.

Chapter summary

Drawing on the opening clinical encounter between Dr. Gulati and Roy Walker, this chapter has illustrated three key points about values in medicine:

1. Values are *wider than ethics* – they extend to needs, wishes, preferences and so forth.
2. Values are *everywhere* – they include the values of clinician and patient, both foreground and background values, and the wider network of values.
3. Values are *action-guiding* – they include anything positively or negatively weighted as a guide to clinical decision-making.

In the next chapter, we follow Dr. Gulati as she turns first to codes of practice and ethics and then to evidence-based practice and decision analysis in trying to decide how to respond to Roy Walker's demands for an off-work certificate. We will find that, although all these are indeed helpful up to a point, when applied to particular individual decisions they raise complex values issues. Neither codes of practice nor ethics guidelines, and neither the tools of evidence-based practice nor those of decision analysis, can resolve these complex issues. Thus, at the point of individual clinical decision-making, there is a clear need for values-based practice.

References

Austin, J. L. (1956–1957). A plea for excuses. *Proceedings of the Aristotelian Society* **57**, 1–30. Reprinted in A. R. White (ed.) (1968). *The Philosophy of Action*. Oxford: Oxford University Press, pp. 19–42.

Corbett, M., Foster, N. and Ong, B. (2009). GP attitudes and self-reported behaviour in primary care consultations for low back pain. *Family Practice* **26**, 359–64.

Fulford, K. W. M. (1989 and 1995). *Moral Theory and Medical Practice*. Cambridge: Cambridge University Press.

Kendall, N., Burton, K., Main, C. and Watson, P. (2009). *Tackling Musculoskeletal Problems: a Guide for Clinic and Workplace: Identifying Obstacles Using the Psychosocial Flags Framework*. London: The Stationary Office.

Hare, R. M. (1952). *The Language of Morals*. Oxford: Oxford University Press.

NICE (2009). *Low Back Pain: Early Management of Persistent Non-specific Low Back Pain. NICE Clinical Guideline 88*. London: National Institute for Health and Clinical Excellence (see also web address below).

Sackett, D. L., Straus, S. E., Scott Richardson, W., Rosenberg, W. and Haynes, R. B. (2000). *Evidence-based Medicine: How to Practice and Teach EBM*, 2nd edn. Edinburgh and London: Churchill Livingstone.

Samanta, J., Kendall, J. and Samanta, A. (2003). 10-minute consultation: chronic low back pain. *British Medical Journal* **326**, 535.

Von Wright, G. H. (1963) *The Varieties of Goodness*. London: Routledge & Kegan Paul.

Websites

- For more on psycho-social yellow flags for chronicity with low back pain see: http://www.kendallburton.com/Flags/flagsindetail.html.
- NICE guidance on chronic low back pain is available as a pdf from: http://www.nice.org.uk/CG88.

"It's my back, Doctor!" (episode 2): applying the tools already in the clinical toolbox for working with values to individuals

Topics covered in this chapter

Continuing the story of Dr. Gulati and Roy Walker, this chapter takes us to the starting point for values-based practice in the complex values involved in individual clinical decision-making.
Other topics include:

- Codes of ethics
- Principles reasoning
- How values and ethics fit together
- Decision analysis
- How values and evidence fit together
- Clinical judgment.

Take-away message for practice

All current tools need the application of individual clinical judgment and up until now there has been little to guide clinicians on processes to find the best solutions for individual cases.

In this chapter, we take the story of Roy Walker and Dr. Gulati a stage further. The doctor turns for help to a number of tools in medicine's values toolbox: first, codes of practice and ethics, then decision analysis and finally evidence-based practice. These all prove helpful but only up to a point, for when applied to the particular circumstances of the patient, each of them raises but fails to resolve a number of complex values issues.

It is these and similar complex values issues raised by clinical decision-making between individual patients and individual clinicians that take us to the starting point for values-based practice.

What to do?

We start this chapter with a suggested reflection aimed at helping us to get away from general ethical theorizing about what Dr. Gulati *ought* to do and to focus rather on what she could do in the *particular*

circumstances in which she found herself on a Monday morning at the start of a busy clinic.

> **Reflection point**
>
> Before reading on, you may want to try imagining what you would do in Dr. Gulati's situation.
>
> You do not have to be a doctor to think about this. But if you are, think about it "for real," i.e. imagine that Roy Walker is consulting *you* and that *you* have responsibility for deciding what to do.

The clinical context

Rather than having an argument with Roy Walker, Dr. Gulati decided that she needed to defuse the situation while at the same time giving herself some time out to think about what to do.

She agreed to issue a certificate for one week, explaining to Roy that what she was making clear in the certificate was that in order to be fair to him she needed to review his medical records and give him a double appointment in a week. They would then have time to go through everything properly and, if appropriate, she would give him a longer certificate. He agreed to this reluctantly as he could see that Dr. Gulati was not going to be bullied into just giving him what he wanted.

Professional codes

The more Dr. Gulati thought about the consultation with Roy Walker over the next day, the more intriguing she found it. She decided to invest a little more time exploring some of the implications of the case, as she had some spare time the next evening. Her first step was to go on the Internet and look up the GMC's Duties of a Doctor. At first this appeared helpful. There was no statement about off-work certificates as such, but, as the first extract given in Fig. 2.1 shows, caring for patients and protecting their health came right at the top of the GMC's list of the duties of a

Extract 1

The duties of a doctor registered with the General Medical Council

Patients must be able to trust doctors with their lives and health. To justify that trust you must show respect for human life and you must:

- Make the care of your patient your first concern
- Protect and promote the health of patients and the public

Extract 2

Work in partnership with patients

- Listen to patients and respond to their concerns and preferences
- Give patients the information they want or need in a way they can understand
- Respect patients' right to reach decisions with you about their treatment and care
- Support patients in caring for themselves to improve and maintain their health

Fig. 2.1. Two extracts from the GMC's *Duties of a Doctor*

All GPs should be able to:

- Recognise the ethical dimension of every healthcare encounter
- Understand the nature of values and how they impact on health care
- Identify the values that patients, families and members of the healthcare team bring to a specific healthcare decision
- Demonstrate moral reasoning skills in the process of choosing an appropriate course of action or resolving conflicting values
- Demonstrate the knowledge skills and attitudes for effective communication in eliciting and understanding the values of patients, negotiating an acceptable course of action and justifying that course of action
- Demonstrate knowledge of the professional ethical guidelines and legal framework within which healthcare decisions should be made
- Recognize their personal values and how these influence their decision-making.

Fig. 2.2. "All GPs should be able to . . ." Extract from the RCGP Curriculum Statement 3.3 on Clinical Ethics and Values-based Practice (version 1.1, February 2009: www.rcgp-curriculum.org.uk/pdf/curr_3_3_Clinical_ethics.pdf).

doctor. Clearly then, she thought, given what was known about the risk factors for chronicity with low back pain (the "yellow flags" we looked at in Chapter 1), her reluctance to give Roy Walker a further off-work certificate was well justified.

A moment's further reflection, however, showed Dr. Gulati that all this had done was to confirm one side of the dilemma in which she found herself, namely her commitment to providing evidence-based care. So far as deciding what to do was concerned, a later section of the same list went on to confirm the *other* side of her dilemma. The second extract she found in the list of a doctor's duties emphasized the importance of being patient-centered as a key component of good practice (Fig. 2.1). True, this part of the list used the language of partnership – a doctor was *not* required to do what a patient wants come what may. But if "responding to (patients') concerns and preferences" meant anything, it meant taking Roy Walker's wishes seriously.

Not only that, but the list (in extract 1) also included a duty to "protect and promote" the health of "the public." This gave a further twist to Dr. Gulati's dilemma, for that phrase "the public" reminded her that, with Roy Walker's suspected history of taking his frustrations out violently on his wife and children, she would have to take the consequences for his family into account as well in deciding what to do.

Next on her list of "favorite sites" on her computer under the subheading "Professional" was the Royal College of General Practitioners (RCGP) site. As her own professional body, the RCGP repeatedly emphasized the importance of "treating the whole family." She looked at the core RCGP Curriculum Statement 1, *Being a General Practitioner*, which is something she often

looked at with trainees. Here she found the guidance on what all GPs should be able to do (see Fig. 2.2).

Clearly, the college attaches importance to some of the processes she had already used in defusing the situation: by allowing herself time out, she felt she had shown good communication skills of conflict resolution. This allowed her to reflect on what to do in an ethically tricky situation rather than jumping in with a quick knee-jerk response, thus demonstrating her degree of values awareness. She was glad of the prompt to revise her moral reasoning skills and her awareness of the professional ethical guidelines and legal frameworks.

These authoritative sources of guidance (GMC and RCGP) thus appeared to endorse *all* the elements of her dilemma about what to do in this particular case, but to some extent this made the problem more acute rather than resolving it.

Professional codes and conflicting values

It might seem surprising that, far from helping Dr. Gulati, the codes of practice to which she turned actually sharpened her dilemma about what to do. After all, such codes are intended to guide practice.

Professional codes of practice make explicit the values by which a given profession defines what it regards as good practice. There is thus no breach of the Trades Descriptions Act in the GMC calling its code "Good Medical Practice." It provides exactly what it says "on the tin." But what is *in* the tin? The "good" in "good medical practice" is a variety of different values, which (as in Dr. Gulati's case) may sometimes come into conflict.

In essence, a code of professional practice, just to the extent that it faithfully *reflects* the values by which good practice is defined within the profession in question, will to the same extent reflect the (potential) *conflicts* that may arise between those same values in practice.

Dr. Gulati's conflicting values

This was exactly Dr. Gulati's experience. Her dilemma (ignoring for the moment the family issues) arose from the fact that, in trying to decide what to do, she found herself caught between two principles of good medical practice, both of which were important but which in the *particular individual circumstances presented by Roy Walker* were pulling her in contrary directions:

- The principle of person-centered practice was pulling her towards *giving* him his off-work certificate.
- The principle of evidence-based care was pulling her towards *withholding* his off-work certificate.

In many situations, these two important principles of good medical practice – person-centered practice and evidence-based care – would be fully aligned. But there is no reason why they should always be aligned; and, as Dr. Gulati tried to decide what to do about Roy Walker's off-work certificate, her dilemma consisted in the fact that the principles of person-centered practice and evidence-based practice were in this case *not* aligned.

From codes to ethics

Dr. Gulati turned next to ethics. A particular approach that she had found helpful both as a medical student and also in her work on bioethics in her Continuing Professional Development (CPD) is called "principles reasoning." This approach was applied to medicine in the early days of bioethics by two North American scholars at Georgetown University, a philosopher and

a theologian, Tom Beauchamp and James Childress, respectively. Dr. Gulati turned to her well-thumbed copy of Beauchamp and Childress's *Principles of Biomedical Ethics* (1989).

Principles reasoning

Principles reasoning involves balancing what are called prima facie principles. It makes a virtue of the fact that values are often conflicting. The idea is that, in any particular situation of a given kind, certain principles are likely to be important (hence prima facie relevant).

Ethical dilemmas then, according to this approach, arise when in any given situation two or more of the relevant prima facie principles are (again as in Dr. Gulati's case) pulling in different directions. Hence, *resolving* the dilemma in question means *balancing* the relevant principles according to the specific circumstances of that particular situation.

Dr. Gulati's principles reasoning

Beauchamp and Childress's prima facie Four Principles of medical ethics are:

- Autonomy
- Beneficence
- Non-maleficence
- Justice.

"That's me," thought Dr. Gulati as she re-read what Beauchamp and Childress had to say about autonomy and beneficence. "I'm caught between Roy Walker's demand for an off-work certificate (autonomy – freedom of patient choice) and my belief based on evidence-based guidelines that his interests are best served by rehabilitation (beneficence)."

However, Dr. Gulati also found the principle of "non-maleficence" (avoiding harm whatever else you do) helpful in clarifying her thinking. As we saw earlier, Dr. Gulati was already concerned about the possible consequences for Roy Walker's wife and children if she refused to renew his off-work certificate. Now, as she re-read the section on non-maleficence, these concerns were brought very much to the front of her mind as key ethical considerations to be weighed alongside the more obvious ethical issues of autonomy and beneficence.

Initially, Beauchamp and Childress's fourth prima facie principle, their principle of "justice," did not seem directly relevant to Dr. Gulati's dilemma about what to do. "Justice" is about fair distribution of limited healthcare resources and is most often discussed in the context of issues of resource allocation (the principle is sometimes called "distributive justice").

But again, as Dr. Gulati re-read what the book had to say about the principle of justice, she realized that it too was relevant to the situation in which she found herself with Roy Walker. True, her decision was not about resource allocation as such, but there was surely something deeply unjust (in this "fair use of resources" sense) in allowing Roy Walker to go on using up healthcare resources (not to mention the benefits budget) inappropriately and at the expense of other perhaps less assertive people who really needed them.

Reflection point

You may find it useful to pause for a moment here to think about how far using principles reasoning has taken Dr. Gulati towards resolving her dilemma.

- How has principles reasoning helped her?
- Where does it fall short?

Strengths of principles reasoning . . .

What Dr. Gulati had found helpful about the Four Principles as a student was the way in which it provided a framework for thinking about ethical problems. Reflecting now on the Four Principles in the context of her problem about how to manage Roy Walker's demand for an off-work certificate had helped her in three distinct ways:

1. It had *clarified and confirmed* the nature of her core dilemma, as a tension between patient choice (autonomy) and best interests (beneficence).
2. It had *reinforced* her thinking of the importance of avoiding harm to Roy Walker's family (non-maleficence).
3. It had *deepened her understanding* of the problem as extending also to issues of fairness in the use of scarce resources (justice).

Going back to the Four Principles had thus helped Dr. Gulati to become clearer about the different elements of her dilemma. Re-reading relevant codes of practice, as we have seen, had started this process. Beauchamp and Childress's more in-depth analysis had now taken it

further by highlighting aspects of the situation of which Dr. Gulati had not previously been fully aware.

We should not underestimate the clinical value of being able to clarify ethical problems through principles reasoning. Mapping out the elements of a complex ethical problem in terms of one or more tensions between relevant prima facie principles helps to make sense of the problem. It can also, as we have just seen, highlight aspects of the problem that may have been overlooked. When we return to the story of Dr. Gulati and Roy Walker in Chapter 14, we will see that reminding Dr. Gulati about two principles (non-maleficence and justice) that had not been at the forefront of her mind in the heat of the moment with Roy Walker demanding "his usual" and a clinic full of patients waiting to see her, turned out in the end to be crucial to how the issues were eventually resolved.

. . . and its limitations

All the same, Dr. Gulati had still only taken a first step towards deciding what to do. She had come to a clearer understanding of the nature of the problem and of its different aspects, certainly. The codes of practice she consulted first had endorsed her concerns: they had told her in effect that by widely agreed standards of good practice she did indeed *have* a problem. The Four Principles had now helped her to map out the nature of the problem more fully.

But helpful as this was, it was only a step in the right direction, showing her that the problem was more complicated than she had originally thought.

General theory and individual cases

Turning back to her copy of *Principles of Biomedical Ethics*, therefore, Dr. Gulati now looked for the section that described how to apply the Four Principles in practice. The general approach as she already understood involved balancing the relevant principles (all four were relevant in her case). But how exactly should she go about balancing the Four Principles appropriately in deciding what to do now? Her question related not to wellness and sickness certificates in general, nor even to patients demanding clinically unjustified certificates, but specifically to the individual circumstances presented by Roy Walker.

She looked eagerly for the relevant passage where Beauchamp and Childress cover how to apply their principles, hoping this would provide the key to deciding what to do.

What Dr. Gulati found was indeed the key to resolving her dilemma about what to do, but it was not the key she expected. What Beauchamp and Childress actually say is that, in themselves, the Four Principles *cannot solve ethical problems.*

Yes, principles reasoning can take us a step towards resolving ethical problems: as just described, they can help to map out and make clear the nature of a given ethical problem in terms of one or more conflicts between relevant principles. But actually *resolving* the problem (on this account) means balancing the principles in question appropriately according to the particular circumstances of a given case. And as Beauchamp and Childress themselves make clear, just how this balancing should be done in practice by a given clinician (Dr. Gulati in this case) in a particular clinical situation (facing a hostile Roy Walker in a busy Monday morning clinic) is not for a philosopher and a theologian to say. There is always, in any given case, *an element of individual judgment* involved in deciding what in those particular circumstances the appropriate balance of principles should be.

From conflicting values to values-based practice

Ethics, in the form of relevant codes of practice and a major textbook, had taken Dr. Gulati so far. It had clarified the nature of her dilemma as a problem of balancing conflicting values appropriately in the particular circumstances in which she found herself.

But here ethics stopped short. Codes and principles reasoning in themselves provided no help with the required *balancing* of the conflicting values they had highlighted. Here Dr. Gulati needed a different, complementary way of supporting clinical decision-making.

Other ethics tools in the medical toolbox

In this section, we will review some of the other ethical tools, besides codes and principles reasoning, to which Dr. Gulati might have turned.

In later chapters, we will consider some of these and other values tools in more detail, looking at how they contribute to the holistic process of values-based practice, which involves the use of many different tools, and used appropriately, the sum of the process becomes more than the parts.

Regulatory ethics

One way of responding to situations where principles are in conflict is to extend our codes of practice to provide more detailed guidance covering situations of different kinds. We have seen something of this in recent years with professional codes becoming ever longer and more detailed.

Code inflation

This "code inflation," as one of us has called it elsewhere (Fulford *et al.*, 2006) is understandable. Faced with the growing complexity of the values bearing on clinical decision-making, it would be a welcome relief if there were a set of rules just telling us what to do. Regulatory ethics, as we will see in the next chapter, has a vital role to play alongside other approaches in supporting clinical decision-making. Dr. Gulati might have hoped to find detailed guidance for example in an update from one or other of her professional bodies in the form of practice guidelines on issuing off-work certificates, extending beyond the rules set out by the Department of Work and Pensions (the relevant government body in the UK).

But regulatory ethics has inherent limitations when it comes to individual clinical decisions. In the first place, there is the risk of defensive practice, a risk that has been much increased in recent years by the quasi-legal model of medical decision-making encouraged by code inflation. Clinical decision-making based not on a given patient's clinical needs but on the clinician's fear of being sued carries an inherent risk of an over-reliance on regulation in medicine.

In the second place, code inflation amounts to chasing the end of the "values rainbow" when it comes to individual decision-making. This is because any set of rules, however detailed and comprehensive, always has to be interpreted and applied to particular cases. This is indeed Beauchamp and Childress's point about the need for judgment in individual cases. It applies to general principles. It applies no less forcefully to more detailed rules.

Individual judgment again

The sheer complexity of the values bearing on Dr. Gulati and Roy Walker's situation is perhaps a sufficient indication that no set of rules could adequately cover all situations. *Applying* the rules "for real," deciding whether this or that rule applies to a particular decision with a particular patient in a particular situation, always requires an individual act of judgment on the part of the decision-maker.

Other ethics

The dominant mode of engagement between bioethics and medicine in practice is through codes and regulation. But other practically useful ethics resources include:

- Utilitarianism, based on "the greatest good of the greatest number."
- Deontology, concerned with rights and responsibilities.
- Virtue ethics, about "good character."

There are also profession-based and subject-specific ethics – nursing ethics, social work ethics and psychiatric ethics, for example, each with distinctive aims, methods and scope relevant to the area in question. (We give examples on the website supporting the series.)

Each of these ethical tools has found one or more important roles in medicine. Utilitarianism is important in health economics, for example, as the basis of the QALY, or quality-adjusted life year. Frequent reference to the NICE guidelines had made Dr. Gulati familiar with these metrics. Deontology is closely connected with medical law, in particular in areas such as human rights and anti-discrimination legislation (we come to an example of this from recent mental health law in the next chapter). Virtue ethics, with its focus on the elements of good character, is relevant to the aims of medical education. The development of subject-specific and professional ethics has gone hand in hand with the rise in importance of clinical governance in different areas of practice.

Other ethical tools and Dr. Gulati's decision

> **Reflection point**
>
> We are coming now to the critical point of transit between ethics as a general theoretical discipline and the individual-focused resources of values-based practice.
>
> Before reading on, you might want to try thinking briefly about two questions:
>
> - Which (if any) of the above ethical tools is relevant to Dr. Gulati?
> - Which (if any) can resolve her dilemma about what to do?

So far as the first of these two questions goes, *all* of the above ethical tools are relevant in one way or another to Dr. Gulati. Remember here the extent of the values network outlined in Chapter 1. Thus:

- *Health economic* considerations have directly determined her resource options (through utilitarianism-based QALYs and their role in the development of clinical guidelines).
- *Medical law* placed clear boundaries around what she could or could not do (reflecting her rights and responsibilities as a doctor and other deontological issues).
- *The virtues* of a good doctor tacitly underpinned her clinical training and hence the attitudes and habits of mind she brought to her consultation with Roy Walker.

As to medicine's particular *professional ethics*, evidence-based prescribing and its importance in local audit and clinical governance was explicitly part of the dilemma she faced.

Yet none of these other tools was, separately or together, sufficient actually to *resolve* her dilemma. As with her earlier fine-grained consideration of codes and principles reasoning, each of these further ethical tools was helpful up to a point: each of them clarified in different ways different aspects either of her dilemma or of the sources of her dilemma. Each of them, furthermore, was the right tool for tackling other aspects of the challenge of values in medicine. Yet as with codes and principles reasoning, so now with these further tools – none of them in themselves actually *resolved* the complex values issues she faced in trying to decide what to do in this particular case.

Other tools in the clinical toolbox for making values-laden decisions

In the remainder of this chapter, we will look briefly at two further tools, decision analysis and evidence-based medicine.

Decision analysis

Decision analysis is a part mathematical, part psychological discipline developed (like values-based practice) as a support tool for complex decision-making. One of our favorite models for decision analysis combines beliefs (evidence) with preferences (values) in an interactive tool developed by Jack Dowie. This tool is available on the Café Annalisa website, where clinicians and lay people can look at the influence of changing beliefs and preferences for decision-making in general and clinical decision-making in particular.

Dowie looks at alternative decisions (e.g. to try for a vaginal delivery or to have an elective cesarean section after a previous cesarean section). He dissects out evidence relevant to a number of factors affecting this decision (e.g. risks to the baby, risks to the mother, length of stay in hospital) and this evidence can be "weighted" according to the strength of evidence. Patients are then invited to weight their preference on each component using graphical "sliders." This reflects their values as, for example, a mother with small children at home might place a lot of weight on early discharge from hospital allowing her to return to her family. As the sliders for the evidence and for the choices are moved, so the emphases on alternative choices for the management decision are changed. Thus, a strong preference for early discharge supports an attempt at vaginal delivery but this might be counteracted by prioritizing reducing risk to the baby over reducing risk to the mother.

Conventionally, decision analysis combines probabilities with values in an applied form of utilitarianism that seeks to balance "utilities" (defined by the *probability* of a given outcome combined with the *value* attached to that outcome). In medicine, the resources of decision analysis have been used widely in relation to issues of resource allocation (see for example, Brown *et al.*, 2005). But it was to a book applying decision analysis directly to clinical decision-making that Dr. Gulati now turned.

As with ethics, Dr. Gulati had read something of decision analysis. The mathematical basis of the methods it offered appealed to her (maths was her favorite subject at school before she decided to go into medicine) and she had particularly enjoyed the clear style of *Decision Making in Health and Medicine* (Hunink *et al.*, 2001). The lead authors, Myriam Hunink and Paul Glasziou, respectively experts in decision analysis and evidence-based medicine, were both clinicians, and the book also had secondary authors from a range of different clinical areas. So, all in all, with its many worked examples, it looked to be just the book she needed.

Strengths of decision analysis . . .

As Dr. Gulati now found, decision analysis certainly had much to offer as a tool for working with values in medicine:

- It was directly on target in being very much about combining values with evidence in clinical decision-making – its subtitle was indeed *Integrating Evidence and Values*.
- It explicitly addressed the challenges of having to make decisions under conditions of uncertainty.
- It recognized that "the decision-maker" varied from situation to situation and that different decision-makers (patients, clinicians, relatives and so on) might bring different values to the same decision.

The book also reminded Dr. Gulati of the range of other disciplines relevant to working with values. Psychological research on values and decision-making has added further tools to the values toolbox, as have other relevant disciplines including anthropology, literary analysis, medical history, various different areas of philosophy, and medical humanities and emergent neuroscience.

The book included a number of practical tips about how to ask about values in a clinical context, and it indicated a number of web-based decision analysis tools that can be used to help decision-makers come to understand their own values better and thus make more informed decisions.

We give examples of some of the above disciplines relevant to working with values in the website supporting this series. These include computer-based aids to combining values and evidence for patients in specific areas of decision-making. We return to the problem of eliciting values, and how web-based decision analysis tools can support this, in Chapter 7 on communication skills and values-based practice.

. . . and limitations

> **Reflection point**
>
> Decision analysis was clearly relevant to Dr. Gulati's situation. Nonetheless, in the event it ultimately failed to resolve her dilemma about what to do in Roy Walker's case.
>
> Why do you think this was so? Clearly, this is not an entirely fair question after such a brief presentation of yet another well-developed and complex area. But try thinking about it for a moment or two before reading on. How would calculating utilities help Dr. Gulati with her core dilemma of resolving the conflicting values in this particular case?

From one to more than one decision-maker

Helpful as Hunink *et al.*'s book was, it failed to get to the heart of Dr. Gulati's problem. There were two main reasons for this. First, the clinical paradigm for decision analysis is of one decision-maker (usually the patient) choosing between different courses of action according to that decision-maker's own values. This was not Dr. Gulati's difficulty, which was instead a conflict between *her* values and *her patient's* values. True, her dilemma was reflected in a number of tensions between the different professional values by which good medical practice is defined in the RCGP and GMC codes. But what drove these tensions was, essentially, that what mattered to *her* (evidence-based rehabilitation) was different from and incompatible with what mattered to *Roy Walker* (getting an off-work certificate). So the problem was not as such a problem of balancing utilities. The problem was that the way Dr. Gulati balanced utilities was different from – and in conflict with – the way her patient, Roy Walker, would balance the same utilities.

From one to more than one type of value

The second reason why decision analysis failed Dr. Gulati in this instance was because it covered too narrow a range of values. The problems of defining values noted in Chapter 1 are evident here. Chapter 4 of Hunink *et al.*'s book entitled "Valuing outcomes" opens with a quote from an economist, Ralph Keeney. "Values are what we care about . . ." the quote starts, and "as such, should be the *driving force* of our actions" (emphasis added). This directly reflects our inclusive "action-guiding" sense of the term "values" in Chapter 1 of this book.

The limitations of decision analysis arising from its restriction to one kind of value (preferences) were pointed out in the early days of the use of QALYs by the Oxford philosopher and ethicist Roger Crisp in 1994. The utilitarian calculation of QALYs, Crisp pointed out, in reflecting the greatest good of the greatest number, inevitably disadvantaged minorities. In decisions about resource allocation, Crisp thus argued, QALYs should be balanced by deontological considerations reflecting rights and responsibilities.

Dr. Gulati was aware of similar considerations bearing on her particular situation with Roy Walker. The whole point of autonomy, after all, she now reflected, was precisely to give patients the right to choose differently from what clinicians might regard as the "best outcome," however obviously right this might appear to be on utilitarian grounds.

Further forward – or not?

Decision analysis, then, Dr. Gulati concluded, was a useful tool, particularly for someone like herself with a rather mathematical turn of mind, in deciding where her responsibility to act in a patient's best interests lay. But in Roy Walker's case, she already knew this from the evidence-based clinical guidelines for managing low back pain. Her problem was rather about squaring the deontological circle between her professional responsibility for evidence-based decision-making and Roy Walker's right to autonomy of patient choice.

But at least, Dr. Gulati thought with an inner sigh of relief, the evidence-base isn't a problem here. So she turned in the last few minutes of her time out to the evidence noted in Chapter 1 with a view to reminding herself of the details of the risk factors for poor outcomes with low back pain.

Evidence-based medicine

> **Reflection point**
>
> As we move from ethics and decision analysis to evidence, you may find it helpful to think again about Dr. Gulati's situation "for real."
>
> This time the question to consider is whether there are any difficulties for Dr. Gulati arising from the evidence base for her decision about what to do. We have focused thus far on her dilemma in the terms in which she herself had understood it, as a problem of conflicting values. The issues here as we have seen are tricky enough. But is the evidence base of her decision really as unproblematic as she thought?

Space permits only a couple of points about evidence and clinical decision-making. First, that values and evidence are not as distinct as is often supposed. Secondly, they both depend on clinical judgment for their application in individual cases.

The relationship between values-based and evidence-based approaches is complex, both theoretically and in practice. We return to some of the practical aspects of this in Part 4 of this book and we include key sources on relevant theory on the website supporting this series.

No sharp separation between evidence and values

Dr. Gulati was a committed evidence-based practitioner who was familiar with the latest research evidence linking chronicity with poor outcomes in patients like Roy Walker. She now went back to this evidence. This, as we saw in Chapter 1, confirmed that Roy Walker did indeed have a full house of "yellow flags," i.e. of evidence-based factors predicting long-term chronicity and disability in patients with low back pain:

- A negative attitude that back pain is harmful or potentially severely disabling.
- Fear avoidance behavior and reduced activity levels.
- An expectation that passive, rather than active, treatment will be beneficial.
- A tendency to depression, low morale and social withdrawal.
- Social or financial problems.

So the relevant evidence-base, it seemed to Dr. Gulati, was indeed unproblematic. There was evidence-based agreement in the literature on the factors predicting chronicity, and Roy Walker showed most if not all of these. But as Dr. Gulati re-read the guidelines with her decision about how to manage Roy Walker specifically in mind, she noticed something that she had previously missed.

Reflection point

As she read through the predictive factors, Dr. Gulati noticed something about them that she now realized might be important in managing Roy Walker's low back pain effectively.

What do you think it was she noticed?

What Dr. Gulati now noticed was that Roy Walker's full house of yellow flags, although at the heart of the evidence-based guidelines on the management of low back pain, was in fact a full house of Roy Walker's *values*.

Values in the guidelines

Fascinated that she had not noticed this before, Dr. Gulati marked up her copy of the guidelines with blue highlighter for explicitly value-laden words (e.g. "negative," "harm," etc.) and underlining for any that were implicitly value-laden – the latter included for example phrases like "fear avoidance" that are not in themselves value-laden but imply a given value, in this case a negative weighting for fear of activities perceived as increasing the risk of low back pain. Her marked-up list is shown below:

- A negative attitude that back pain is harmful or potentially severely disabling.
- Fear avoidance behavior and reduced activity levels.
- An expectation that passive rather than active treatment will be beneficial.
- A tendency to depression, low morale and social withdrawal.
- Social or financial problems.

So what Dr. Gulati noticed was that the values issues in the problem she faced were not just in how to *manage* the clinical problem presented by Roy Walker against a background of essentially value-free evidence. Values were also there, right up front, in *the problem itself* as defined by the evidence on chronicity.

Values everywhere

The literature on decision analysis as we have seen standardly assumes a model in which there is a clear separation between the facts (evidence-based probabilities of a range of outcomes) and the values (preference-based utilities) bearing on a given decision-maker's choices in a given situation. But what Dr. Gulati now recognized was that here at least, with the factors predicting chronicity for low back pain, there is no such clear separation. The problem she faced was not merely one of Roy Walker's values getting in the way of her management of his low back pain. Here, the patient's values were intrinsically problematic in the practice of patient-centered medicine. The problem *itself* was Roy Walker's values.

We will pick up further on this point in the next chapter. One of our three key points about values (see Chapter 1) is that values are everywhere.

Individual clinical judgment

Feeling that she had not made much progress in deciding how to manage Roy Walker, and with the second consultation getting closer, Dr. Gulati turned finally to one further book she had first read as a student, David Sackett and colleagues' (2000) *Evidence-based Medicine: How to Practice and Teach EBM*. Dr. Gulati recalled Sackett and his colleagues addressing the challenge of thinking about patients' values in evidence-based decision-making with individual patients. So she still had hopes of a solution here.

Initially, she was disappointed. Innovative as it was in its day, the practical guidance it gave about applying evidence-based medicine in individual cases followed very much the same lines as Hunink *et al.*'s *Decision Making in Health and Medicine*. Both books employed decision analysis with its essentially utilitarian values, and in a paradigm that had the patient (or clinician or carer as surrogate patient) as a sole decision-maker. Neither therefore fully served her current purpose.

But then, as she was closing the book, Dr. Gulati's attention was caught by the definition of evidence-based medicine that Sackett and his colleagues gave on the very first page of their introduction.

Reflection point

We give Sackett's definition of evidence-based medicine in full in Fig. 2.3.

Before reading on, have a look at this definition. What do you think caught Dr. Gulati's eye?

There is something there that has been left out of the account thus far. What do you think this is?

Clinical expertise and clinical judgment

Thus far, Dr. Gulati had understood her problem about Roy Walker's demand for an off-work certificate in terms of the standard duo of evidence and values. As Fig. 2.3 shows, evidence and values were indeed both represented in the Sackett definition (the definition of patients' values is, as just noted, that given earlier, in Chapter 1). But between evidence and values in the Sackett definition came a third term, *clinical expertise*.

This was not the first time Dr. Gulati had read the Sackett definition of evidence-based medicine. Its inclusive nature, as against more narrowly focused evidence-only definitions, had been one of the things that had inspired her to read the book as a student. But her previous reading had all been in a more or less theoretical frame of mind and she had taken the middle term in their definition, clinical expertise, largely for granted.

Back with Dr. Gulati

Now, reading Sackett's definition for the first time "for real," with a real decision to be made with a particular

---

Evidence-based medicine (EBM) is the integration of best research evidence with clinical expertise and patient values.

- By *best research evidence* we mean clinically relevant research, often from the basic sciences of medicine, but especially from patient-centered clinical research into the accuracy and precision of diagnostic tests (including the clinical examination), the power of prognostic markers, and the efficacy and safety of therapeutic, rehabilitative, and preventive regimens. New evidence from clinical research both invalidates previously accepted diagnostic tests and treatments and replaces them with new ones that are more powerful, more accurate, more efficacious, and safer.
- By *clinical expertise* we mean the ability to use our clinical skills and past experience to rapidly identify each patient's unique health state and diagnosis, the individual risks and benefits of potential interventions, and the patient's personal values and expectations.
- By *patient values* we mean the unique preferences, concerns and expectations each patient brings to a clinical encounter and which must be integrated into clinical decisions if they are to serve the patient.

When these three elements are integrated, clinicians and patients form a diagnostic and therapeutic alliance which optimises clinical outcomes and quality of life.

Fig. 2.3. Definition of evidence-based medicine from Sackett *et al.*, 2000.

---

patient in a particular concrete situation, Dr. Gulati realized that clinical expertise, sitting as it did between evidence and values in the Sackett definition, was the missing link she had been looking for in using her clinical judgment to apply evidence and values in this (or any other) particular case.

This "Ah ha!" moment triggered for Dr. Gulati a memory of the last time she had felt really empowered to tap into her tacit reserves of clinical expertise. That was when she "discovered" narrative-based medicine. Prompted by an article in the *British Medical Journal* entitled "Why study narrative?" (Greenhalgh and Hurwitz, 1999), she had first bought their book (Greenhalgh and Hurwitz, 1998) and then avidly read John Launer's book on the same topic (Launer, 2002). Narrative, she now realized, is also crucial to empathic understanding of values. As Giovanni Stanghellini says in *The Grammar of the Psychiatric Interview* (2007), "Narratives are the natural forms through which people attempt to express and order the feelings and the meanings of their experiences. They are personal, individual reconstructions of one's experiences which are also based on general (i.e. impersonal), culturally shared patterns of meanings."

So it was her expertise that underpinned the *clinical judgment* she had to exercise in bringing values and evidence together "for real" in an individual case. With hindsight, this was clear from Beauchamp and Childress's insistence that applying principles reasoning in individual cases always involved an element of judgment. Sackett's three-part definition (evidence, experience and values) of evidence-based medicine amounts to a generalization of the same point. As Dr. Gulati now recognized:

- *Clinical* judgment is crucial to deciding whether a given ethical rule (however detailed) applies in a particular case: this requires skills and experience.
- *Clinical* judgment is no less crucial to deciding whether a given body of evidence (however comprehensive it may be) applies to a particular case: this too requires skills and experience.

Planning her repeat consultation with Roy Walker, Dr. Gulati was fully aware that her decision, if it was to be consistent with current principles of good medical practice, had to be made in partnership with Roy Walker. (We return to the nature of partnership in values-based practice in Chapter 13.) She had a number of tools more or less readily to hand that could be helpful to her in deciding what to do with Roy Walker. But what she now realized was that actually *using* those tools "for real," actually making this (or any other) particular decision in partnership with this (or any other) particular patient, was a matter for *her* clinical judgment.

It was at this stage that Dr. Gulati decided to look once again at the RCGP website. This time she wanted to look particularly for what help is available for developing clinical judgment. She came across the curriculum statements for general practice, and one in particular caught her eye; it was the curriculum statement on clinical ethics and values-based practice, and here, at last, she felt that there was something that spoke to her learning needs. Fig. 2.4 shows the headline learning outcomes that she selected as relevant to her "stuck point."

Primary care management

By the end of the GP training the specialty registrar (GP) should demonstrate:

- Awareness of the range of values that may influence a patient's behaviour or decision-making in relation to his or her illness
- How to integrate knowledge of patients' values with the relevant scientific evidence and clinical experience to achieve the best outcome for the patient
- Ability to recognise the ethical issues raised by public health programmes and develop appropriate approaches to their implementation
- Ability to recognise the needs and values of carers and their impact on patient care.

Person-centred care

By the end of GP training the specialty registrar (GP) should demonstrate:

- Skills to achieve meaningful consent by a patient to a plan of management by seeing the patient as a unique person in a unique context

Fig. 2.4. Extract from the RCGP Curriculum Statement 3.3 on *Clinical Ethics and Values-based Practice* (version 1.1, February 2009: www.rcgp-curriculum.org.uk/pdf/curr_3_3_Clinical_ethics.pdf).

Back to "Go" a final time

On our journey with Dr. Gulati, we have once again reached the starting point for values-based practice in the complex and conflicting values that arise when individual clinical judgment has to be exercised in taking decisions for real with particular individual patients. Fig. 2.5 shows diagrammatically the role of clinical judgment in decision-making and how this is supported on the one hand by evidence-based practice and on the other by values-based practice.

Squaring down

One of us, from whose work this diagram is taken (Peile, 2011), has called the role of clinical judgment in individual decision-making "squaring down." The idea is this. When we see a patient with a new problem, we gather a good deal of information that may potentially be relevant to diagnosis or treatment. Much of the art of clinical decision-making is to focus on the more relevant information rather than the less relevant information arising from history, examination and

1. **Information about the patient** expands
with clinical process

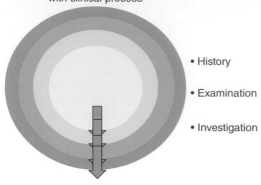

- History

- Examination

- Investigation

2. Clinicians "square down" on **diagnosis**,
narrowing the possibilities as they
accumulate information

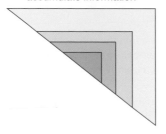

3. At the same time, as they accumulate information,
clinicians "square down" on **management and treatment
decisions**, focusing on the most important first steps

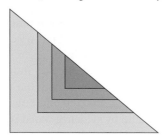

Fig. 2.5. Squaring down.

4. In "squaring down", bringing the focus onto the most likely
diagnoses and the most important treatment decisions,
evidence-basing is vital to clinical process

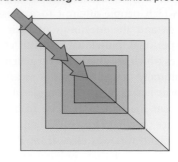

5. So too is **values-basing**
Discovering more about the values sharpens the focus onto
the relevant diagnostic and treatment issues for
this particular patient in this particular situation

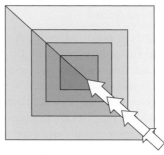

6. The round peg in the square hole!
What we have learnt about the patient fits into
our 'squared down' focus on **diagnosis and management**

Where does it fit?
=
**Professional
judgment**

investigations. All models of clinical decision-making (for example hypothetico-deductive reasoning, pattern recognition and scheme-inductive reasoning) emphasize this. Diagnosis and treatment are, of course, not independent. In any given clinical situation, we may reach the point where we are ready to help the patient make a decision about management before we have arrived at a finite diagnosis. For example, "We don't yet know what's wrong, but we do know this is potentially serious. I would advise you to let me put a cannula in your arm and call an ambulance."

Conversely, we may reach a point of certainty about diagnosis before we are ready to decide on treatment, for example, "Now that we know that you have got rheumatoid arthritis, we need to look at the options for treating this together." The information we have gathered thus has to be progressively "squared down" as we focus in on the best way to help the patient in question.

It is to this process of squaring down that clinical judgment based on skills and experience is crucial. In the growing complexities of current practice, clinical judgment increasingly has to be supported by the resources of evidence-based practice. But the complexities bearing on clinical judgment in current practice are equally in the *values* base as in the evidence base of decision-making. Hence, just as there is a growing need for *evidence*-based practice to support clinical judgment in decision-making with individual patients, so too is there is an equal and counterpart need for *values*-based practice.

Chapter summary

In this chapter, we have followed Dr. Gulati during a period of time out, as she worked her way through a number of tools in what we have called medicine's values toolbox: ethical codes and principles reasoning, the more mathematical decision analysis, and evidence-based practice.

Each of these tools Dr. Gulati found helpful in different ways and up to a point. Each of them has its own distinctive and important place among medicine's growing resources for working with values. Yet none of these tools, separately or together, actually resolved Dr. Gulati's dilemma about what to do when they were applied for real with an individual patient, Roy Walker, in a particular clinical context:

- Codes simply *reflected* Dr. Gulati's dilemma as a tension between different "goods" in "good medical practice."
- Principles had to be *balanced* in individual cases.
- Decision analysis, although it focused on individual cases, did so from the perspective only of the decision-maker (whereas Dr. Gulati's problem was *between* her and Roy Walker) and in terms mainly of utilitarian values (whereas Dr. Gulati's problem was a tension *between* utilitarian and deontological values).

The focus on clinical expertise as a crucial third term between best evidence and patients' values finally helped Dr. Gulati make progress. She had not as yet actually decided what to do. But what she now realized was that informed as she might be by ethics, decision analysis and other similar tools, the decision about what to do was, in the end, between her and Roy Walker as the two individuals directly concerned. In exercising her clinical judgment, Dr. Gulati, as we will see when we return to her story in Chapter 14, would draw equally on evidence-based practice and on values-based practice as she "squared down" on a decision about what to do.

In the final chapter of this part, we give an outline of values-based practice. It is our claim that values-based practice adds an important new dimension to clinical practice that will be illustrated by the clinical narratives in the rest of the book.

References

Beauchamp, T. L. and Childress, J. F. (1989). *Principles of Biomedical Ethics*, 3rd edn (6th edn, 2009). Oxford: Oxford University Press.

Brown, M. M., Brown, G. C. and Sharma, S. (2005). *Evidence-based to Value-based Medicine*. Chicago: American Medical Association Press.

Crisp, R. (1994). Quality of life and health care. In K. W. M. Fulford, G. Gillett and J. Soskice, eds., *Medicine and Moral Reasoning*. Cambridge: Cambridge University Press, pp. 171–83.

Fulford, K. W. M., Thornton, T. and Graham, G. (2006). From bioethics to values-based practice. In K. W. M. Fulford, T. Thornton and G. Graham, eds., *The Oxford Textbook of Philosophy and Psychiatry*. Oxford: Oxford University Press.

Greenhalgh, T. and Hurwitz, B. (1998). *Narrative Based Medicine: Dialogue and Discourse in Clinical Practice*. London: BMA Books.

Greenhalgh, T. and Hurwitz, B. (1999). Why study narrative? *BMJ* **318**, 48–50.

Hunink, M., Glasziou, P., Siegel, J. *et al.* (2001). *Decision Making in Health and Medicine: Integrating Evidence and Values*. Cambridge: Cambridge University Press.

Launer, J. (2002). *Narrative Based Primary Care: a Practical Guide*. Oxford: Radcliffe Medical Press.

Peile, E. B. (2011). Teaching with patients. Available at: http://www.epigeum.com/component/programmes/?view=programme&programme=21 (in press).

Sackett, D. L., Straus, S. E., Scott Richardson, W., Rosenberg, W. and Haynes, R. B. (2000). *Evidence-based Medicine: How to Practice and Teach EBM*, 2nd edn. Edinburgh and London: Churchill Livingstone.

Stanghellini, G. (2007). The grammar of the psychiatric interview. *Psychopathology* **40**, 69–74.

Websites

- The "Duties of a doctor" are given in the GMC's Good Medical Practice at http://www.gmc-uk.org.
- The Royal College of General Practitioners' website is http://www.rcgp.org.uk.
- Café Annalisa decision support is at http://www.cafeannalisa.org.uk.

An outline of values-based practice: its point, premise and ten-part process

Topics covered in this chapter

This chapter gives an initial overview of values-based practice by way of preparation for the case studies that follow in the rest of the book. We cover:

- The *point* of values-based practice: balanced decision-making within a framework of shared values
- The *premise* of values-based practice: mutual respect for differences of values
- *Ten elements of the process* of values-based practice:
  - Four areas of clinical skills
  - Two aspects of professional relationships
  - Three links with evidence-based practice
  - Dissensus: a basis in partnership.

Take-away message for practice

*Values-based practice is a **process** that supports **balanced decision-making** within a **framework of shared values** where complex and conflicting values are in play.*

In this chapter, we give an outline of values-based practice by way of preparation for the detailed case studies that follow in the rest of the book. We will be drawing in this instance not on a specific clinical scenario but rather on a number of brief examples, mainly from mental health and primary care.

Values-based practice aims to support balanced decision-making within a framework of shared values, based on a premise of mutual respect and relying for its practical effectiveness on good process rather than pre-set right outcomes. We start with the point of values-based practice by looking in more detail at what balanced decision-making within a framework of shared values really means.

The point of values-based practice – balanced decision-making

The need for balanced decision-making on individual cases where complex and conflicting values are involved became clear as we followed the story of Dr. Gulati and Roy Walker in the last two chapters. The values involved here were clearly complex – we found that every component of what we called the network of values was reflected explicitly or implicitly in the brief clinical scenario with which we opened Chapter 1.

But the values involved were also conflicting. When Dr. Gulati took time out to re-read her ethics books, she came to recognize that her difficulty in deciding what to do was, precisely, a difficulty about balancing a variety of conflicting values. A number of tools from medicine's values toolbox then proved helpful to Dr. Gulati up to a point, but none actually resolved her dilemma about what to do in this particular case. She found that ultimately the decision had come back to roost with her as a matter for her own clinical judgment. The processes of values-based practice are designed to assist that judgment.

Values, values everywhere

It is important to recognize first just how pervasive in health care are difficulties of the kind experienced by Dr. Gulati. The Four Principles of Beauchamp and Childress (1989) actually characterize ethical problems as a whole in this way. It is in the very nature of ethical problems, they argue, that they arise from conflicts or tensions between two or more "prima facie principles" (or values), each of which is important in its own right but neither of which is clearly pre-eminent in the particular situation in question. Hence, values are in conflict one with another.

Beauchamp and Childress may or may not be right that ethical problems can always be characterized as conflicts between prima facie important principles. There is much theoretical debate in philosophy about the nature of ethical problems. But they are surely right that a great many ethical problems in health care arise from complex and conflicting values. The aim of values-based practice is to assist balanced decision-making in individual cases.

An example from mental health

An example of balanced values-based decision-making in practice is provided by the training materials produced for the UK government's Department of Health to support the implementation of new legislation covering the use of compulsory (non-consenting or involuntary) admission and treatment for mental disorders (Care Services Improvement Partnership (CSIP) and the National Institute for Mental Health in England (NIMHE), 2008).

By its very nature, the use of compulsion involves conflicting values – the patient concerned wants one thing, *not* to receive treatment, while almost everyone else wants the opposite, that he or she *does* receive treatment. Compulsory treatment is correspondingly an ethically problematic area of mental health practice on which there is a large and well-established bioethical and legal literature (see, for example, several chapters in Bloch *et al.*'s seminal *Psychiatric Ethics*, 1999).

Shared values and guiding principles

As might be expected, therefore, the process of public consultation that preceded the introduction of the new legislation was both protracted and contentious. What emerged from this consultation, however, was a set of *shared values* – that is, a number of aspects of the way this or any other similar legislation should be used that all stakeholder groups (including patients, carers, clinicians, lawyers and legislators) agreed were important. It was these shared values that in the form of a set of Guiding Principles were the foundation for the values-based approach adopted in the training materials produced to support implementation.

The law, a Code of Practice and the Guiding Principles

This is broadly how the approach worked:

- The law defined what could be done.
- An accompanying Code of Practice set out more detailed rules about how to do it.

- The Guiding Principles provided a framework of shared values within which balanced decisions on the use of compulsion could be made in individual cases.

The Guiding Principles are reproduced in Fig. 3.1. As you can see, each of the principles is in itself complex – the Principle of Respect for example means different things to different people in different contexts. Equally important, though, the Guiding Principles taken together are, like Beauchamp and Childress's principles to which Dr. Gulati referred in Chapter 2, inherently in tension one with another.

Balanced decision-making within a framework of shared values

> **Reflection point**
>
> At this point, you may find it helpful to think from your own experience of how the Guiding Principles set out in Fig. 3.1 might come into tension and hence have to be balanced in an appropriate way when applied to an individual case.
>
> You don't have to be a doctor to think about this. Think about it from your own point of view and drawing on your own experience, whether as a clinician (perhaps as a GP, for example, or a social worker), a patient or an informal carer.
>
> Also, think about it "for real," i.e. as the Guiding Principles might apply in a real concrete situation involving particular individuals, rather than in a general theoretical way.

Many examples may spring to mind here. The Resources Principle, for example, which includes a value of efficient use of resources, may be in tension with the Principle of Respect (there being a limit to how far resources can efficiently be tailored to individual needs); or again, the Purpose Principle, which includes a value of "protecting other people from harm," may be in tension with the Principle of Least Restrictive Alternative. As with Beauchamp and Childress's principles, therefore, the Guiding Principles in the Code of Practice to the new Mental Health Act amount to a framework of shared values within which the provisions of the Act have to be applied in a balanced way according to the particular circumstances presented by each individual situation.

Purpose	Decisions under the Act must be taken with a view to minimising the undesirable effects of mental disorder, by maximising the safety and well-being (mental and physical) of patients, promoting their recovery and protecting other people from harm.
Least restrictive alternative	People taking action without a patient's consent must attempt to keep to a minimum the restrictions they impose on the patient's liberty, having regard to the purpose for which the restrictions are imposed.
Respect	People taking decisions under the Act must recognise and respect the diverse needs, values and circumstances of each patient, including their race, religion, culture, gender, age, sexual orientation and any disability. They must consider the patient's views, wishes and feelings (whether expressed at the time or in advance), so far as they are reasonably ascertainable, and follow those wishes wherever practicable and consistent with the purpose of the decision. There must be no unlawful discrimination.
Participation	Patients must be given the opportunity to be involved, as far as is practicable in the circumstances, in planning, developing and reviewing their own treatment and care to help ensure that it is delivered in a way that is as appropriate and effective for them as possible. The involvement of carers, family members and other people who have an interest in the patient's welfare should be encouraged (unless there are particular reasons to the contrary) and their views taken seriously.
Resources (effectiveness, efficiency and equity)	People taking decisions under the Act must seek to use the resources available to them and to patients in the most effective, efficient and equitable way, to meet the needs of patients and achieve the purpose for which the decision was taken.

Fig. 3.1. The Guiding Principles for the UK Mental Health Act 2007.

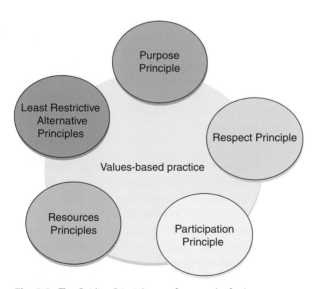

Fig. 3.2. The Guiding Principles as a framework of values.

Fig. 3.2, which is taken from the training materials produced to support the Mental Health Act 2007, shows the approach diagrammatically. The Guiding Principles are represented as a "round table" at which none is pre-eminent – there is no "top value" as it were. There is a

need, therefore, for what Beauchamp and Childress called "situational judgments," that is, judgments about how to balance the conflicting demands of the Guiding Principles appropriately in the particular concrete situation presented by a given case (Beauchamp and Childress, 1989, 3rd edn, p. 53; the corresponding discussion in the 2009 6th edn comes on p. 15). It is here, as the round-table diagram shows, that values-based practice provides the skills and other resources for balanced decision-making in individual cases.

We include on the website supporting this book the Foundation Module from the training manual, which gives a number of worked examples of how values-based practice supports this process of balanced decision-making in applying the Act.

Human rights as a framework of values

There are precedents for this round-table approach to balanced decision-making. In a lecture to the British Academy in 2002, Lord Woolf, at the time the UK's most senior lawyer, described the Human Rights Act in similar terms. The rights embodied in the Act, he said, should not be understood in the way that rights are generally understood by lawyers. They are not a checklist of legal "must haves" (not his term). Rather they represent a framework of values that have to be used in a balanced way in particular cases (reproduced in Hansard, the proceedings of the UK Parliament – see Woolf, 2002).

The premise of values-based practice – respect for differences of values

Dr. Gulati, you will recall from Chapter 2, was at one stage in her "time out" hoping to find ethical authority, initially in various codes of practice and then in Beauchamp and Childress's *Principles of Biomedical Ethics*, to resolve the conflict of values she faced.

This is natural enough. Wherever there are conflicting values, it is natural that the search should be on for an authority to define a rule or "top value," a moral anchor that will prevent us being blown on to the rocks. This is reflected in the way we talk about "strong values," about being "clear about the bottom line," or being "confident in your faith." The rise in ideologically based religions, similarly, reflects a widespread need for an "authority," for someone who will just get on and tell us "exactly what *is* the right thing to do." Without such strong values, so this approach assumes, ethical reasoning is toothless and we risk sliding into relativism and moral chaos.

My values today! Your values tomorrow!

Values-based practice, in being premised on mutual respect for differences of values, is vulnerable to these concerns. "Ha! My values today! Your values tomorrow!" we heard someone quip in a workshop on values-based practice, thus neatly capturing the absurdities of a moral relativism in which "anything goes." Beauchamp and Childress, whose balanced approach through principles reasoning is vulnerable to similar concerns, note that there are well-grounded moral theories based on "top values."

We do not have the space here to argue the theoretical issues (although for more on this, see sources on the accompanying website). From a practical perspective, the key point to emphasize is that deeply held personal religious (or other) beliefs are entirely compatible with values-based practice.

Take, for example, His Holiness the Dalai Lama's exposition of Buddhist "Right view: right conduct" in

The Leader's Way (2008): "The right view is of no value if it does not lead to the right action – and taking the right action is obviously fundamental for success. . . . Leadership is about making decisions, and not just any decisions – the right ones." The Dalai Lama, importantly, does not *prescribe* the right view or the right action: what he does (consistently with values-based practice) is to suggest *processes* conducive to finding them for any particular situation. There is thus no conflict with the premise of values-based practice in this teaching. We return to this point in connection with the Christian tradition of spiritual direction in Chapter 12.

For the moment, though, a more immediate way of putting the issues in perspective is by comparing the mutual-respect-based values-based practice with the equally mutual-respect-based political democracy.

Democracies for and against

> **Reflection point**
>
> Think for a moment about political democracies and values-based practice. Are there any parallels to be drawn here?
>
> In particular, is there a parallel between the key principle underpinning a parliamentary democracy ("one person, one vote") and the starting point for values-based practice in its premise of mutual respect for differences of values?

The parallels between a political democracy and values-based practice should not be stretched too far, of course. Neither should such parallels as there are be taken as a knock-down argument for the values-based premise of respect for differences of values. For one thing, democracy itself is far from being universally accepted. There are many who believe that at least the "Western" model of democracy has gone too far towards individualism. As the social psychologist Barry Schwartz has pointed out, in his aptly titled *The Paradox of Choice* (2004), it is very far from clear that people are happier the more autonomy they have. Few would disagree with the Egyptian psychiatrist Ahmed Okasha (2000) that those living in industrially developed countries have much to relearn from more traditional cultures about the values of family and community.

Unique individuals and good process

Nonetheless, for good or ill, values-based practice is in at least two respects very like a political democracy:

- Both start from the *unique individual* – "one person, one vote" in a political democracy; "one person, one value (or at any rate unique set of values)" in the values democracy of values-based practice.
- Both rely on *good process* rather than preset "right outcomes" to guide decision-making.

We come to the process of values-based practice in a moment. First, it will be worth looking briefly at how a "values democracy" works out in practice with a second example from mental health. This example will show that, far from being ethically toothless, the premise of values-based practice in mutual respect for differences of values carries with it clear and definite implications for policy and practice.

A second example from mental health – the NIMHE Values Framework

In the early 1990s, the UK's Department of Health set up the NIMHE to support implementation of mental health policy. NIMHE's first task was to agree and set out an explicit set of values to which all stakeholders – service users as well as service providers – subscribed and that would therefore provide a clear and strong basis from which to develop and implement policy. To understand how the NIMHE Values Framework ultimately emerged as a democracy of values, it will be worth a brief historical detour.

Diversity of needs

The need for an agreed set of values underpinning NIMHE's work had been identified by the (then recently appointed) National Director for Mental Health, Professor Louis Appleby, a psychiatrist with a background in epidemiology. Appleby set up a website to which he invited everyone concerned with mental health to contribute, service users and service providers alike. He was overwhelmed with "hits." But what particularly impressed Appleby was the extent to which service users clearly felt that what they were being offered failed to coincide with their real needs. A wide diversity of needs was expressed. But a common theme was that what service providers genuinely

believed to be what their clients and patients wanted, all too often was not.

There was at the time a growing body of evidence suggesting an endemic mismatch between real and perceived service needs in mental health (see, for example, Rogers *et al.*, 1993). But what should NIMHE do? One way forward was for those responsible for NIMHE to set out a list or statement of "core values" – such lists were being produced by everyone who was anyone in health care at the time from voluntary organizations to pharmaceutical companies, and NIMHE did indeed produce such a list. Useful as these lists were up to a point, however, rather than guiding decision-making, they tended to be forgotten – "gathering dust on the CEO's desk," as one CEO put it at the time.

From prescribed values to democratic process

A different way forward was to go through a process of consultation with stakeholders to define their respective value perspectives and to see to what extent they could come up with an agreed values framework to guide NIMHE's work. This was the approach that NIMHE adopted. Anthony Sheehan, NIMHE's first Director, convened a Values Project Group chaired by a service user and expert on recovery, Piers Allott. The group, which included representatives of each main stakeholder group, produced a draft framework, which was then revised and refined through an extensive process of consultation.

NIMHE's framework of shared values

The full text of the NIMHE Values Framework is given in Fig. 3.3. As you can see, it is both brief and very different in form from any "list of core values." The first half of the framework gives what we might call the "three Rs" of values-based practice – recognition, raising awareness and respect. These three Rs cover three features of values-based practice that were particularly important in guiding the development of the framework and hence of NIMHE's work:

- *Recognition* is about recognizing the importance of values as a partner alongside evidence in all areas of policy and practice. This corresponds with the Two-feet Principle of values-based practice described below in this chapter and illustrated in Chapter 10.
- *Raising awareness* highlights the importance of awareness of values and of diversity of values as the

first and, as we will see later in this chapter, foundational clinical skill for values-based decision-making.

- *Respect* is a direct reference to the premise of values-based practice. We return to the implications of this shortly.

Specific policy and practice implications

The second half of the framework then follows through with specific policy implications of a values-based approach. The extent and detail of these implications gives the lie to the idea that the principle of respect is a recipe for relativism and chaos. This list, applied here in the context of mental health, shows that the premise of respect supports a whole series of well-defined policy and practice objectives. Examples include the importance of services being person-centered and multidisciplinary.

No top value?

The NIMHE Values Framework is premised on the democratic principle of mutual respect and is very far from being empty of content.

Reflection point

You may want to pause here for a moment to think about that claim. The claim is that, although carrying specific implications for policy and practice, the NIMHE Values Framework is premised like values-based practice on respect for differences of values.

Certainly, this is what the framework *says*. But is there in reality a "top value" implicit in the drafting?

Try looking through the framework again in Fig. 3.3 and see what you think.

There are at least two potential candidates for top value here: "service-user centrality," which is described as the "starting point," and "anti-discrimination," which is given particular prominence with a whole paragraph to itself. It will help us in understanding the premise of values-based practice to spend a few moments looking at why in fact neither of these candidates is a (hidden) top value in the framework.

Service-user centrality

Perhaps the most obvious candidate for top value in the framework is the principle of "service-user centrality." This principle is made explicit in the principle of respect and is emphasized later in the framework as

---

The work of the National Institute for Mental Health in England (NIMHE) on values in mental health care is guided by three principles of values-based practice:

1. **Recognition** – NIMHE recognises the role of values alongside evidence in all areas of mental health policy and practice.
2. **Raising Awareness** – NIMHE is committed to raising awareness of the values involved in different contexts, the role/s they play and their impact on practice in mental health.
3. **Respect** – NIMHE respects diversity of values and will support ways of working with such diversity that makes the principle of service-user centrality a unifying focus for practice. This means that the values of each individual service user/client and their communities must be the starting point and key determinant for all actions by professionals.

Respect for diversity of values encompasses a number of specific policies and principles concerned with equality of citizenship. In particular, it is anti-discriminatory because discrimination in all its forms is intolerant of diversity. Thus, respect for diversity of values has the consequence that it is unacceptable (and unlawful in some instances) to discriminate on grounds such as gender, sexual orientation, class, age, abilities, religion, race, culture or language. Respect for diversity within mental health is also:

- *user-centred* – it puts respect for the values of individual users at the centre of policy and practice;
- *recovery oriented* – it recognises that building on the personal strengths and resiliencies of individual users, and on their cultural and racial characteristics, there are many diverse routes to recovery;
- *multidisciplinary* – it requires that respect be reciprocal, at a personal level (between service users, their family members, friends, communities and providers), between different provider disciplines (such as nursing, psychology, psychiatry, medicine, social work), and between different organisations (including health, social care, local authority housing, voluntary organisations, community groups, faith communities and other social support services);
- *dynamic* – it is open and responsive to change;
- *reflective* – it combines self monitoring and self management with positive self regard;
- *balanced* – it emphasises positive as well as negative values;
- *relational* – it puts positive working relationships supported by good communication skills at the heart of practice.

NIMHE will encourage educational and research initiatives aimed at developing the capabilities (the awareness, attitudes, knowledge and skills) needed to deliver mental health services that will give effect to the principles of values-based practice.

Fig. 3.3. The NIMHE Values Framework.

the first of the specific policy implications. So "service-user centrality" is clearly important. But is it a top value for NIMHE in the sense that it is a value trumping all others?

What is important here is the precise wording drafted by Simon Allard for the NIMHE Values Project Group. Simon had had earlier personal experience as a service user and thus had more reason than many to make the interests of service users a top value. But what his drafting so carefully captures is the difference between a consumerist "patient as God" model and the balanced mutual respect model of values-based practice.

The consensus in mental health, as in other areas of medicine, is that particular weight *should* be given to the values of patients and carers as the actual users of services. Simon Allard's drafting of the NIMHE Values Framework specifies that ". . . the principle of service-user centrality [should be] a unifying focus for practice." What this means, the framework continues, is that the values of individual service users (and where relevant their communities) should be ". . . the starting point and key determinant for all actions by professionals." Note therefore the careful wording here: the principle of service-user centrality is the "starting point" but not the *only* point, and it is the "key" but not the *only* determinant, of actions by professionals. Service-user *centrality*, then, is fine; but this does not mean service-user *totality*.

Racism and relativism

A second, less obvious candidate for a top value in the framework is the importance of being "anti-discriminatory." Like the principle of service-user centrality, this is given some prominence in the framework. In contrast to what the framework says about service-user centrality, the wording leaves no room for a balanced approach. Discrimination of *any* kind, the framework says unequivocally, ". . . is unacceptable (and unlawful in some instances) . . ."

So is there a limit to the principle of respect for diversity? Is discrimination, at least, out? Yes it is, because, as the framework makes clear earlier in the same paragraph, ". . . discrimination in all its forms is intolerant of diversity." In other words, discrimination is "out" because it is, by definition, *inconsistent with the premise* of values-based practice in mutual respect.

Two reasons to be cheerful

There are respectable bodies of moral opinion advocating a top value, and arguing that without one we

inevitably slide into the chaos of a moral relativism in which "anything goes." The NIMHE Values Framework has now given us two clear reasons why, in the values democracy of values-based practice, as in political democracy, the chaos of moral relativism has not resulted from following a premise of mutual respect.

Reason 1: shared values

The first reason is simply that people's values, although indeed individually unique, are very far from being chaotic. Thus, "service-user centrality," although not a top value in the sense of a value trumping all others, is nonetheless a value that is widely shared among everyone involved in health care. It is a value that *should* be given particular weight in decision-making by health-care professionals (among others).

A similar use of shared values underpinned the incorporation of the Guiding Principles for the UK's Mental Health Act 2007 into the training materials described earlier in this chapter.

In Chapter 14, when we come back to how Dr. Gulati used a values-based approach to resolving her dilemma, we will again demonstrate the importance of shared values.

Reason 2: values excluded by definition

The second reason why having no top value in a democracy does not lead to "anything goes" is simply that some values are ruled out by being inconsistent with the premise of mutual respect as one of the defining features of values-based practice. Values that involve discrimination, of which racism is a particularly pernicious example, are a case in point. Anti-discrimination is emphasized as a main principle in the NIMHE Values Framework because discrimination is inconsistent with respect for diversity.

The limits of tolerance are always contestable in a democracy. To this extent, therefore, the fear of a limited form of relativism is well founded, although – as one of us has argued elsewhere – we have perhaps more to fear from absolutism (Fulford *et al.*, 2003). But in the democracy of values represented by values-based practice, the premise of mutual respect puts racism at least, and with it any other form of discrimination, firmly beyond the pale.

The NIMHE Values Framework and Dr. Gulati

The NIMHE Values Framework was produced as a direct response to the extent of the complex and often conflicting values at play in mental health. We will see in Chapter 14 how a similar process of developing a shared framework for values-based practice can help Dr. Gulati to move forward in a different clinical domain.

Making effective use of such a framework of shared values depends, in our view, on developing the skills and practicing the elements of the process of values-based practice. It is to this process, therefore, that we turn now.

The ten-part process of values-based practice

In the rest of this chapter, we introduce the ten key elements of the process by which values-based practice, starting from a premise of mutual respect, supports balanced decision-making in health care.

A *ten*-part process may sound a bit complicated. But a degree of complication is inevitable in a complex area like clinical decision-making (think of the complexities of evidence-based practice). Moreover, as with any skills-based activity, values-based practice is used much of the time (once it has been learned) on "automatic." And although working together as a whole overall, the different parts of the process of values-based practice apply in different ways and to different extents in different areas of decision-making.

In brief then, the process of values-based practice includes four areas of clinical skills, two aspects of relationships, three principles of the relationship between evidence and values, and a particular take (dissensus) on partnership in clinical decision-making.

Four areas of clinical skills

The four areas of clinical skills underpinning values-based practice are awareness of values, reasoning, knowledge and communication skills. Each of these is crucial right up front, as it were, in the clinical encounter. Here, as with other clinical skills, it is important to differentiate between learning and doing. We have to reflect on a skill when we are acquiring it. But it fails *as* a skill if eventually we are unable to use it for real in a natural and unselfconscious way.

In Part 2, therefore, we will focus on the importance for values-based decision-making, respectively,

of awareness of values in relation to recovery in schizophrenia (Chapter 4), reasoning about values as illustrated by the problems of managing teenage acne (Chapter 5), knowledge of values in a case involving a long-term smoker with chronic obstructive pulmonary disease (Chapter 6), and last but not least in Chapter 7, on the crucial importance of communication skills as illustrated by the challenges of maintaining blood sugar control in an adolescent girl with type I diabetes.

Relationships in values-based practice

Clinical skills can never be detached from the quality of our professional relationships, and the next two elements of the process of values-based practice are correspondingly about person-centered practice and multidisciplinary teamwork.

There are *two-way* interactions between values-based practice and both person-centered practice and multidisciplinary teamwork. Values-based practice both depends on and in turn contributes to person-centered practice. Similarly, values-based practice both depends on and in turn contributes to multidisciplinary teamwork. The significance of these two-way relationships will be illustrated, respectively, with a case of early breast cancer (person-centered practice) in Chapter 8, and child safeguarding (multidisciplinary teamwork) in Chapter 9.

Science and values-based practice

Values-based practice, as the subtitle of this book reminds us, is all about linking science, as represented particularly by evidence-based practice, with the unique values of individual people. But the relationship between science and values is itself highly complex and much contested. This part of the process of values-based practice thus highlights three principles covering aspects of the relationship between science and values that are particularly crucial in the context of the clinical encounter.

Clinically, each of these principles can be thought of as a values "red flag", a danger signal that we may be missing some important aspect of a presenting problem:

- *The Two-feet Principle* (Chapter 10, on essential hypertension) picks up the point made in Chapter 1 that *all* decisions, whether overtly value-laden or not, are based on the two feet of values and evidence. Clinically, what this means is that, if a problem appears to be nothing more than a matter of establishing the facts, a red flag should go up – look out for hidden values. The warning is "Think evidence, think values too!"

- *The Squeaky-wheel Principle* (Chapter 11, on unexplained abdominal pain) picks up the point that we tend to notice values when they cause trouble. In the analogy, the expert haulier does more than just apply a spot of oil to a "squeaky wheel": he thinks about why this wheel is squeaking and what is going on with the axles and the other wheels. Clinically, this translates into the opposite of the Two-feet Principle, namely that if a clinical problem appears to be nothing more than a matter of values (as in an ethical dilemma), the red flag should warn us to look for hidden matters of fact. So here the warning is the opposite: "Think values, think evidence too!"
- *The Science-driven Principle* (Chapter 12, on infertility treatment) is about advances in medical science and technology driving the need equally for values-based as for evidence-based practice. We will look at why this is so in Chapter 12. But the clinical bottom line is that, with problems arising in high-tech areas of medicine (like IVF), look out *both* for hidden values *and* for hidden evidence. So in high-tech areas, the red flag warning is: "Think both evidence *and* values!"

Dissensus: a basis in partnership

Values-based practice brings a particular concept, dissensus, to the idea of partnership between clinicians and patients and their families in decision-making. Despite its name, "dissensus" as we will see in Chapter 13, is not about disagreement in the sense of dissent (falling out). Dissensus can be thought of rather as a particular values-based take on "agreeing to disagree." In the more familiar consensus, those concerned *come to an agreement* on whose values are right. In dissensus, differences of values, instead of being resolved, *remain in play* to be balanced according to the circumstances presented by particular decisions.

We will be looking in detail at dissensus and how it links up with the more familiar consensus in Chapter 13. Drawing on a case of partnership in decision-making in palliative care, we will see that dissensus builds directly on (and thus helps to draw together) the other elements of values-based practice.

Values-based practice in practice

In this chapter, we have presented the main features of values-based practice from a somewhat theoretical perspective, emphasizing its underlying premise and how this relates to balanced decision-making as the point of the whole thing. In practice, however, it is the *process* of values-based practice that is crucial in getting us from premise to point. As Fig. 3.4 indicates, it is the ten process elements of values-based practice that, building on the premise of mutual respect, support balanced clinical decision-making within frameworks of shared values.

Time is against us

It is correspondingly the ten process elements of values-based practice on which we will be focusing in the rest of the book. But by now you may well be asking "given the pressures under which most healthcare workers have to work, do we really have time for all this?" True, the elements of values-based practice can be used to good effect separately as well as together: simply raising awareness of values such as strengths, for example, as we will see in the next chapter, can make an immediate difference to assessment and care planning. But all the same, with indeed *ten* process elements in play, isn't this all rather unrealistic?

This is an important question on which to finish this overview of values-based practice. Issues of resourcing are crucial in health care, particularly in the current climate of budget cuts, and our most precious (and surely most limited) resource is time.

Work smarter, not harder

The quick answer is that values-based practice is about working smarter, not harder. This means that, as with evidence-based practice, some up-front investment of time and training is needed, but that this investment, once made, pays off in terms of better targeted and more effective use of resources. As a skills-based approach, values-based practice once learnt is about doing the same things, only better.

Saving time and making time

One of the ways in which values-based practice helps us to do the same things better is by improving our communication skills. We will be looking at the communication skills for values-based practice in more detail in Chapter 7. But the point for now is that good communication skills can convert *saving time*

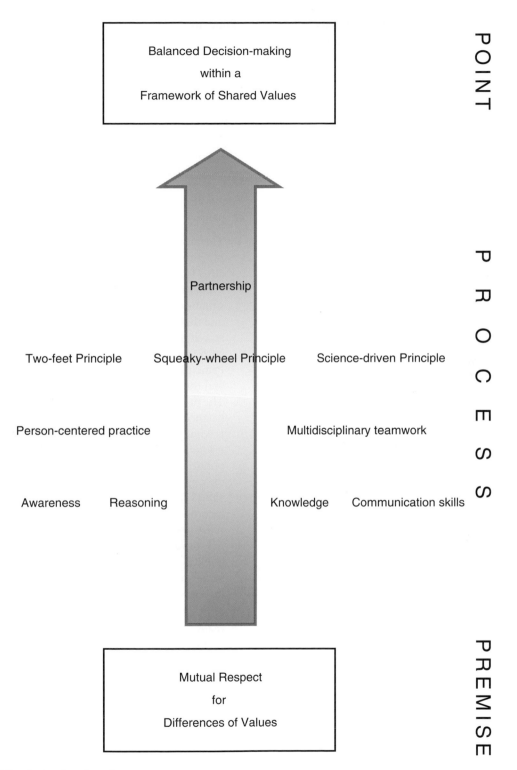

Fig. 3.4. Map of values-based practice.

(experienced by patients as time contracting) into *making time* (experienced as time expanding).

Thus, it might *save time* to stand at a patient's bedside while you talk with them rather than drawing up a chair and sitting down. But two minutes spent talking with that patient sitting down will feel to the patient like ten minutes standing. So a 30-second investment in sitting down effectively pays off with a fourfold increase in the patient's "experienced time." From the patient's point of view, you have, quite literally, *made time*.

"Time out" for reflective practice is "time made"

One of the distinctive features of values-based practice is the attention it pays to clinicians' values. Yet reflective practice including reflection on one's own values is a common casualty of budget cuts.

Once again, this is an example of saving time at the expense of making time. Dr. Gulati in Chapter 2 gained important insights into her own values in her time out to think through what to do about Roy Walker and his demands for an off-work certificate. Other characters in other chapters have similar experiences. So if you want to make good use of your scarce resource of time, hang on to reflective practice and take time out to understand your own values as well as those of others.

Donald Schön makes the point that "reflection on action" can inform subsequent "reflection in action" (Schön, 1983).

The value of care

"But," the hard-pressed practitioner may now persist, "does this matter? The warm glow of feeling that your doctor or nurse cares enough to make time to listen to you is all very well but I have targets to meet. So, sadly, these soft outcomes are a luxury I can't afford."

Understandable as this "but" might be, the implied distinction between soft and hard outcomes is not as well founded as many might think. A case in point is the GP in Chapter 10 whose lack of insight into her own values has the direct consequence of increasing rather than reducing her patient's cardiovascular risk. This case is consistent with a growing evidence base supporting the clinical experience that feeling cared for pays off in terms of the hardest of hard outcomes such as bed-occupancy times and recovery rates.

A recent report from the NHS Confederation (which is the NHS employer's organization) describes a number of initiatives in Hospital Trusts in the UK showing how developing a culture of care actually improves effective use of resources in improving clinical outcomes. The report also cites a number of more formal research studies from the USA showing similar findings (NHS Confederation, 2010). There is, as the NHS Confederation report puts it, a "win–win" case for care.

We return to the value of care in our postscript.

Chapter summary

The outline of values-based practice given in this chapter has covered:

1. The aim of values-based practice. Values-based practice, rather than giving us answers as such, aims to support *balanced decision-making within frameworks of shared values* appropriate to the situation in question. An appropriate framework is one that reflects the values shared by the stakeholder group in question. We looked at two such frameworks, the "round table" of Guiding Principles supporting the Mental Health Act 2007, and the NIMHE Values Framework.

2. The premise of values-based practice. The basis for balanced decision-making in values-based practice is what we called the "democratic" premise of *mutual respect for differences of values*. Like a political democracy, this premise avoids the chaos of "anything goes" partly by excluding certain values (racism, for example, being by definition incompatible with mutual respect) and partly by its reliance on shared values.

3. The process of values-based practice. Again, like a political democracy, the values democracy of values-based practice supports decision-making through good process rather than prescribing pre-set right outcomes. We introduced the *ten key elements of the process* of values-based practice covering clinical skills, professional relationships, the links with evidence-based practice and dissensus as the basis of partnership in decision-making.

It is the ten-part process of values-based practice that will be the focus of the further case studies that follow in the rest of the book.

References

Beauchamp, T. L. and Childress, J. F. (1989). *Principles of Biomedical Ethics*, 3rd edn (6th edn, 2009). Oxford: Oxford University Press.

Bloch, S., Chodoff, P. and Green, S. A. (1999). *Psychiatric Ethics*, 3rd edn. Oxford: Oxford University Press.

Care Services Improvement Partnership (CSIP) and the National Institute for Mental Health in England (NIMHE) (2008). *Workbook to Support Implementation of the Mental Health Act 1983 as Amended by the Mental Health Act 2007*. London: Department of Health.

The Dalai Lama, Van Den Muizenberg, L. (2008). *The Leader's Way*. London: Nicholas Brealey Publishing.

Fulford, K. W. M., Morris, K. J., Sadler, J. Z. and Stanghellini, G. (2003). Past improbable, future possible: the renaissance in philosophy and psychiatry. In K. W. M. Fulford, K. J. Morris, J. Z. Sadler and G. Stanghellini, eds., *Nature and Narrative: an Introduction to the New Philosophy of Psychiatry*. Oxford: Oxford University Press, pp. 1–41.

NHS Confederation (2010). *Feeling Better? Improving Patient Experience in Hospital*. London: NHS Confederation.

Okasha, A. (2000). Ethics of psychiatric practice: consent, compulsion and confidentiality. *Current Opinion in Psychiatry* 13, 693–8.

Rogers, A., Pilgrim, D. and Lacey, R. (1993). *Experiencing Psychiatry: Users' Views of Services*. London: Macmillan Press.

Schön, D. (1983). *The Reflective Practitioner: How Professionals Think in Action*. Boston: Arena Publishing.

Schwartz, B. (2004). *The Paradox of Choice*. New York: HarperCollins Publishers.

Woolf, Lord (2002). Lecture to the British Academy, 15/10/02, quoted in Hansard 28/10/02 col. 607.

Websites

- Royal College of General Practitioners (2005) Curriculum Statement: Ethics and Values Based Medicine:http://www.rcgp.org.uk/gpcurriculum/pdfs/ethicsAndVBPsfRCGPCouncilDec2005.pdf.
- Further reading on the theory and empirical basis of values-based practice and of developments in mental health and primary care is given on the website supporting this series. As noted in the chapter, this includes downloadable training materials.

Introduction to Part 2

With Part 2, we come to the first and foundational group of process elements of values-based practice: the four key areas of clinical skills.

- Chapter 4 introduces awareness. Without awareness of values and of the often-surprising diversity of values, none of the other process elements of values-based practice can get any purchase. In this chapter, the story of how a young woman, Sally Coombs, reaches a turning point towards recovery from schizophrenia illustrates the importance of raised awareness of values as the basis of effective clinical care. Later chapters will illustrate the importance also of developing tools for self-awareness.
- Chapter 5 describes reasoning. In Chapter 2, Dr. Gulati applied "top-down" principles reasoning in trying to work out what to do about Roy Walker's demand for an off-work certificate. This chapter shows how "bottom-up" case-based reasoning (sometimes called casuistry) helped a different GP, Dr. Charles Mangate, in managing a case of teenage acne.
- Chapter 6 discusses knowledge. This chapter focuses the narrative primarily on knowledge of values for training and research. It shows, through the story of a nurse practitioner, Trish Butler, and her patient, Sandy Fraser, with chronic obstructive pulmonary disease, what we can learn but also what we cannot learn about values by searching electronic databases.
- Chapter 7 describes communication skills. Where Chapter 6 focused on training and research, this chapter brings us back to the challenges of clinical work. Through the story of a teenager, Vicky Bartlett, with type I diabetes, it illustrates the importance of communication skills, particularly for eliciting values and in conflict resolution.

The skills illustrated by the stories in this part of the book are foundational not only to values-based practice in isolation but also to its relationships with evidence-based practice (focusing on research evidence) and narrative-based medicine (focusing on clinical expertise). We will be looking in detail at three particular aspects of the relationship between values and evidence from both research and clinical experience in Part 4.

The broader message here is that, by mastering learnable clinical skills, clinicians can develop a process for values-based practice that works in partnership with evidence-based and narrative approaches in linking science with people.

Balanced Decision-making
within a
Framework of Shared Values

Partnership

Two-feet Principle   Squeaky-wheel Principle   Science-driven Principle

Person-centered practice   Multidisciplinary teamwork

Awareness   Reasoning   Knowledge   Communication skills

Mutual Respect
for
Differences of Values

Map of values-based practice – awareness.

4

Recovery in schizophrenia: a values wake-up call
Values-based practice element 1: awareness of values

Topics covered in this chapter

The importance of raised awareness of values is illustrated by a story of recovery in schizophrenia.

Other topics include:

- Crises and shared values
- NICE guidelines
- Person-centered and multidisciplinary assessment
- Assessment of strengths (StAR values)
- WRAP (Wellness Recovery Action Plan).

Take-away message for practice

In assessing a patient's problems, always think about their **strengths, aspirations and resources** *(their* **StAR values**), *as well as their needs and difficulties.*

The first process element of values-based practice is raised awareness of values, including one's own values, and raised awareness of the diversity of values. In this chapter, we explore the importance of this first element through the story of a young woman, Sally Coombs, following her admission to the acute care ward of her local psychiatric hospital.

We noted in Chapter 1 the importance for values-based practice of raising awareness of positive as well as negative values. It turns out that at the heart of Sally Coombs' story were positive and previously unrecognized aspects of her own values including a number of strengths, aspirations and resources. We call these StAR values. Raising awareness of these StAR values through an ongoing process of person-centered and multidisciplinary assessment is a crucial element of this story.

The clinical context

Sally Coombs, a 21-year-old art student, was brought to the acute admissions ward of her local psychiatric hospital by two police constables. PCs George Abrams and Brenda Jones had found Sally sitting on the pavement outside a day center she had been attending after the day center staff had called for help. The background was that Sally Coombs had walked out of the day center after "going berserk" in the OT (occupational therapy) room, slashing her art work, shouting and breaking up the easels and other equipment. The day center staff had confirmed that she had not gone home and they had been understandably very concerned that she was not in a fit state to be wandering the streets.

By the time the officers arrived, Sally Coombs was quiet, but she was withdrawn and appeared not to know where she was. She refused to talk to them or to go back into the day center and, although unlikely to hurt anyone else (her outburst had been directed at things rather than people), her own safety was clearly at risk. The day center staff accordingly called the Duty Charge Nurse of the acute care ward with whom they worked closely, and it was agreed that, as Sally was unable or unwilling to communicate with anyone, the ward would accept her on a Section 136 order for assessment. (Section 136 is a short term "holding" section of the UK's Mental Health Act that allows a person with a mental disorder to be taken to "a place of safety.")

Crisis management

> **Reflection point**
>
> Before going on, you may find it helpful to think for a moment about the immediate priorities in this situation.
>
> You don't have to be a health professional to think about this question. Indeed, the idea is to think about it specifically from *your own background and perspective*. If you are a health professional, then

imagine Sally Coombs is your patient or client. If you are not, imagine you are one of Sally's parents or friends, or imagine you are Sally herself.

Take whichever view point is closest to your own experience (of course, you may have experience of more than one of these perspectives) and think "for real" what your priorities would be.

Shared values in the foreground

In an acute situation of the kind presented by Sally Coombs at this stage in her story, the immediate priority for everyone involved is to get on and deal with the situation in hand. So this is a situation in which, although values are driving what is done, the values in question are the largely *shared values* of containment and safety and other aspects of effective risk management. Those responsible for Sally Coombs, either professionally or as a relative or friend, are likely to be concerned with containing the situation and ensuring that as far as possible neither she nor others are put at risk.

Those concerned, including Sally Coombs, were of course not thinking "values" at the time. Shared values, to the extent that they are unproblematic, tend to go unnoticed, as we saw in Chapter 3. This is the idea behind the Squeaky-wheel Principle of values-based practice to which we return in Chapter 11. As with any other generalization, there are exceptions to the rule of shared values driving acute situations. But in general an acute crisis situation is one in which the foreground values are the shared values involved in dealing decisively with the situation in hand.

Some background complications

That said, even in this scenario there are a number of background values of which it is clinically important to be aware. These background values include both *conflicting* and *complex* values.

Two kinds of conflicting values

One important area of conflicting values in mental health is between what the person concerned wants *and what other people believe is in their best interests.* The UK's Mental Health Act 2007 covers the use of involuntary admission and treatment for mental disorder. Thus, the Act, as we noted in Chapter 3, is by definition concerned with situations in which the patient

wants one thing (*not* to be admitted to hospital and/or treated) while almost everyone else wants the opposite (that they *should* be so admitted and/or treated).

Sally Coombs was neither assenting to nor dissenting from an emergency admission, and her decision-making capacity was not at issue (in the UK, the Mental Health Act 2007 takes precedence over capacity legislation). We return below to what it turned out later Sally Coombs actually wanted at that stage. But at the time, the use of the Mental Health Act was motivated primarily by the protections it offered her as a short-term "safety and containment" measure.

A second and perhaps even deeper conflict of values arising widely in mental health is between what the person concerned wants *and the interests of others.* This second kind of conflict, like the first, is reflected in mental health legislation: the Mental Health Act 2007 (in common with other similar legislation around the world) covers the use of involuntary admission and treatment not just (as above) in *the interests of the patient* but also in *the interests of others.*

A concern for the interests of others was in play in at least two ways in the background to the use of the Mental Health Act in Sally Coombs' case. First, when the staff at the day center initially called the police for help, it was as much for the safety of other people (other patients and staff) as for that of Sally with which they were concerned. Similarly, when PCs Abrams and Jones arrived, even though Sally had by then settled down, there was still a concern that she might "flare up again." From their perspectives as police officers therefore, in addition to Sally's own safety, the protection of others was certainly an important factor in the background to their decision to use Section 136.

There was no real practical difficulty involved in balancing the relevant values (the interests of Sally Coombs and the interests of others) in this case. Yet it remains important in values-based practice not to lose sight of the fact that a balancing of values is needed on the part of the decision-makers. This is in part because some of the worst abuses of involuntary treatment have arisen from a failure of balanced decision-making on involuntary treatment where there is an actual as opposed to merely a potential conflict between the interests of the patient and the interests of others (we give examples on the series website). But balanced decision-making is also important for the influence it has on *how those involved do what they do.*

We will see later in this chapter that what mattered to Sally Coombs in the longer term was not so much *what* was done when she was in crisis (i.e. *whether or not* the Mental Health Act was used) but *how* it was done (i.e. *how* the Mental Health Act was used). The Mental Health Act requires that the Guiding Principles (as a framework for balanced decision-making) apply not just in difficult cases, but to *every* decision taken under the Act.

Many complex values

If the complication of conflicting values was somewhat in the background at this period in Sally Coombs' story, the complication of complexity of values was very much more in the foreground. You will recall from Chapter 1 that many values, even though shared, are complex in the sense that they are capable of very different interpretations by different people and in different situations. "Best interests," for example, means very different things in different situations, to different individuals and in different cultures. But are the values of risk management (of containment and safety), as represented in Sally Coombs' emergency admission, complex in this sense? And does this matter clinically?

> **Reflection point**
>
> Before reading on, you may like to think about these questions for a moment.
>
> How might the shared risk-related values of containment and safety be interpreted differently from the different perspectives of those involved in the clinical scenario outlined at the start of this chapter? What perspectives could it be helpful to be aware of here? And why might awareness of these different perspectives be important clinically?

The acute care ward team involved in Sally Coombs' admission was multidisciplinary and each of its members brought a different set of professional values to their interpretation of their shared concerns for safety and containment of risk. One way to see this is in

| Purpose | Decisions under the Act must be taken with a view to minimising the undesirable effects of mental disorder, by maximising the safety and well-being (mental and physical) of patients, promoting their recovery and protecting other people from harm. |

Fig. 4.1. The first of the Guiding Principles of the Mental Health Act, 2007

terms of the Guiding Principles governing the use of the Mental Health Act 2007, whereby the team's shared risk-related values are directly reflected in the first of the Guiding Principles, the Purpose Principle (reproduced here as Fig. 4.1). The issues of risk management reflected in the Purpose Principle are likely to have been interpreted to some extent differently, for example by the mental health state-registered nurse on the team, SRN Brenda Matthews, and the psychiatrist, Dr. Alyson Brown:

- *Brenda Matthews.* As a nurse who had recently qualified as one of the new Approved Mental Health Professionals (AMHPs), Brenda Matthews was concerned that taking too restrictive an approach now might adversely affect Sally Coombs' chances of recovery later on when she returned to independent living. In terms of the Purpose Principle then, she was in effect balancing the negative issues of risk reduction embodied by the principle against the positive considerations of "maximising the safety and well-being . . . of patients (and) promoting their recovery" that are also embodied within the Purpose Principle. She could also be understood as balancing the Purpose Principle as a whole against the claims of the Least Restrictive Alternative Principle, which requires that clinicians should ". . . attempt to keep to a minimum the restrictions they impose on the patient's liberty" (see Fig. 3.2).
- AMHPs were created by the Mental Health Act 2007 to extend the range of professionals able to give a second opinion on decisions about the use of compulsion in individual cases. Previously, this role had always been occupied by someone trained as a social worker, and this ensured that there was a balancing of social with medical perspectives, the first opinion being a medical opinion. Training for the AMHP role included the latest evidence on the social factors (housing, employment, friendships and so forth) supporting recovery, and this social perspective continues to provide a valuable contribution to balanced decisions about the use of the Act. (The importance of a balance of perspectives generally in mental health has, of course, long been recognized; see, for example, Pattison *et al.*, 1965; Rogers *et al.*, 1998.)
- *Dr. Brown.* As a psychiatrist, on the other hand, Dr. Brown was more aware than Brenda Matthews and other non-medical team members of the medical aspects of risk. The Purpose Principle,

which emphasizes the importance of "physical" as well as "mental" well-being, refers to "minimising the undesirable effects of mental disorder."

- Like all psychiatrists in the UK, Dr. Brown had a good basic training in medicine including neurology (in which she had done one of her junior house jobs). She had noted that Sally Coombs seemed disoriented to the two police officers who found her outside the day center, and her continuing withdrawn state was punctuated by brief startle reactions, followed by periods of apparent confusion.
- Dr. Brown recognized a probable reaction by Sally to her "voices" and as such this was consistent with an acute relapse of her schizophrenia. But the story was also consistent with a number of organic disorders – perhaps the effects of illegal drugs she may have taken, as the day center staff reported that Sally had taken cannabis in the past and they were concerned that she may have started again. Less likely, but vital to exclude, was a developing metabolic disorder, such as high blood sugar from undiagnosed diabetes (which is more common in schizophrenia). In addition to a mental state assessment therefore, Dr. Brown was concerned to carry out a careful physical examination and get a number of tests done as soon as possible.

We have looked at the perspectives of Nurse Matthews and Dr. Brown in some detail to bring out the extent to which, even in the context of an emergency admission where there are a number of shared values (like risk management) in play, there may still be important differences between team members with different professional backgrounds in the way they *interpret* those values.

Nurse Matthews and Dr. Brown were both concerned about the possible risks to Sally Coombs or others arising from her mental disorder. However, the risks that concerned them reflected the different training and disciplinary perspectives of the two professionals: risk to her chances of longer-term recovery on the one hand and physical health risks on the other.

The acute care ward team and values-based practice (the "delusion of sameness")

If you work in a team yourself, you may think it unlikely that two members of this acute care ward team, who had no doubt worked together for some time and in some challenging situations, should approach the situation presented by Sally Coombs from perspectives representing such a different balance of priorities.

We will see in Chapter 9, however, when we look at team working in more detail, that such differences of perspective are the norm. So, too, is it the norm that differences tend to go unrecognized for what they are. This "delusion of sameness," as it might be called, is indeed particularly active among people who have worked closely together for some time – precisely *because* when we have worked closely with someone we assume we share the same or at any rate similar values. As we will see in Chapter 9, this is simply not the case.

How these differences of values play out depends on whether or not they are recognized for what they are. We will be looking at this in more detail in Chapter 9, but briefly:

- If differences of values between team members, including those from the same profession, are *not* recognized (if the delusion of sameness has hold), then, as was the experience particularly in the early days of multidisciplinary mental health teams, the result is apparently inexplicable disagreements between team members, miscommunications and failures of shared decision-making (Colombo *et al.*, 2003).
- If, on the other hand, they *are* recognized for what they are (if the delusion of sameness is broken), then, by contrast, the same differences of values between team members cease to be a source of difficulty and become instead a positive resource for balanced values-based decision-making.

This is one area, then, in which the first element of values-based practice – raised awareness of values – has a key purchase on decision-making. What is important here is indeed not just to raise awareness of values but, as this element specifies, to raise awareness of the *diversity* of values. This is important between people meeting for the first time (as with a first medical consultation, for example) and in intercultural medicine (where, as we describe in Chapter 11, there are well-recognized differences of values). But this first element of values-based practice reminds us that values diversity is also important much closer to home in the often surprising extent to which the values of those with whom we work most closely differ from our own.

The acute care ward team and evidence-based practice (the NICE guidelines)

The importance of balancing Nurse Matthews' and Dr. Brown's different perspectives at this stage in Sally Coombs' story becomes clear if we turn to current best evidence about the factors supporting recovery in schizophrenia.

In the UK, revised guidelines on the management of schizophrenia in adults were published by the National Institute for Health and Clinical Excellence (NICE, 2009). We will be returning to NICE's 2009 guidance on schizophrenia at several points in this chapter. Two aspects of the guidance are directly relevant to understanding the clinical significance of Dr. Brown's and Nurse Matthews' different priorities for the initial management of Sally Coombs' admission to the acute care ward team:

- *Nurse Matthews' concern* to avoid inevitably intrusive interventions at this early stage with a young woman who was already clearly frightened and agitated is supported by the emphasis in the NICE guidelines on the importance for recovery of positive early engagement and trust as the foundations on which to build a strong therapeutic alliance.
- *Dr. Brown's concern* to exclude serious underlying pathology such as undiagnosed diabetes is supported by the emphasis in the NICE guidelines on the importance (i) of ensuring the physical health of patients with schizophrenia in general and (ii) of monitoring regularly for specific conditions such as diabetes and heart disease from which patients with schizophrenia are known to be at increased risk. In Sally Coombs' case, Dr. Brown's awareness of the increased risk of undiagnosed medical conditions was further justified by the fact that Sally Coombs had gained weight as a side effect of her medication.

The point here, then, is not who is right, Nurse Matthews or Dr. Brown. Both will be concerned for risk and safety as reflected in the Purpose Principle (above). But the differences of perspective between them in how they understand the issues of risk and safety reflect different aspects of best (evidence-based) management as reflected in the NICE guidelines. On current best evidence, that is to say (as summarized in the NICE guidelines) *both* are right in the sense that

their respective perspectives reflect *different priorities based on the same evidence.*

In terms of values-based practice then, Nurse Matthews and Dr. Brown brought different value bases to the interpretation of the same evidence base. Once their different value bases are recognized for what they are, they may cease to be a source of conflict and difficulty and become a resource for balanced decision-making. Focus too exclusively on the *medical aspects* and the key opportunity for engagement presented by "first contact" will be lost. Focus on the other hand too exclusively on *engagement* and serious underlying pathology will (rarely but with potentially tragic consequences) be missed.

The question is how to balance these two perspectives appropriately in the particular circumstances presented by Sally Coombs. This question brings us back to the need for values-based practice standing alongside and as a partner to evidence-based practice in clinical decision-making.

Back to Sally Coombs

So how did values-based practice and evidence-based practice come together at this early stage of the relationship between the acute care ward team and Sally Coombs?

Reflection point

You may find it helpful in understanding what the acute care ward team decided to do if you think for a moment about what *you* would do in this situation (if you were professionally responsible for Sally Coombs), or what you would *want* to happen next (if you were personally concerned for her, as a parent for example).

Think about this in light of the different value perspectives outlined above and how these might support a way forward that balances the immediate medical risks with the importance of establishing a strong therapeutic alliance as the basis for longer-term recovery.

The acute care ward team members in this story had good working relationships. They discussed their different concerns and agreed that, as Sally Coombs appeared by that time to be more settled and in touch (if still uncommunicative), their first step should be to "wait and watch": this would allow them to monitor Sally Coombs' mental state carefully and to act quickly at the first sign of any change for the worse (suggesting a developing underlying medical condition); but at the same time they would have avoided rushing in with potentially invasive investigations that, from her reactions thus far, would be likely to increase her evident fear and level of agitation. Close monitoring would also reduce the risks of possible self-harm.

Jenny Khan

It is at this point that a team member who is to prove crucial to Sally Coombs' eventual recovery first comes on the scene. Jenny Khan was a 30-year-old Support Time and Recovery (STR) worker. Jenny had joined the acute care ward team shortly after STR workers were first introduced into mental health services in England and Wales (Department of Health, 2000). STR workers have no professional qualification (they are "non-professionally aligned") but are given training before joining multidisciplinary teams to provide (as their title suggests) support in delivering recovery-oriented services.

In this instance, Jenny Khan had already taken the lead by sitting quietly with Sally Coombs after she had arrived on the acute care ward. It was thus natural that she should take the "wait and watch" role – supported by other team members – for a further period. In the event, Sally Coombs continued to settle and gradually became calmer and more accessible to the point where she started to talk with Jenny about what had happened. We return to what Sally Coombs told Jenny Khan below.

From crisis to on-going assessment

Over the immediate period that followed Sally Coombs' arrival on the acute care ward, her mental state improved further and she became less distracted by her voices. Her Section 136 had been rescinded now that she was in a "place of safety" and she seemed willing to stay on the ward as a voluntary patient for a few days to "see how it goes." Among other reasons for this, it turned out that she had been worried about her health as she had gained weight on her medication and she was pleased that someone was "checking her out" (her tests all proved to be fine).

Sally Coombs' parents (with whom she was living) were contacted by Dr. Brown on the first day and came to see her that evening. They wanted to take her home initially, but when Sally Coombs herself made it clear she wanted to stay on for a few days, they agreed to

this. They were also reassured that the team all seemed happy to talk to them and that there was an open and welcoming feel when they arrived on the ward. Sally Coombs' family doctor, her GP Dr. Jones, had been contacted by the day center staff to let him know what had happened. Dr. Brown rang Dr. Jones later that day to reassure him that Sally Coombs was settling well and to check on her medication. The situation having thus been safely contained, the acute care ward team began to put together the background to Sally Coombs' emergency admission.

Several stories, one assessment

Besides Sally Coombs herself, the acute care ward team spoke to several people to build up a picture of what had happened to her. In this section, we outline some of the key points from what they were told.

> **Reflection point**
>
> As you read through the following accounts of Sally Coombs' story, think what may have gone wrong. You will see that a number of people all did their best to help Sally Coombs. Yet she ended up with an acute (if brief) psychotic episode in the day center.
>
> Why? Was it inevitable, schizophrenia being after all traditionally a relapsing condition? Or was there a chance this could this have been avoided? If so, what are the implications for Sally Coombs' ongoing care?

The story from Sally Coombs' GP, Dr. Jones

Dr. Jones confirmed that Sally Coombs was diagnosed with a first episode of psychosis two years ago, while at an art college, and had been diagnosed as suffering from schizophrenia. The first sign of any problem was when her art had gone from original and challenging to "disturbing," with vivid images of death and dying. She was believed to have started taking increasing quantities of drugs at this time, but it was not clear whether this was cause or effect. In any case, these images then spread from her artwork to invade her everyday world in the form of vivid and distressing visual and auditory hallucinations. She began to withdraw, and after some months of progressive isolation and self-neglect, was found by her parents cutting the wall paper in her room and her bed with a kitchen knife and shouting as if someone was attacking her. They brought her to Dr. Jones and agreed to her being admitted to the psychiatric ward of their local hospital on a "section."

She had been an inpatient for some weeks but was eventually discharged back to her parents, apparently symptom-free on oral medication. Dr. Jones had seen her every few months and her medication had been supervised on a more frequent basis by the practice nurse. Initially, Dr. Jones had felt she was doing well at the day center, where she had opportunities to pursue her art. But there had been worrying signs recently that she had become increasingly reluctant to take her medication, and he wondered if she had started taking drugs again (although she had denied this).

The story from Sally Coombs' first psychiatrist, Dr. Hastings

Dr. Rodney Hastings remembered the family from Sally Coombs' time on the ward. Sally Coombs' father was a teacher (he told Dr. Brown when she telephoned him) and a church elder. Her mother was a care assistant in a nursing home.

Dr. Hastings said that he had always felt Sally Coombs' parents had never fully accepted the reality of her illness and he was concerned that they still did not really believe she needed medication. He had found himself feeling quite defensive when they came on the ward – they were often, in his view, unnecessarily hostile and aggressive. They had even complained ("kicked up a fuss") about some of the other patients' behavior and insisted on Sally Coombs getting a single room. He could not help wondering to what extent they had made things worse by their constant criticisms. He felt that they would be unlikely to tell the team about any symptoms suggestive of a relapse and warned Dr. Brown not to trust their superficial politeness.

> **Reflection point**
>
> To what extent do you think that Dr. Hastings' viewpoints could result from a certain lack of *self*-awareness?
>
> If you were Dr. Hastings' therapeutic supervisor, can you think of any questions you might suggest he asks himself in order to reveal more of his own values to himself?
>
> What difference do you think it would make to his interactions with patients, relatives and colleagues if Dr. Hastings became more self-aware?

When asked by Dr. Brown what he thought might have led to Sally Coombs' psychotic episode, Dr. Hastings said it reflected in his view everything that had gone wrong with psychiatry in recent years (at 62, he had seen many changes in psychiatry and he "couldn't wait to retire!"). First, although he recognized the importance of the growing awareness of rehabilitation and social functioning, he had found working in the community increasingly like being a social worker. He still believed that the proper place for treating serious mental illness is in an inpatient setting where his role and authority were clear.

Secondly, he still had a strong belief in the role of antipsychotic medication if used correctly. This was one reason why he believed the ward with its consistent relationships and the calm environment it could offer was the right place to establish treatment: "It's much harder to treat patients effectively when they're back home, often in chaotic lives and with poor adherence to medication." Yes, the NICE guidelines talk about offering psychological treatments – but this is still in limited supply in the NHS, and anyway the guidelines ". . . were written by a psychologist!" (The Chair of the NICE Guideline Development Group was Elizabeth Kuipers, Professor of Clinical Psychology at the Institute of Psychiatry in London.)

Dr. Hastings always did what he could to ensure patients took their medication as prescribed – if Dr. Brown really had Sally Coombs' best interests at heart, she should use a community treatment order to make sure Sally complied with her treatment. "My Community Nurse" (Brendan Farley, see below) "tells me this is coercion. He's a good chap but what he doesn't seem to realize is that the reason patients won't take medication is because they lack insight – it's all part and parcel of their illness." Dr. Hastings went on to explain that he respected his nursing colleagues for their role, which he saw as complementary to but different from his own. "Medication decisions and diagnoses are *my* responsibility. It's what I came into medicine to do!"

The role of others in developing self-awareness

When Dr. Brown was listening to her consultant colleague, Dr. Hastings, she was actually thinking that he had a bit of a blind spot, but this, she thought, was neither the time nor the place to point this out. Her focus was on Sally Coombs. Nonetheless, she was unwittingly an agent for change in Dr. Hastings' thinking. Something about her communication on the telephone – maybe an inflexion in her voice suggesting a question mark – was enough to cause a little turbulence in Dr. Hastings' mind after their conversation.

He was left feeling uncomfortable and he shared this (creative) discomfort later with a colleague, Toby Minton, the Clinical Director, who was himself an experienced psychiatrist. "So you think that Alyson Brown was surprised at your views? Why do you think that was?" Toby asked. "I suppose I may have been coming across as a little old-fashioned," replied Dr. Hastings. "Mmm, do you think there is anything wrong in old-fashioned?" asked Toby. "No, sometimes experience can contribute something valuable." Then, after a pause, Dr. Hastings opened up further, revealing something he had not recognized before this moment. "You know, Toby," he said, "I think her reaction, and my own reaction now, is one of surprise at my apparent intolerance. Looking back on it, my words were the defensive words of an old fogey feeling on the back foot in the brave new world! I guess I'm getting to the point where I have either got to get out, or I have to learn how to bring my experience to bear in a way which is contributory rather than destructive. I haven't always been like this – I think I'm just feeling marginalized by the way things have moved on."

This little side story illustrates something about self-awareness. For the most part, we have to become more aware of our own values by self-reflection, but others may still be our allies if we let them. If we look out for the raised eyebrow or listen for the question mark as we reveal our values, two things may happen. First, we may become aware that not everyone does share our values (questioning the implicit assumption that everyone thinks like I do). Secondly, we have rich material for our reflective practice. "I wonder why she reacted this way? How might I have elicited a different reaction? Now that I am no longer feeling defensive, do I want to stand up for those values, or perhaps modify them?"

The story from Sally Coombs' Community Mental Health Nurse, Brendan Farley

Sally Coombs' Community Mental Health Nurse, Brendan Farley, who had been reviewing Sally Coombs fortnightly, was contacted by the acute care ward nurse, Brenda Matthews. Brendan Farley's reaction to the news that Sally Coombs had relapsed was that he was not surprised.

He had been increasingly anxious about Sally Coombs and her family recently. He had seen some evidence of ongoing psychosis, which Sally Coombs was adept at hiding in superficial conversation, and had been worried that the family were colluding with her in denying that there was a problem. He had also been concerned that, although her parents had previously supported him in insisting that she take her medications, they now seemed to be siding with Sally

Coombs about coming off them. Although he had some sympathy with this, he believed that in her case it could be "hazardous," putting her at risk of another acute episode, especially if she started smoking cannabis again (which he suspected she had, although as with others she had always denied this).

Given the growing problems with Sally Coombs and her parents, Brendan Farley had scheduled a family appointment for them in the joint clinic he now ran with Dr. Hastings, the psychiatrist. When asked whether he thought this would have helped, Brendan replied that, like everyone else in the community team, he respected Dr. Hastings' clinical judgment and knew that his patients and their families greatly appreciated the care and attention he gave them. But Brendan admitted that, from his perspective, he found Dr. Hastings at times frustratingly old-fashioned. Brendan had trained in an early-interventions team where they worked in a more flexible way with which he felt more comfortable (Spencer *et al.*, 2001). "It is more important," he said, "to understand a patient's illness in the context of their lives than to insist on them accepting diagnostic labels."

He saw his nursing approach as being within a recovery model of mental disorder in which social functioning rather than simply control of symptoms was one of his main goals in working with patients. (This is, of course, also the model with which many psychiatrists work; see, for example, Slade, 2009 and Harland *et al.*, 2009.)

The story from Sally Coombs' parents

Sally Coombs initially refused permission for the team to talk with her parents. She said that Brendan, her community nurse from the other hospital, had respected her confidentiality and she expected the same from them. After some discussion, however, she accepted that her parents were entitled at least to an assessment of their own needs. It was thus agreed that the social worker attached to the acute care ward team, Jim Rankin, who was not directly involved with her care, should offer to see her parents on a basis of mutual confidentiality; i.e. Jim would neither tell her parents what Sally Coombs had said nor tell Sally Coombs what her parents had said.

Sally Coombs' parents jumped at the chance to talk with Jim Rankin, although they felt hurt by Sally's insistence on confidentiality. They believed that, as her parents and carers, and those who lived with her and her illness, they had a right to any information that they felt would help her, and they resented the way in which Brendan (the Community Mental Health Nurse) had sometimes withheld information because of "confidentiality" (Tuck *et al.*, 1997).

They remained devastated by their daughter's illness. They felt they had lost "their pretty, bright girl" and all their hopes for her future. They still saw glimpses of the "real Sally" at times but did not know how to deal with the very different person into which the illness and her medication had turned her.

Worse still, they felt they had betrayed her by agreeing to the "section" when she first became ill; and they still blamed themselves for not having just taken her home at half-term when the first signs of her "breakdown" were developing. They now thought that the spell in the hospital had just made things worse. They had hoped to be able to find her somewhere "to be made better, to be safe." It had felt anything but. They were appalled by the ward – it was always "full of shouting and people who seemed disturbed and dangerous." When Sally Coombs told them about finding a man at the foot of her bed one night, they had been horrified and tried to get her a room of her own so she could be safe.

They were an intensely private family who had always been close and would rather not have others involved. They resented the intrusion of the psychiatrist and the mental health team into their home and family life. They did not now think that medication was the answer, either. They had tried being strict with Sally and insisting that she took her medication as prescribed. They had always trusted medical advice and this was what Dr. Hastings seemed to think was important for their daughter. But it had resulted in many arguments and all it had done was to turn her into a "zombie." The day center had been better, but the risk was that she might "get in with a bad crowd" and start taking drugs again.

The story from Sally Coombs

Sally Coombs' story as she gave it initially to Dr. Brown added little to what the team had learned from others or were able to infer from what they had been told. Essentially, she felt that her life seemed to stop when she became unwell. She remembered her time in hospital as a hazy, distorted nightmare period in her life. She had not been back to college since. Her college friends – even her old school friends – had had nothing to do with her. She had gone home to live with her parents, but this was a source of considerable stress, and stress made her voices worse.

She admitted to Dr. Brown that, as they had suspected, she had started smoking cannabis again lately with a couple of people from the day center. But she felt that this was a "totally normal" thing to do: most of her old friends also smoked and nothing had happened to them, and she enjoyed the experience. She also liked the feeling that she had got friends again. She was aware that smoking cannabis was something she had been warned against but felt that it calmed her down. She had been feeling quite "worked up" recently and had been very distressed by the increasing aggressiveness of the voices and how they had begun to invade her life again.

Sally Coombs hated having to take her medication. Although she welcomed the release it offered from some of the distressing hallucinations she experienced in hospital, and the fact that it made the voices kinder and easier to cope with, she hated feeling so dull, so like a "zombie" (the term her parents had used). The weight she had put on since she first became ill did not bother her initially, when she was too ill to care, but it had now become another source of distress and a reminder of another thing she had lost – her appearance. She had looked at service user "blogs" and spoken to other patients at the day center and had become convinced that her current medication was little better than poison. She had not tried to discuss this with her doctor because "He'll see it as a sign that the dose needs to be increased, or put me on injections to make sure I don't stop it."

A values-based assessment

The assessment process carried out by the acute care ward team to this point showed two key features that, as we outlined in Chapter 2, support values-based practice: it was person-centered (it reflected Sally Coombs' priorities as much as the team's priorities) and multidisciplinary (it was multiperspective as well as multiskilled).

It will be worth spending a few moments looking in a little more detail at these two features and how they fit with recent work on what is important in assessment in mental health:

- *Person-centered assessment.* The information from Sally Coombs, although largely confirming what the team already knew or had suspected (notably that she had started taking cannabis again), also included important information about how Sally Coombs herself felt about what had been happening to her.

- Again, the team could have inferred this information but what was important from Sally Coombs' perspective and also vital in terms of building engagement between her and the team was that she now felt for the first time that she had *really been listened to*. The assessment had been a genuinely two-way process focusing as much on what Sally Coombs (from her personal perspective) wanted to tell the team as on what the team (from their professional perspectives) wanted to know about Sally Coombs.
- *Multidisciplinary assessment.* Assessment from different disciplinary perspectives is of course normal in modern health care: no one claims to be an expert radiologist, for example, as well as a bacteriologist. The assessment carried out here following Sally Coombs' emergency admission drew similarly on different professional skill sets (of medicine, nursing, social care and so on). Importantly, however, for values-based practice, the assessment also drew on different professional *priorities and perspectives* (notably medical and social perspectives).
- We will see in Chapter 8 (which focuses on team work) that this multiperspective as well as multiskills approach to assessment is important in helping to bring out (to move from the background to the foreground) aspects of the values bearing on a situation that may be central to understanding what has happened and hence to guiding us about what to do next.

The three keys

In being person-centered and multidisciplinary, the acute care ward team's assessment reflected two of the three "keys" to assessment in mental health identified in a recent national consultation in the UK (see Fig. 4.2, reproduced from National Institute for Mental Health in England (NIMHE) and the Care Services Improvement Partnership, 2008).

The Three Keys consultation included a wide range of stakeholders in mental health (patients and carers, as well as GPs, nurses, psychiatrists, psychologists, social workers, occupational therapists, pharmacists and ward managers), and the report (which is repro-duced in full on the series website) includes many examples of good practice from front-line services. We will see in a moment that the third key given in Fig. 4.2, strengths assessment, was to prove even more important to Sally Coombs' recovery. But to set the

The three keys to the shared approach are:

1. *active participation* of the service user concerned in a shared understanding with service providers and where appropriate with their carers
2. input from *different provider perspectives* within a multidisciplinary approach, and
3. a person-centered focus that builds on the *strengths, resiliencies and aspirations* of the individual service user as well as identifying his or her needs and challenges.

Fig. 4.2. Extract from the three keys to assessment in mental health, reproduced from the National Institute for Mental Health in England.

context for this, we need to look first at what had gone on in the build-up to her crisis as now revealed by the reports that the acute care ward team had pulled together.

Awareness and lack of awareness of values

Reflection point

Before looking at what the acute care ward team made of the information they now had about the background to Sally Coombs' emergency admission, you may find it helpful to go back to the questions we raised above.

From what you have read of the various reports why do *you* think Sally Coombs ended up in crisis? Clearly, it is not always possible to prevent a relapse. But how might the perspectives of those concerned, as brought out by these reports, have (inadvertently) contributed to her crisis?

One point that stands out clearly from the reports is that everyone had done their best for Sally Coombs as they saw it. The problem was that those concerned brought a different balance of perspectives to their understanding of what was "best," and Sally Coombs ended up in effect falling between the cracks. This was particularly the case between the psychiatrist Dr. Hastings (medical > social perspective) and the Community Mental Health Nurse Brendan Farley (social > medical perspective).

In terms of values-based practice, the situation to this point was thus similar in this respect to that which Sally Coombs later encountered when she was first admitted in crisis to the acute care ward team. There was a crucial difference, however, in the extent to which those concerned in the two situations were aware of their respective differences of perspective:

- Dr. Hastings and Brendan Farley were largely *unaware* of their respective medical and social perspectives. True, they both *expressed* respect for the other's role and abilities. But there was no real understanding of each other's position. The result, as we have seen, was misunderstandings and failures of shared decision-making. We know that this occurred widely in the early days of Community Mental Health Nurses (Colombo *et al.*, 2003).
- Dr. Brown and Nurse Matthews in the acute care ward team, by contrast, in being *fully aware* of each other's respective medical and social perspectives, were able to use these in coming to a balanced decision about what to do, namely their "wait and watch" initial phase, reflecting, you will recall, the corresponding balance of medical and social priorities in the relevant evidence-based NICE guidelines. (This again is the key point about values and multidisciplinary team work that we will pick up in Chapter 9.)

Sally Coombs was thus caught in the unacknowledged tensions between the medical and social perspectives represented, respectively, by Dr. Hastings and Brendan Farley. So too, and importantly, were her parents. There were clearly additional factors at work here: a perhaps rather authoritarian approach from Dr. Hastings that resulted in Sally Coombs' parents feeling excluded from ongoing decisions about their daughter's care while at the same time being expected to carry out the role of principal carers. This de facto exclusion also meant that they had no opportunity to work through their sense of guilt about their part in Sally Coombs' original "section." It was small wonder, then, that a vicious cycle built up in their relationship with the ward staff. But the net result for Sally Coombs was that (again contrary to NICE guidelines) she ended up living at home but in a deteriorating relationship with her parents.

The care plan

So far, so easy (with hindsight). But the challenge for the acute care ward team was where to go from here. They felt that they had established a trusting relationship with Sally Coombs who now seemed positively keen to stay on the ward. This was not a long-term option, nor in their view would it be helpful to her.

They were conscious here of the evidence of the importance of social factors in recovery – employment, independent living, friendships and so forth (Copeland, 2005; Slade, 2009). Accordingly, they began to map out a care plan for discussion with Sally Coombs that included:

- *A review of her medication and diet.* Remember in this respect the social as well as medical significance for Sally Coombs and her parents of the side effects of her current medication: that it made her into a zombie and had also resulted in unacceptable weight gain.
- *Supporting her in developing her talent as an artist.* The team saw this as being clearly at the heart of Sally Coombs' priorities and hence a potential foundation on which to build on the following:
  - Helping her to re-establish her social world (friends, independent living, employment, etc.).
  - Establishing cognitive–behavioral therapy to help her cope better with her voices.
  - Through both of these, supporting her in coming off and avoiding illicit drug use (which in Sally Coombs' case was motivated both by trying to establish new friendships and by the need to mitigate the unpleasant intrusiveness of her voices).

Working with Sally Coombs' parents presented more of a challenge for the acute care ward team given her continued refusal to involve them, but they would liaise with the social worker attached to the acute care ward team, Jim Rankin, who now had an established link with them.

A values-based and evidence-based care plan

On the face of it, this care plan thus had both a sound values-base and a sound evidence-base. On the values side, it primarily reflected Sally Coombs' priorities but also those of her parents as her principal carers. On the evidence side, it reflected key elements of the NICE guidelines: these included the importance of social functioning as well as of medication, the need for engagement with the patient and (while respecting confidentiality) the carers (Sally Coombs' parents), the use of cognitive behavioral therapy (CBT) as an evidence-based psychological intervention and art therapy (also specifically endorsed by the Guidelines for use in schizophrenia).

It was at this point, however, that Jenny Khan, the STR worker we introduced earlier in the chapter, made her key contribution. Jenny had not previously spoken in the case review, but what she came up with now completely changed how Sally Coombs' story was understood. This, in turn, transformed her care plan from one that would have (unwittingly) repeated the unintended mistakes of her previous care into a very different care plan that would lead to her eventual recovery.

Vital missing information

> ### Reflection point
>
> Again, you may find it useful to try to anticipate what Jenny Khan contributed at this point in the case review meeting.
>
> Essentially, she came up with an aspect of Sally Coombs' story that had previously been completely misunderstood and that turned out to be the missing link in her recovery.
>
> What do you think this missing link was?

What Jenny Khan told the team was that, far from art being Sally Coombs' number one priority and hence a foundation on which to build, it was *art that was her problem*.

You will recall that, when Sally Coombs was admitted in crisis, it was Jenny Khan, as the STR worker, who took the lead in sitting quietly with her in the initial "watch and wait" period of close observation. This was pivotal for Sally Coombs. In her previous admission, she had been put through a whole series of rushed and (to her) meaningless assessment procedures that had (again to her understanding) little relevance to the way she was ultimately treated (i.e. put on medication). On this occasion, by contrast, her first experience of the team was of care and attention (Jenny Khan sitting with her). Instead of increasing her fear and agitation (with the clear risk of a further intrusive experience in the form of "emergency sedation"), she was thus allowed to settle and to gain confidence in the environment in which she found herself.

One result of this initial positive engagement was that, as noted earlier, when Dr. Brown saw her the next day, Sally was actually relieved that someone was going to "check her out" medically. A second positive result was that Sally gradually opened up to Jenny Khan in a way that she had not previously felt able to with anyone else.

There was no formal assessment process here. But what emerged from their conversations, many of which took place when Jenny Khan went out with Sally Coombs for walks in the local park, was that Sally had done well at a variety of subjects at school but, because of her particular talents as an artist, "everyone" had wanted her to pursue this as a career. The "everyone" here included her parents to whom as an only child she had been particularly close. Also, as a teacher and care worker, respectively, her father and mother had to make significant financial sacrifices to support her at college. So, one way or another, she had felt that her parents would be very let down if she "dropped out" of a career in art.

Similar considerations were driving her concerns about confidentiality. She had not previously told anyone about her lack of interest in following a career as an artist. But she knew that she would have to do so eventually and did not want to disappoint her parents when they found out that this was how she was feeling. For the same reason, Sally Coombs had initially asked Jenny Khan not to pass on this information. But by the time of the case review, her confidence in the team as a whole had reached the point where she agreed that it was "now or never."

So, what did Sally really want to do? This was not clear, Jenny explained, because Sally had never had a chance to consider other career options. Sally's own self-assessment was that, although she was indeed a good artist and capable, as had been said, of some original work, she was "not *that* good." One thing at least was clear – that by "supporting" her to get back to a career in art, far from building on a foundation of her own strengths, the team would have been digging Sally Coombs in even deeper with her problems.

A revised care plan and WRAP

With this new information in place, it was clear that a very differently focused care plan was needed. The basis of this new plan, consistent with the well-recognized links between recovery and values (Allott *et al.*, 2002; Slade, 2009), was to work with Sally Coombs on what she herself really wanted to do while at the same time helping her talk with her parents about how she felt. Much of the resulting new care plan was similar to the previous care plan (the need for a review of her medication and diet, the work with her parents, the use of CBT and so forth). But the breakthrough in understanding Sally's true aspirations led to the introduction of a number of crucial new elements. In particular:

- *A joint occupational therapy and psychology assessment.* This helped to clarify Sally Coombs' potential employment options; it also strengthened her confidence by confirming her intelligence and broad areas of competence.
- *A personal recovery plan.* Working further with Jenny Khan, Sally Coombs developed her own WRAP, a Wellness Recovery Action Plan.

StAR values and recovery

WRAPs were developed by service users for service users and are available in the form of web-based resources (Copeland, 2005; Slade, 2009; see also the series website). Understanding a person's values and in particular their strengths is central to developing an effective WRAP (Allott *et al.*, 2002; Copeland, 2005). This point came through clearly in the consultation that led to the publication of the three keys (see above). It is natural that clinicians should concentrate on problems in assessment – this is, after all, what people come to us about. But the Three Keys consultation showed that it is important in assessment to look at the positives as well as at the negatives.

This is why the third of the three keys is about looking at strengths, aspirations and resources (StAR values as we call them), as well as at needs and difficulties. Of these StAR values, furthermore, as many respondents emphasized, aspirations are the most important for recovery. As with Jenny Khan in Sally Coombs' story, it is the non-professionally aligned STR workers who are often best placed to understand an individual's true aspirations.

Developing a WRAP based on her own aspirations certainly proved helpful to Sally Coombs at a number of levels:

- It allowed her to manage her voices more effectively and consistently with her more pressing objective of re-establishing her social world: "recovery" in this context means finding a good quality of life, which may include living with rather than totally suppressing symptoms.
- Sally Coombs was supported further in this by a self-help group run by a service user organization, Hearing Voices (see website for details).
- It helped to turn the broad objectives of her overall care plan into a manageable one-step-at-a-time journey towards recovery. One of these steps was to open up with her parents who, in the event, were fully supportive of her wish to give up her career in art.

- It reinforced the work she was now doing through CBT in developing her own positive skills for self-management of her symptoms.

It was Jenny Khan, the non-professionally aligned STR worker, who in recognizing Sally Coombs' true aspirations had provided the "key of keys" to her recovery. To build effectively on the insight gained into the patient's strengths would require all the different skills and perspectives of the team as a whole, working together with Sally Coombs and her family.

Chapter summary

In this chapter, we have illustrated the importance of the first of the skills area supporting values-based practice – raised *awareness* of values and of *differences* of values – with the story of a young woman, Sally Coombs, as she went from an emergency admission to the local acute care ward team through an assessment process that led to the first steps towards her eventual recovery.

Raised awareness of values was important at each step in this story:

- *On admission*, the mutual understanding of initial priorities between Dr. Brown (the acute care ward psychiatrist) and Brenda Matthews (the AMHP) allowed Sally Coombs to build a positive engagement with the team.
- *In developing an initial care plan*, the team drew on a person-centered (participatory) and multidisciplinary (including multiperspective) process of assessment that allowed them to balance the medical and social priorities of care, as reflected in the relevant NICE guidelines.
- *The revised care plan* built directly on the team becoming aware through her relationship with the team's STR worker, Jenny Khan, of Sally Coombs' true aspirations (*not* to become an artist).

Sally Coombs' story thus amply demonstrates the importance of values (as well as evidence) in building what David Sackett (in Chapter 2) called the "diagnostic and therapeutic alliance" between clinicians and patients that in evidence-based medicine (no less than in values-based medicine) is at the heart of effective clinical care. As the Three Keys consultation demonstrated, attention to positive strengths, aspirations and resources (StAR values) as well as negative needs and difficulties is important here; and of these, in mental health at least, it is the patient's individual aspirations that are often the key to recovery.

Along the way, we have also started to look at tools for developing *self*-awareness, which is a vital aspect of awareness. We will return to this later.

References

Allott, P., Loganathan, L. and Fulford, K. W. M. (2002). Discovering hope for recovery. In *Innovation in Community Mental Health: International Perspectives. Canadian Journal of Community Mental Health* (special issue), 21, 13–33.

Colombo, A., Bendelow, G., Fulford, K. W. M. and Williams, S. (2003). Evaluating the influence of implicit models of mental disorder on processes of shared decision making within community-based multi-disciplinary teams. *Social Science & Medicine* 56, 1557–70.

Copeland, M. E. (2005). *Wellness Recovery Action Plan*. Liverpool, UK: Sefton Recovery Group.

Department of Health (2000). *Mental Health Policy Implementation Guide: Support Time and Recovery (STR) Workers*. London: Department of Health.

Harland, R., Anatova, E., Owen, G. S. et al. (2009). A study of psychiatrists' concepts of mental illness. *Psychological Medicine* 39, 967–76.

National Institute for Mental Health in England (NIMHE) and the Care Services Improvement Partnership (2008). *3 Keys to a Shared Approach in Mental Health Assessment*. London: Department of Health.

NICE (2009). *Schizophrenia: Core Interventions in the Treatment and Management of Schizophrenia in Adults in Primary and Secondary Care*. NICE clinical guideline 82 (an update of Guideline 1). Developed by the National Collaborating Centre for Mental Health. London: National Institute for Health and Clinical Excellence.

Pattison, S., Hannigan, B., Pill, R. and Thomas, H. (1965). *Emerging Values in Health Care: the Challenge for Professionals*. London/Philadelphia: Jessica Kingsley Publishers.

Rogers, A., Day, J. C., Williams, B., et al. (1998). The meaning and management of neuroleptic medication: a study of patients with a diagnosis of schizophrenia. *Social Science and Medicine* 47, 1313–23.

Slade, M. (2009). *Personal Recovery and Mental Illness: A Guide for Mental Health Professionals (Values-based Medicine)*. Cambridge: Cambridge University Press

Spencer, E., Birchwood, M. and McGovern, D. (2001) Management of first-episode psychosis. *Advances in Psychiatric Treatment* 7, 133–140.

Tuck, I., du Mont, P., Evans, G. and Shupe, J. (1997). The experience of caring for an adult child with schizophrenia. *Archives of Psychiatric Nursing* 11, 118–125.

Websites

- The publication of the Three Keys consultation, which includes examples of the role of non-professionally aligned STR workers (like Jenny Khan in this story) in working with patients' strengths (their StAR values) and thus supporting their recovery, is given in full as a downloadable PDF on the series website. The website also includes links to web-based resources for WRAP planning.
- The website of the self-help group Hearing Voices is: http://www.hearing-voices.org/.

CHAPTER 5 begins on following page

POINT

PROCESS

PREMISE

Balanced Decision-making
within a
Framework of Shared Values

Partnership

Two-feet Principle   Squeaky-wheel Principle   Science-driven Principle

Person-centered practice   Multidisciplinary teamwork

Awareness   Reasoning   Knowledge   Communication skills

Mutual Respect
for
Differences of Values

Map of values-based practice – reasoning.

Teenage acne: widening our values horizons
Values-based practice element 2: reasoning about values

Topics covered in this chapter

The role of reasoning in values-based practice is illustrated by the use of case-based reasoning (casuistry) in the management of a case of teenage acne.
   Other topics include:

- Evidence-based medicine and management of teenage acne
- Cosmetic and medical treatments
- Values and communication skills
- Principles reasoning
- Other methods of ethical reasoning (utilitarianism and deontology).

Take-away message for practice

*You can use case-based and other ways of reasoning about values to **explore your own and other's values as they as they impact on practice**.*

Where awareness of values as the first skills element of the process of values-based practice provides a wake-up call to values, reasoning about values as the second element is about expanding our values horizons. Reasoning skills in values-based practice are not used to derive particular moral or other evaluative conclusions (to "prove" what is right or wrong). In values-based practice, reasoning skills are used rather to explore and come to understand better our own and other's values as these bear on and influence a given situation.

Expanding our values horizons with case-based reasoning (casuistry)

The importance of expanding our values horizons in this way is illustrated in this chapter by following a consultation between a GP, Dr. Charles Mangate, and his patient Jane Brewer, a 17-year-old aspiring model with mild acne.

We run the consultation twice. First time round, there is a values gap (a values gulf, really) between patient and doctor, with the result that the consultation – although unexceptionable in terms of clinical guidelines – leaves Jane Brewer feeling patronized and mistrustful of further involvement with conventional medicine. This prompts an exercise in case-based reasoning (also called casuistry) with Dr. Mangate. Case-based reasoning in this instance helps to bridge the gap of values in the consultation by extending Dr. Mangate's understanding of his own values, and hence in the re-run of the consultation, his ability to understand and engage with those of Jane Brewer.

From one tool to many

Case-based reasoning is only one among a number of ways of reasoning about values, each of which has its own strengths and weaknesses and each of which is useful in different contexts in medicine. We noted one of these other ways of reasoning, principles reasoning, in Chapter 2: Dr. Gulati, you will recall, used the Four Principles approach in her time out to consider how to respond to Roy Walker's demands for an off-work certificate for low back pain. In the final section of the chapter, we look briefly at principles and at a number of other ways of reasoning about values.

The clinical context

"So you are not going to help me." There is an awkward pause. Dr. Mangate, aged 35, stares rather miserably at his computer screen as though hoping for inspiration. He is aware that he is losing this one: he has done his best to explain things and the consultation is already running over time. But what else can he say? There is no treatment he can offer that would be acceptable to the patient and prescribable within the locally agreed formulary. This does all seem a lot of fuss about a pretty mild case of acne. Jane Brewer, aged 17, is angry and embarrassed. Her mum had said how nice Dr. Mangate was (when she had her "breast scare"), but all her friends will say, "Told you so!" Well, never again.

First run of the consultation

How did Dr. Mangate and his patient Jane Brewer get to this impasse?

The background to the consultation

Jane Brewer had turned up at the surgery asking to see someone about "a personal thing." The practice nurse, Sue Barnes, was available and offered to talk with her. Jane and her mother were long-term patients of the practice and Sue Barnes had seen Jane occasionally when she was a child.

Jane Brewer explained that she was now at the local college doing a course in Fashion and Design. Her tutor had encouraged her to try for an annual photo shoot run by the college, which might result in some part-time work as a model. She had been keen to do this (she had very little money) and then disaster had struck – she had developed acne on her face and neck. Sue (who was herself smartly dressed) began to run through the standard advice that the practice had prepared on acne, based on the NHS Clinical Knowledge Summary (CKS) *Acne vulgaris – Management. Scenario: Mild acne.*

But Jane stopped her, saying that she had tried all the usual self-help approaches and her last hope was that she could get a prescription for one of the stronger treatments.

At this point, Jane Brewer had produced a cutting from a magazine article about a girl whose acne had eventually been cured by laser treatment combined with various prescription medications in a private clinic. This worried Sue Barnes. She suspected that Jane Brewer did not have the resources for expensive private treatments and was anyway doubtful of the efficacy (let alone safety) of the treatment described in the magazine. But it was clear that Jane Brewer had grown up into a determined and independent-minded young woman who was at risk of going her own way and getting involved with potentially dangerous alternative treatments if she did not get the right advice and support at this stage.

So Sue Barnes decided to refer Jane Brewer to one of the doctors in the practice sooner rather than later. Jane had not been seen by any of the doctors recently (her last appointment had been a long time ago when she came as a child with her mother). But Jane explained that her mum had told her how kind Dr. Mangate had been when she had had a "breast scare" and she wondered if he would see her. Sue Barnes thus made an appointment for her with Dr. Mangate while offering to see Jane herself afterwards if she wanted to talk things over again.

Dr. Mangate's first reaction

Dr. Mangate was not very pleased when he read the note from Sue Barnes on his computer before seeing Jane Brewer. His last patient had been a young mother with what he suspected would turn out to be breast cancer. The contrast cut against all his principles. He did not go into medicine to deal with "photo shoots." In fact, he blamed the cosmetics industry for causing a lot of unhappiness with its "celeb" culture making young women so appearance-conscious. And why ever was Sue (an experienced nurse practitioner) landing him with having to deal with this when she knew full well that, as a nurse prescriber, she was perfectly capable of prescribing the first-line topical retinoid or benzoyl peroxide.

Right on cue, and as if to rub salt in the wound, as Dr. Mangate reflected crossly on the referral, an email popped into his inbox from the practice manager congratulating them all on once again "... leading the PCT [primary care trust] in responsible prescribing with lowest cost per doctor and lowest cost per patient; highest generic proportion and only 1.2% of all prescriptions on the PCT "less desirable" list." "Well done – keep it up," the email continued, "Our prescribing incentives money is enough to fund our homeless outreach service for yet another year." Reining in his irritation, Dr. Mangate pressed the buzzer for Jane Brewer to come in.

How the consultation went

CM Come and have a seat, Jane. What can we do for you today?

JB (*Looking uncomfortable as she sits down*) It's like I said to the nurse, I need treatment for my spots.

CM (*Kindly*) Well, sometimes spots don't need any treatment, they get better on their own; and there are lots of things you can get from the chemist nowadays.

JB I've tried things from the chemist and they haven't helped. I need proper treatment.

CM I see. What treatments have you tried, Jane?

JB I got some wash stuff – panoxyl, I think it was – and that just made it worse. My skin went like beetroot and so itchy – I had to stay in for three days – couldn't even go to college. My mum bought me some Clearasil™ Max but that didn't any good either.

CM I wonder, Jane – do you need to do anything at all? You know, spots are quite normal at your age – it's just the phase that your hormones are in. They get a little unbalanced as far as your skin is concerned. Leave it alone, don't worry about it and the chances are that your skin will be right as rain in a year or two ...

JB *(Stung)* But, they're gross.

CM Perhaps we should have a look at them. I see a lot of spots, you know, and the ones you have on your face aren't that bad. By our standards, we would call that mild acne *(he leans over and looks at her face)*; yes, a few whiteheads and papules but no real pustules. If you saw some of the people that I see you wouldn't be worrying about this, honestly. This is not going to scar. Have you got any anywhere else?

JB *(Embarrassed)* Well, er, my chest is OK but I've got them on my back.

CM *(Looks at the back of her neck)* Well, I see – there's one little pustule here, but there again, you really shouldn't be worrying about that.

JB *(Tries to cover herself up again and shifts round, terminating the examination)* So you're not going to help me then? I'm a student. I can't afford to go private.

CM It's not a question of affording, Jane, it's about needing. I am trying to say that you don't *need* to do anything. Your skin is not that bad, you know. I realize it may feel awful to you, but it's really very normal. I want to help you just ignore the problem and it will all settle down.

JB *(Producing her* Daily Mail *article rather desperately)* But look what this girl had to go through. Her spots ruined her life until she got to a private clinic, but at least her doctor gave her some proper treatment first.

CM *(Skim reads the article)* Yes I see . . . roaccutane . . . dianette . . . You see, Jane, these are what I call "heavy-duty treatments." I hardly ever prescribe them: in fact, I can't prescribe the roaccutane . . . only dermatologists can prescribe that. It's quite toxic, you see. Can cause permanent harm to your liver, and you don't want that. As for dianette, I can't remember the last time I prescribed that – it significantly increases the risk of a blood clot and you don't want to end up with a stroke or something just to treat a few spots. No, Jane *(rather firmly now)*, you are better off with nothing.

JB But I'll get nowhere in the photo shoot if I don't get something to help me.

CM *(Not unkindly)* What's this about photo shoots, Jane?

JB We've got this photo shoot coming up at college and that could be my chance.

CM *(A little incredulous)* Would you really want to be a model, Jane? It's not all it's cracked up to be, you know. The whole fashion industry is just a form of corporate abuse – mega industrial companies trying to get your money for cosmetics you would be better off without, clothing manufacturers operating third-world sweatshops and trying to create markets by selling new lines as this season's fashion.

Do you really want to get caught up in that world?

JB So you are not going to help me?

Casuistry and the consultation

Standing outside this consultation, it is easy to be critical of Dr. Mangate's communication skills. But that would be too simplistic. The question is why an experienced and clearly caring GP working in a high-performing practice should "lose it" so easily in this situation. It is not a matter of his knowledge and use of evidence – he is right about the indications for treating mild acne in an otherwise healthy teenager. Nor is it a matter of ethics – there is no malpractice here: consistent with GMC guidelines (see Chapter 2), Dr. Mangate is courteous throughout and he does his best to explain why it would be unprofessional for him to give Jane Brewer what she is asking for.

In this section, we look at how the failure of this consultation was driven by values: not by negative values (such as lack of commitment, knowledge or skills) but by the positive values of two strong-minded and committed people, Dr. Mangate and Jane Brewer, meeting without mutual understanding. Later in the section, we will see how casuistry can help improve understanding of our own and other people's values. First, it will be worth reviewing briefly the clash of *positive* values that (being unacknowledged) led to the failure of this consultation.

Initial (positive) values mapping

> **Reflection point**
>
> You may want to think about the positive values in play in this consultation for yourself before seeing what we have to say about them.
>
> From what you have heard thus far about Jane Brewer and Dr. Mangate, what values do you think were driving the consultation? What was important to both of them? And how did their respective values bring them into misunderstanding and conflict?
>
> Think about both foreground and background values, and about the wider network of values (Chapter 1). And think particularly about positive values (Chapter 4).

If you tried this for yourself, the values you thought of are likely to be similar to ours in some respects and different in others (see below). This diversity of values is important: it reflects similarities and differences in our respective values that in turn will influence the way we use casuistic (case-based) and other ways of reasoning about values. As noted at the start of this chapter, the aim of reasoning about values in values-based practice is not to decide "who is right" ("who has the *right* values") but rather to expand our understanding of the values in play in a given situation. It is this expanded understanding that is needed to support the consultation between Dr. Mangate and Jane Brewer, and different value perspectives can be helpful in achieving this.

We return to the role of different professional value perspectives in Chapter 9 (on team working). For now though, the question is how do the values of Jane Brewer and Dr. Mangate play out in the consultation? Again, there are many possible combinations here, and we will not try to spell all of them out. But here are a few examples:

- Dr. Mangate, working under pressure [*positive value* – efficient use of time] finds himself caught (as he sees it) [*positive value* – multidisciplinary team work] with having to deal with a request [*positive value* – person-centered care] with which he thoroughly disapproves [*positive values* – evidence-based prescribing; well-being; fair trade; sustainable development]. So, Dr. Mangate rushes in, making assumptions and in effect telling Jane Brewer that there will be "nothing doing" almost before she has sat down.
- Jane Brewer is thus put on the defensive from the start. She is already nervous (remember this is her first time "driving solo" with a doctor) [*positive value* – establishing independence] and instead of "the kind doctor" her mother talked of [*positive value* – respect for her mum], she feels she has not been listened to, still less understood; she thus has to fight [*positive value* – determination] to get her agenda, including her *Daily Mail* article [*positive value* – information-based decision-making], appearance [*positive value* – looking good] and career and work [*positive value* – strong work ethic], into the consultation at all.

Casuistry and clinical experience

So how can casuistry help? Rather than approaching this directly, we will start with a re-run of the background to the consultation but with one key difference. This time we will give Dr. Mangate a chance to

think about the referral for a minute or two before Jane Brewer comes in. As we will see, this breathing space gives him an opportunity to reflect on a case he saw the day before and to compare his reaction to that case with his reaction to Jane Brewer.

Comparing cases is one of the most powerful ways in which, as professionals, we draw on our clinical experience (one of the three essential elements, you will recall from Chapter 2, of evidence-based medicine). Comparing cases is also the essence of casuistry as a way of reasoning about values. After following Dr. Mangate's reflection on his earlier case then, and thinking a bit more about it as an exercise in casuistry, we will see how this changed his consultation with Jane Brewer.

Rewinding the spool

We are back with Dr. Mangate in his surgery. This time, his previous patient turned out to be straightforward (a check on blood pressure and repeat prescription) and, being generally rather good at time management, he is a little ahead of his list. He sees, as before, the note from the nurse practitioner – about Jane Brewer insisting on seeing him about acne because of a photo shoot; as before he picks up the email thanking everyone for their success in sticking to prescribing guidelines; and as before, his first reaction is to think "What a waste of NHS resources."

But here the story takes a new turn. For this time, in his brief space for reflection, he suddenly recalls a patient he saw the day before who, like Jane Brewer, presented with a "cosmetic" problem but to whom he had reacted quite differently.

Dr. Mangate reflects

Dr. Mangate might have stopped right there, of course. But his habit of imaginative honesty took over and he found himself wondering, "Well, what *was* the difference? Why did I feel OK about that patient but not about Jane Brewer?"

Reflection point

Try sharing Dr. Mangate's reflection here. Think of cosmetic cases from your own experience: which cases do you think justify the use of medical resources and which in your view do not?

What are the differences between them (again, in your view)?

Many different cases will come to mind for each of us, but we give here part of Dr. Mangate's thinking as he reflected on his two cases.

"What a waste of NHS resources," he thought. "Another self-absorbed wannabe 'celeb' expecting me to spend our prescribing budget on cosmetics! Not like that poor child I saw yesterday, that eight-year-old boy with a strawberry birth mark on his face . . .

"But hang on. Wasn't that a cosmetic problem too? Well, yes, but that was different – after all, we can treat strawberry marks – laser treatments are more or less routine and offer a pretty harmless way of removing them. Then again, though, laser treatments are certainly not a cheap option . . . so why *do* we use them for a cosmetic problem? The child I saw yesterday was being bullied. I know how ghastly that can be from what happened to our son at his first school – heartbreaking for his mother as well . . . and his school work was suffering. But what if that mother yesterday had come asking for her son's birth mark to be treated so he could compete in a photo shoot for child modeling? Would I have been sympathetic? I doubt it . . .

"Am I being unfair to Jane Brewer, then? After all, it's not like Sue Barnes to make a fuss about nothing. Well, let's see what Jane has to say for herself . . ."

He presses the buzzer for Jane Brewer to come in.

Casuistry and self-understanding

We touched on the importance of reflective practice for developing self-awareness in the last chapter. We emphasized the importance of using others as a "mirror" to help us see our own values when they might not be obvious to us. Dr. Mangate's casuistry is an extension of this. Here, he is subjecting himself to a fairly rigorous analytic process in order to understand more about the "grey areas" of his values.

Reflection point

We will see shortly how the re-run of the consultation between Dr. Mangate and Jane Brewer went. First, think for a moment about Dr. Mangate's reflection. Exactly what was it that changed his attitude to Jane Brewer in advance of seeing her?

Was there a material difference between the two presenting conditions (strawberry birth marks and acne)? Was it the evidence (of a difference in treatment safety and effectiveness)? Was it new self-understanding (of the values he brought to the consultation)?

As we noted earlier, reflecting on similarities and differences between cases is a powerful way of exploring any aspect of clinical decision-making. But in this instance at least, it is clear that Dr. Mangate's change of attitude in advance of his consultation with Jane Brewer was driven by a new self-understanding of how his own values were shaping his attitude towards her. There was no material difference between the presenting problems: both were cosmetic problems. True, there was a difference in the availability of effective evidence-based treatments (strawberry marks really can be removed by laser treatments); but being *able* to change something does not in itself *justify* changing it (certainly not using NHS resources – think of the arguments over cosmetic surgery).

So we come with Dr. Mangate to his own values. We have seen already that as a doctor he was strongly committed to evidence-based prescribing and was deeply skeptical of the pharmaceutical industry. By way of further background, it is worth adding that he and his wife had always tried to be green and eco-friendly (his wife wore no cosmetics). Also, their two children (a boy and a girl) were still young and doing well at school, although the bullying episode had been a setback for their son. Small wonder, then, that Dr. Mangate's initial reaction to Jane Brewer's acne in this re-run of the build-up to the consultation was to compare her unfavorably with the eight-year-old that (in this version of the story) he had seen the previous day with a strawberry mark and who was being bullied at school (as his own son had been). But as we saw earlier when we looked at the values in play in the first run of the consultation, Dr. Mangate was also strongly committed to both patient-centered practice and multidisciplinary teamwork. Once he recognized the extent to which his adverse reaction to Jane Brewer reflected his own values, he readily switched to a more open-minded approach to the consultation.

Re-running the consultation

CM   Come and have a seat, Jane. What can we do for you today?

JB   (*Looking uncomfortable as she sits down*) It's like I said to the nurse, I need treatment for my spots.

CM   OK, what have you tried for yourself?

JB   I've tried things from the chemist and they haven't helped. I need proper treatment.

CM   I see. What did you try from the chemist?

JB   I got some wash stuff – panoxyl I think it was – and that just made it worse. My skin went like beetroot and so itchy – I had to stay in for three days – couldn't even go to college. My mum bought me some Clearasil™ Max but that didn't do any good either.

CM   Perhaps we should have a look at them; slip your jacket off (*taking her over to the examination couch; she is wearing a jacket over a T-shirt*). Yes, I see what you mean (*examining her cheek and forehead*). Have you got any anywhere else?

JB   (*Embarrassed*) Well, er, my chest is OK but I've got them on my back . . .

CM   (*Looks carefully at the back of her neck and shoulders*) Yes, I see – apart from these spots your skin is very good (*and noting her firm shoulder muscles and good physique, he adds*). You must look after yourself.

JB   (*Pleased*) I gave up chocolate and "smokes" two years ago when one of my friends got really bad acne.

CM   That was a good idea – you would have had a lot more trouble if you didn't take care of your health. OK, that's fine, pop your jacket on again (*returning to his desk and indicating she should do the same*).

CM   The nurse you talked to, Sue Barnes, tells me you're worried about a photo shoot at your college – is that part of your course?

JB   It's not part of the course, but my Mum thinks I could be a model and it's a chance to earn some money . . . and it would be good experience – I want to train as a beautician. My Mum's a beautician.

CM   Yes, I can see it's important. Look, I'm going to be straight with you, Jane, there really is no safe treatment for acne.

JB   (*Producing her* Daily Mail *article rather tentatively*) But look what this girl had to go through. Her spots ruined her life until she got to a private clinic; I can't afford to go private but at least her doctor gave her some proper treatment first.

CM   (*Looks at the article attentively as he skim reads it*) Yes . . . I see . . . roaccutane . . . dianette . . . You see, Jane, these are what I call "heavy-duty treatments." I hardly ever prescribe them: in fact, I can't prescribe the roaccutane . . . only dermatologists can prescribe that. The problem is that these treatments are very unlikely to get rid of your spots and they could really damage your health.

JB   You mean like the panoxyl, only worse? Even the girl in that article got depression.

CM   Exactly. It's really bad luck about the spots and the photo shoot, Jane, but there really isn't anything more than you are already doing that would help.

JB   (*Smiling now*) That's what my Mum said – beauticians have to be very careful too about what they recommend, asking about allergies and things – must be a bit like being a doctor . . .

CM   Sue Barnes knows a lot about cosmetics – would you like to have another talk with her?

JB   No, that's fine. I just wanted to be sure. Thanks for seeing me.

Follow-up (positive) values mapping

This re-run of the interview clearly went very differently. This time Dr. Mangate's communication skills were fully and effectively engaged: he got to the same bottom line (no prescription) but with Jane Brewer understanding the issues and unlikely to rush into potentially harmful alternatives. Dr. Mangate's brief reflection before seeing Jane Brewer, comparing her case with the child with a strawberry mark he had seen the day before, thus meant that the positive values that had worked *against* them in the first run of the interview now worked *for* them.

Reflection point

Do you agree with this claim?

The claim is that (i) a brief (casuistic) reflection by Dr. Mangate on the similarities and differences between Jane Brewer's problem with acne and a child with a strawberry mark he had seen the previous day made him more aware of how his own values were shaping his approach to the consultation; (ii) this radically improved his ability to draw on his (already well developed) communication skills; and (iii) this in turn resulted in an engaged rather than enraged response from Jane Brewer at his inability to offer any actual treatment.

Go back for a moment to our initial values mapping we carried out above and think how the positive values we identified there played out in the re-run consultation.

As with our initial values mapping above, there are different ways in which the values involved might have played out in the re-run consultation between Dr. Mangate and Jane Brewer; but here is our interpretation:

- Dr. Mangate, with a couple of minutes for reflection before seeing Jane Brewer [*positive value* – efficient use of time], realizes his initially adverse reaction to her cosmetic problem (of acne) is at odds with his positive response to another child with a cosmetic problem (of a strawberry birth mark) that he had seen just the day before, and he wonders why; after all, it is not as if one condition (the strawberry mark) is a "proper" medical problem while the other (acne) is not – to the contrary, they are *both* cosmetic problems.

- True, the evidence base for his decision is that there is a safe and effective treatment for the one (strawberry mark) and not for the other (acne) [*positive values* – evidence-based prescribing; well-being].
- However, he realizes that his decision to actually *offer* treatment for the strawberry mark was driven not by the availability of an evidence-based treatment but by his *values* – essentially he disapproves of the "celeb culture" [*positive values* – fair trade; sustainable development] while identifying with a mother's concerns about her son being bullied at school and failing academically [*positive value* – person-centered care].
- He thus recognizes that he is at risk of pre-judging Jane Brewer [*positive value* – person-centered care] and in consequence approaches the consultation with an open mind.
- His open-minded approach is further reinforced by his reflection that the practice nurse, Sue Barnes, is not in the habit of making inappropriate referrals [*positive value* – multidisciplinary team work].

Dr. Mangate's more open approach means that right from the start Jane Brewer gets the message that she is being taken seriously (he listens carefully to what she has to say) and he builds on this good start throughout the consultation (he takes an interest in her *Daily Mail* article; he makes an appropriately thorough, rather than cursorily dismissive, examination of her spots; he is straight with her about the lack of safe treatments; and so on).

- Jane Brewer, instead of being put on the defensive, thus feels that her decision to ask for medical help has been endorsed [*positive value* – establishing independence].
- She feels that her mother (who had encouraged her to see Dr. Mangate) had got it right, while her skeptical friends had got it wrong [*positive value* – respect for her mum].
- She feels that her ideas and sources of information (including her *Daily Mail* article) have been

accepted alongside medical knowledge [*positive value* – information-based decision-making].
- She feels that her values, notably the importance she attaches to her appearance [*positive value* – looking good], but also including her hopes and aspirations (her intended career) [*positive value* – strong work ethic], have been respected (you will recall the significance of patients' aspirations from Chapter 3).
- Finally, although Dr. Mangate hadn't been able to give her any new treatment, she now feels satisfied that she has done all she can in order to do well in the photo shoot [*positive value* – determination].

What Jane Brewer learned from Dr. Mangate

Instead of leaving the consultation feeling embarrassed and mistrustful of future contact with doctors, Jane Brewer thus gained confidence in standing on her own feet; and while she could see that Dr. Mangate was not really "into" fashion (he consults in cords and a sweater), she shared some of his priorities (notably about health – it really wouldn't help her career as a beautician to be left scarred with the wrong treatment); and his support and endorsement mattered to her – not quite a dad (her dad left them when she was three years old and hadn't been seen since), but . . . at least he was someone she could trust in the future.

What Dr. Mangate learned from Jane Brewer

Dr. Mangate, too, took away many positive outcomes from the consultation. He learned much that was positive about Jane Brewer as one of his rapidly growing-up patients: her unexpected strengths (the way she looked after her health); her commitment and determination; and her relationship with her mum.

He also felt encouraged that he had been able to relate apparently effectively with a teenage girl – never a "ladies man," he had not had much to do with teenagers and was dimly aware of a growing anxiety in his role as a father as his own daughter (now aged 9) was beginning to mature. He gained a more balanced and less stereotyped view of the fashion world as the basis of his own values – Jane Brewer was clearly very far from his image of the "evil empire of the cosmetics industry," and hadn't he read something recently about the therapeutic value of make-up (which he had laughingly thought of at the time as a "touch of lipstick") in women with cancer?

More about casuistry

This was truly a win–win situation, then, for doctor as well as patient. As with any other powerful technique, however, casuistry should be used carefully and with awareness of its down sides as well as potential benefits. In this final section of the chapter, we thus look in a bit more detail at casuistry as case-based reasoning, at its strengths and weaknesses, and at how it fits together with principles and other ways of reasoning about values.

Casuistry in clinical practice

The term "casuistry" often has negative connotations in everyday usage, meaning a cynical molding of cases to fit one's own purposes. Casuistry, however, was rehabilitated for use in clinical contexts in the early days of bioethics by two American scholars, A. R. Jonsen and S. Toulmin (1988), building on their experience serving on an American Presidential Commission on Bioethics.

What they noticed was that, on most of the ethical issues under discussion, the members of the commission generally agreed on what it was right or wrong to do but often for very different reasons: in other words, they agreed on the "*what*" but not on the "*why*." So, Jonsen and Toulmin concluded, the way to think about ethical issues in medicine is by immersion in the details of cases (on *what* is done) rather than worrying about theories (on *why* it is done).

In practice, "immersion in cases" (or casuistry) means asking two questions:

1. What *changes in the case* in question would make it clearer what to do?
2. What *related cases* would be more or less clear-cut ethically speaking?

In values-based practice, values reasoning is used primarily to open up understanding of the values in play in a given situation rather than to close down on an ethical "solution." But the approach is the same. Dr. Mangate in effect used both the above questions in coming to a better understanding of how his own values were shaping his initial adverse reaction to Jane Brewer.

Use with care

Given the importance of case-based reasoning in general to the professional skills base of medicine, casuistry might seem a harmless enough method to use for reasoning about values. But there are no "free lunches" in values reasoning.

> **Reflection point**
>
> In the final reflection in this chapter, think for a moment what dangers there might be in casuistry and how these could be mitigated. (Clue: think about exactly how and why casuistry got rehabilitated by Jonsen and Toulmin.)

The main danger of casuistry is also its strength, i.e. that it taps into shared values. Recall Jonsen and Toulmin's key observation that members of the Presidential Commission on Bioethics *agreed* on the right thing to do in particular cases. Fine, but to the extent that this agreement reflected already-shared values, casuistry inevitably carries with it, as the American philosopher Loretta Kopelman (1994) first pointed out, the risk of endorsing bias and prejudice; and this risk is much increased if the values concerned (as in case-based reasoning) are largely implicit.

One way to mitigate this danger is thus by using casuistry alongside and in partnership with other methods of values reasoning that are less dependent on implicit values. Principles reasoning, as used by Dr. Gulati in Chapter 2, offers one effective counterbalance to casuistry in this respect (and vice versa). Casuistry is bottom-up reasoning based on largely implicit values; principles reasoning is top-down from high-level general principles that are largely explicit.

Other explicit methods of reasoning about values include utilitarianism (balancing good and harm, as in health economics), deontology (based on rights and responsibilities, and the basis of codes and medical law) and virtue theory (with a growing role in medical education). We provide further reading on these and other methods of ethical reasoning on the series website.

A second way to mitigate the danger of casuistry reinforcing bias and prejudice is by including a range of diverse perspectives in the way it is used. We will see the importance of this in later chapters: in relation to multi-disciplinary teamwork in Chapter 9 (when we look at risk management), and in relation to patients and carers working alongside professionals in Chapter 14 (when we look at values-based approaches to developing practice policies in areas such as commissioning and the efficient use of resources). As we will see, casuistry is a powerful way of establishing a framework of shared values within which balanced decisions can be made on individual cases.

Chapter summary

In this chapter, we have shown how reasoning about values by comparing cases (casuistry) helped a GP, Dr. Mangate, to reflect on his own values and hence to use his already well-developed communication skills to better effect in a difficult consultation on acne with a 17-year-old patient, Jane Brewer.

Dr. Mangate's reflection took a minute or two. But the net result was a win–win outcome for the therapeutic relationship:

- Jane Brewer still had to cope with her acne, but she left the consultation feeling that she had been listened to and with her ambitions on hold but intact.

- Dr. Mangate gained in confidence in dealing with teenagers (his own daughter was fast approaching this stage) and with a more balanced (because less stereotypical) understanding of the cosmetics industry.

As we indicated in the final part of the chapter, casuistry is only one of a number of different ways of reasoning about values (we introduced principles reasoning in Chapter 2). None of these ways of reasoning offers a sinecure. Each has strengths and weaknesses. Used with care, however, values reasoning, as in Dr. Mangate's consultation with Jane Brewer, can help to improve mutual understanding as the basis of good clinical care.

References

Jonsen, A. R. and Toulmin, S. (1988). *The Abuse of Casuistry: a History of Moral Reasoning*. California: University of California Press.

Kopelman, L. M. (1994). Case method and casuistry: the problem of bias. *Theoretical Medicine* 15, 21–38.

POINT

Balanced Decision-making
within a
Framework of Shared Values

PROCESS

Partnership

Two-feet Principle   Squeaky-wheel Principle   Science-driven Principle

Person-centered practice   Multidisciplinary teamwork

Awareness   Reasoning   Knowledge   Communication skills

PREMISE

Mutual Respect
for
Differences of Values

Map of values-based practice – knowledge.

Chapter

6

A smoking enigma: getting (and not getting) the knowledge

Values-based practice element 3: knowledge about values

Topics covered in this chapter

Trish Butler, a research-oriented practice nurse who runs a smoking cessation clinic, explores a variety of sources of knowledge of values as she tackles the clinical, training and research problems raised by her patient, 68-year-old Sandy Fraser, who continues to smoke despite the fact that both he and his wife, Ivy, have severe smoking-related disorders (chronic obstructive pulmonary disease and a stroke, respectively).

Other topics include:

- Stuck points and how we learn
- Explicit and tacit knowledge
- Motivational interviewing
- PUNs and DENs in clinical learning
- Values literature retrieval: clinical purposes
- Values literature retrieval: training and research purposes
- A variety of values research methods
- Knowledge of values from research and unique individuals.

Take-away message for practice

*A wide variety of methods (including retrieval of research evidence from electronic databases) can be used to learn about the values likely to be in play and influencing a given clinical situation – but the **individual is always unique**.*

This chapter is different. The story line is still narrative in form – we follow an experienced nurse practitioner, Trish Butler, as she tries to understand why one of her patients, Sandy Fraser, refuses to give up smoking. But Trish Butler in addition to her clinical concerns has

also a particular interest in training and research. Hence, if your interests are mainly clinical, you may want to "skim and skip" some of the more technical detail in this chapter and concentrate on the clinical sections.

Getting and *not* getting knowledge of values

The other way in which the chapter is different is that, as its title suggests, it is as much about *not getting* as about getting knowledge of values. One reason for this is that, as Trish Butler finds, learning about values from research presents particular challenges. Standard medical databases (such as PubMed, a free database accessing primarily the MEDLINE database of references and abstracts on life sciences and biomedical topics) are not well set up for retrieving research on values. For clinical purposes, a quick Google search is often just as helpful.

There are, of course, many other ways of getting knowledge of values besides searching electronic databases. We cover some of these briefly as they relate more particularly to the demands of clinical work in the first section of the chapter. Communication skills, for example (the subject of Chapter 7), are vital in this respect.

A second reason why this chapter is about not getting as well as getting knowledge of values has to do with the uniqueness of our values as individuals. What this means clinically is that values research has a strictly limited role. Research can help us understand the values that are *likely to be in play* in a given situation. This can be important (we come to an example of this with Tony Colombo's work on team values in Chapter 9). But the bottom line clinically is that, whatever the research findings, the individual (clinician as well as patient) is always unique. So research can never in itself tell us what values are *actually in play* between the particular (and always values-unique) individuals concerned. Sandy Fraser indeed remains at the end of this chapter an enigma.

The clinical context

Trish Butler, practice nurse, relaxing over a cup of coffee in her room after the morning's smoking cessation clinic, was running over her latest encounter with her patient Sandy Fraser. Sandy, she reflected, was an enigma. Now aged 68 and a retired bus driver, he was referred to her clinic as a life-long smoker when he was first diagnosed with chronic obstructive pulmonary disease (COPD). This was three years earlier, and in the interim, his wife, Ivy, at 66 a little younger than him and also a smoker, had suffered a major stroke. This had left her disabled and needing full-time care, the burden of which fell on Sandy, supported by visits from the district nurses. The Frasers had no children.

Trish Butler was disappointed that Sandy Fraser had not given up smoking, as she had had good reason to believe that he would. The practice had recruited her a few years earlier to run the smoking-cessation clinic they had set up in response to persuasive new evidence of the clinical value of giving up smoking for patients with COPD, even when they had been long-term smokers (Edwards, 2004). Using motivational interviewing techniques (see below), Trish Butler had proved very effective in this, and her experience had given her considerable first-hand knowledge of the factors that prompt even dedicated smokers to give up.

True, living with a partner who smokes (as Sandy's wife, Ivy, did) could be a problem (Monden et al., 2003) and giving up could have a negative impact on social networks (Ritchie et al., 2010). But a serious health scare of the kind that Sandy Fraser appeared to have had was, in Trish's experience, often enough. And in Sandy's case, he had the further motivation of wanting to provide care for Ivy following her recent stroke. As a couple, she knew they were very close and Sandy had refused point blank any suggestion that Ivy might have to go into a care home. Yet even the argument that Sandy needed to remain fit for as long as possible if he was to continue to care for Ivy at home had failed to persuade him to reduce let alone give up his smoking. "I just can't understand where he's coming from," she thought. "Perhaps, if he would open up a bit . . .?"

Sandy Fraser, moreover, was not her only problem patient, although he was perhaps the most inexplicable, and there had been growing discussion within the practice about how to manage their remaining die-hard smokers. This was another worry, Trish Butler thought. Their work in the smoking-cessation clinic risked being undermined by the inconsistent attitudes emerging among the doctors, ranging from a laissez-faire *resignation to what she regarded as an equally unproductive tougher and more aggressive line.*

Tom Peters, the GP registrar (in the final year of his general practice training), was a case in point. Tom had been sitting in on her clinic that morning and had clearly been unhappy with how she had handled things with Sandy Fraser. If he had had his way, he had said to her later, he would have told Sandy to stop wasting their time and to come back when he was "ready to see sense." "That might be OK in a hospital clinic," Trish had replied, "but Sandy and Ivy are our patients, come what may, and the fact that Sandy keeps his appointments despite no doubt expecting "another lecture" shows that at some level he is aware that he needs our help. Besides," she had concluded, "you can never tell when a breakthrough will come . . ."

She had been aware that Tom Peters was not impressed by her argument. "And he does have a point," she thought. "As a practice, we really are getting stuck with where we go from here with patients like Sandy Fraser – and I'm the one," she remembered, "who offered to run a discussion on smoking cessation for our next protected learning time (PLT) session!"

Trish Butler was proud of her status as a practice-based teacher for student nurses and she normally enjoyed the challenge of inter-professional teaching. But her sense of having failed to get her message across to Tom Peters, set against the emerging difficulties about smoking cessation across the practice as a whole, now made the impending PLT session look more challenging. "However am I going to get that sorted," she thought, "when I haven't even started the outline research proposal to send to my MSc tutor by the end of the month?"

Stuck points and new learning

In this extended opening scenario, Trish Butler has come up against a situation that does not fit with her own experience and knowledge – she has reached what we call a "stuck point." These "stuck points" are often potent routes to learning, whether scientific and technical, or as in this case about values.

Reflection point

In this chapter, we will be following Trish Butler as she moves on from her "stuck point." But before reading about this, you may find it helpful to reflect for a moment on where Trish Butler is starting from:

- What kinds of problems does she face?
- What knowledge does she already have to build on?
- Where does the mismatch come between problems and knowledge (thus leaving her at a "stuck point")?

Problems in clinical practice, training and research

Three kinds of problem face Trish at her stuck point. They all contribute to her determination to explore further knowledge about values:

1. *A clinical problem* – how to help her patient Sandy Fraser (and others like him) to stop (or at any rate cut back on his) smoking.
2. *A team-development problem* – the PLT session offers an opportunity to tackle the growing inconsistencies within the practice in how different clinicians tackle problems of smoking cessation, but she has to find a way of ensuring that the session is productive rather than simply stirring up more disagreement.
3. *A research problem* – although struggling to find time and inspiration to write an outline research proposal for her MSc, Trish is aware that values is something that interests her.

Explicit and tacit knowledge

Trish Butler's reflections on her morning clinic demonstrate that she already has a considerable knowledge base on which to draw in tackling the problems she faces. In the first place, she has clinical knowledge: she knows a great deal about smoking-related disorders and in particular about the problems faced by patients who want or need to stop smoking.

As with any other area of knowledge, Trish Butler's clinical knowledge base is in part explicit but also importantly tacit (Polanyi, 1967; Thornton, 2006). Explicit knowledge is mainly knowledge of facts of the kind that can be learned from other people, from books and from the Internet; it includes the knowledge we derive from empirical research (including, as we will see, research on values). Tacit knowledge, by contrast, is gained mainly through experience and includes knowledge expressed in the exercise of skills. Thus, someone who knows how to ride a bike has explicit knowledge (for example of the correct side of the road on which to ride) and tacit knowledge (for example of how to balance and how to steer round a corner).

Trish Butler's explicit clinical knowledge is derived partly from her nurse training including the additional courses she took in respiratory disorders before taking on the smoking-cessation clinic, together with her regular reading of journals and professional update bulletins (note here her knowledge of relevant research). But she also has all the tacit knowledge and skills she has gained through her experience of running her clinic.

That both kinds of knowledge are important clinically is reflected in David Sackett and colleagues' definition of evidence-based medicine that we looked at in Chapter 2 (Fig. 2.3). Sackett's definition, you will recall, started with best research evidence but extended also to include "... the ability to use our clinical skills and past experience ..."

From "stuck point" to new learning

So why is Trish Butler as a knowledgeable practitioner at a "stuck point"? In a word, *values*. Again, Sackett's definition from Chapter 2 reminds us of the importance of values. Evidence-based medicine, he said, must integrate three things: research evidence (explicit knowledge), clinical experience (tacit knowledge) and values. Sackett's definition specified patients' values. But as we saw in Chapter 2, the relevant values include those also of clinicians. For Trish Butler, her knowledge of motivational interviewing made it natural for her to formulate her stuck point in terms of her own and other values.

Motivational interviewing

In training to run the smoking-cessation clinic, Trish Butler had read William Miller and Stephen Rollnick's (2002) *Motivational Interviewing: Preparing People for Change*. This book, which she sometimes referred to as her "bible on motivational interviewing," built on Carl Rogers' work on counseling and a careful analysis of the "non-specific factors" in successful counseling, i.e. the factors that relate to the personality and communication style of a given counselor rather than to the particular therapeutic method he or she employs.

Motivational interviewing and values

Thus, motivational interviewing, Miller and Rollnick write, starts from "... the person's own experiences and values" (motivational interviewing is in this sense a person-centered approach). The willingness to change depends in motivational terms on there being a "... discrepancy between status and goal, between what is happening at present and what one values for the future." Indeed, "a change process kicks in ... when things are sufficiently discrepant from the desired or expected ideal ..." and, contrary to confrontational interviewing, "... change seems to arise when the person concerned connects it with something of intrinsic value, something important, something cherished," so that, finally, the "... way out of the forest has to do with exploring and following what the person is experiencing and what, from his or her perspective, truly matters."

Motivational interviewing made sense to Trish Butler within her own scale of values. Miller and Rollnick's carefully evidence-based "more carrot than stick" approach fitted well with her positive problem-solving approach to life (see, for example, in the smoking-cessation literature, Butler *et al.*, 1998 and Richards *et al.*, 2003).

This, too, was consistent with her experience of seeing clinicians with Tom Peters' "more stick than carrot" approach succeeding with patients who were ready and able to change their health-damaging behaviors but simply frightening off or demoralizing those who were not. By contrast, she found motivational interviewing offered a powerful resource for activating people's own motivations to help them achieve sustainable changes in their behavior.

Self-awareness first

"Well," Trish Butler thought, reflecting on motivational interviewing, "what about values here? I clearly don't understand where Sandy Fraser is coming from. And given Tom's reaction to me this morning, I probably don't really understand where he and some of my colleagues are coming from." Trish Butler thus recognized that before she went any further she had to get in touch with her own values. Values awareness starts at home!

After a little deliberation, she identified some pertinent values in herself:

- I have always enjoyed feeling fit – looking after myself is important to me.
- I am interested in evidence. I respond to evidence. I would now like to contribute towards developing evidence, because I believe evidence is vital for good patient care.
- I derive considerable job satisfaction from helping patients in the smoking-cessation and other clinics gain the skills they need to improve their own health.
- I embrace change.

It was not then difficult to identify mismatches between her values, both personally and as a clinician, and those of her patient, Sandy Fraser. It made sense of her comment to herself over her cup of coffee that she "... just can't understand" how anyone in Sandy Fraser's situation could want to continue smoking. Similarly, it explained her (as she saw it) ineffective feedback session with Tom Peters after their morning clinic.

So, where to go from here? How can Trish Butler learn more about the values underpinning her stuck point? Before looking at what research can offer, it will be worth reviewing briefly what Trish Butler could learn from other elements of values-based practice.

Knowledge of values – a values-based practice reprise

> **Reflection point**
>
> From what you have read already, which elements of values-based practice do you think involve learning about values?

Values-based practice, as we outlined in Chapter 3, builds on learnable clinical skills in the four key areas. Each of these four skills areas, taken separately or together, can help to improve our understanding of the values in play in a given situation. Let us take a moment to see how knowledge fits with the other three clinical skills – awareness, reasoning and communication skills – in the particular situation facing Trish Butler.

- *Awareness of values and the diversity of values.* Trish was unusual among clinicians in that her interest in motivational interviewing meant that it came naturally to her to formulate her problems explicitly in terms of values. She thus had no need of the "wake-up" call embodied in this first and foundational skills area for values-based practice. Nonetheless, like the mental health team in Chapter 4, Trish Butler might gain further understanding of Sandy and Ivy's smoking values by asking for knowledge from one or other of the district nurses who visit them at home. Their more intimate day-to-day contact with Sandy and Ivy in their own home could shed light on the couple's strengths (their StAR values, as we called them in Chapter 4). "Situated knowledge" (both biomedical and social) has its place in medicine, and values are a vital component (Maudsley and Strivens, 2000).

- *Reasoning about values.* Trish Butler might expand her "values horizons" by exercising one or more of the ways of reasoning about values outlined in Chapter 5. Principles reasoning, for example, could show her that, in addition to the "autonomy versus beneficence" differences between herself and Tom Peters, there were complex issues of (distributive) justice involved in the way they deploy the resources of the practice with apparently recalcitrant patients. This line of thought might require a little bit more knowledge of resource allocation than Trish currently had at her fingertips, something that could perhaps be addressed by looking at some of the background material for "World-class commissioning" (a statement of intent put forward by the UK Department of Heath for the NHS)?

- Drawing on her own knowledge, Trish might also have found "bottom-up" case-based reasoning helpful, as we saw with Dr. Mangate in Chapter 5. Case-based reasoning accesses tacit knowledge and could be useful for working with the GP registrar, Tom Peters. Tom clearly found Sandy Fraser's attitude difficult to take. Yet Trish had seen him respond in a far more supportive way with men of a similar age to Sandy Fraser who had drinking problems. Case-based reasoning might help to clarify the differences between the two kinds of case in terms of Tom Peter's experience and values. This might help him find a way of extending his person-centered approach to patients with whom he felt less natural sympathy.

- *Communication skills.* Tapping into knowledge requires communication skills – especially drawing on the knowledge of others. Even web-searching is a form of communication skill, especially when we try to develop our knowledge in discussion forums. We return to communication skills as the fourth skills area for values-based practice in Chapter 7.

Now let us turn to knowledge of values as a distinct skills area in its own right.

Accessing knowledge

In this section, we will look first at what is known about how clinicians in general go about seeking new knowledge and then follow Trish Butler as she tries various ways of accessing knowledge of values.

> **Reflection point**
>
> Trish Butler now has to decide how far to go in framing and answering further questions for herself about the clashes of values behind her stuck point with Sandy Fraser.
> How would *you* go about this?

PUNs and DENs and Slotnick's cycle of learning

Clinical learners go as far as they need to in order to satisfy their own assessment of the PUNs (patient's unmet needs) and DENs (doctor's educational needs) described and copyrighted by Richard Eve (Eve, 2003). Thus, in her clinical role, only Trish Butler can decide what is a "good enough answer."

Hank Slotnick's research into physician learning has shown that learning episodes follow four definite stages: scanning for problems, deciding whether to pursue the learning task, acquiring new knowledge and skill, and gaining experience with what has been learned (Slotnick, 1999). Although we focus in this chapter with Trish Butler only on the first three of Slotnick's stages, it is important to consider all of them. Learning is not just about the acquisition of new knowledge and skills and gaining experience with their use. The key point is this: without the decision to pursue a learning task, in-depth learning does not take place. Slotnick points out that numerous potential questions crop up in everyday clinical practice. As the questions float past on the river of clinical practice, the decision to wade in and catch one for closer examination is an active decision.

Slotnick's cycle and learning about values

Think about the implications of Slotnick's work for the knowledge base of values. A working clinician is unlikely to set out like a researcher to explore the values around obesity, disfigurement or end-of-life care by reading numerous original papers. More likely, a clinical case with an interesting values dimension will prompt a quick look at the Internet or a re-thumbing of a well-loved book. It is really important then, that this initial, tentative approach to exploring values knowledge is rewarded by at least a glimpse of what is out there in the world of values. So how did Trish Butler get on?

A quick first Google search

In the first instance, Trish Butler did as perhaps most of us would do in her situation and turned to our twenty-first-century oracle, the Internet. Trish Butler was an experienced web user and had accessed its resources successfully in her role as both a clinician and a clinical trainer. She had found it a ready source of information on topics ranging from new medications and other areas of scientific and technical update through ethical guidelines to local and national policy publications. Up to this point, though, she had had no experience of searching the web for knowledge of values. As we will see, this was to present particular challenges.

Reflection point

Before reading on, you may find it helpful to ask yourself, if you were in Trish Butler's situation, how you might go about searching for values on the Internet.

If you have access to the Internet, you may even want to try a couple of quick searches to see what you come up with.

Google

As most of us might do, Trish Butler started with the "lowest cost of entry" approach and ran a Google search. She knew well enough that to get anything useful she had to make her search reasonably specific. Just searching on "values and smoking," for example, would pick up large numbers of papers using the term "values" in scientific and technical senses (in phrases like "... study samples yielded a P value of 2.14×10^{-9}," "the mean values of," "changes in ghrelin values," and "predictive value of"). So she tried entering the search string "understanding why people keep smoking."

Google returned over 44 million "hits"! Reading down the first screen of results she thought, "Well, OK, but there isn't much here I haven't heard a hundred times in my clinic." The "hits" were mostly to individual blogs and other materials expressing a range of views about smoking (from very positive to

very negative) broadly consistent with the views that Trish Butler or any other clinician working with smoking cessation will hear day in, day out in their clinics.

We will return to what Trish Butler made of this material later as a resource for training and research. But for the moment, it gave her little in the way of new information on what made Sandy Fraser's behavior so inexplicable: he was neither an ardent pro-smoker (as evidenced by his willingness to continue attending the clinic) nor strongly motivated to change, despite serious smoking-related health issues.

Google Scholar

One of Trish's academic mentors, a social scientist, had encouraged her to use Google Scholar rather than getting caught up in more complex searches. Going to http://scholar.google.co.uk, she tried a search on "understanding why people keep smoking" and one on "qualitative, smoking, persistent, reasons, values." Both threw up a number of papers, and looking down the list, she spotted a couple that looked useful. She looked at the journals they were published in as a rough guide to quality. She was also looking for studies where the research population was similar to those with which she was having difficulty, and where the cultural context was similar, picking out UK-based studies with older people. One interesting article (about the "potential of teachable moments" in smoking cessation) caught her eye. "I'll come back to that later," she thought.

She also noted that, corresponding with the range of personal views she had seen expressed in her first Google search, there had been a good deal of research on "positive mental aspects of smoking." "Perhaps," she reflected, "I've been so focused on the negatives I've lost track of these positives a bit. They're obviously relevant to motivation. They might be a topic for my research." As with her first Google search, however, the specifics mentioned (the belief that smoking helps people relax, reduce stress, feel more comfortable with other people, keep their weight down, etc.) were not news to her and they did not seem immediately illuminating to her more immediate problem of understanding Sandy Fraser.

Two papers by the same authors reporting qualitative studies of older people and smoking attracted Trish's attention. The two papers in question are shown as they appeared in her search in Fig. 6.1. "That's the sort of study I'd like to do," she thought,

3 Cultural context, older age and **smoking** in Scotland: **qualitative interviews with older smokers with arterial disease**
[HTML] from oxfordjournals.org
O Parry, C Thomson . . .– Health promotion international, 2002 – Oxford Univ Press . . .The paper draws upon a Scottish **qualitative** interview study to explore life course changes in **smoking**-related beliefs and behaviours, in current smokers between the ages of 65 and 84 years with arterial disease. . . .The **reasons** for **persistent smoking** are complex and it is . . .Cited by 14 – Related articles – All 6 versions

10 Dependent behaviours and beliefs: a **qualitative** study of older long-term smokers with arterial disease
O Parry, C Thomson . . .– Addiction, 2001 – Wiley Online Library
. . .of a larger **qualitative** study of Life Course Influences on Patterns of **Persistent Smoking**. . . .**Qualitative** semi-structured interviews explored how respondents described their relationship to **smoking**, using . . .smokers with arterial disease defined their relationship to **smoking** in either . . .
Cited by 12 – Related articles – Get This in Print at – BL Direct – All 4 versions

Fig. 6.1. Two of the first ten results from Trish Butler's Google Scholar search using "qualitative, smoking, persistent, reasons, values."

"and these are UK-based researchers so perhaps I could contact them at some point."

What Trish Butler learned from her quick Google search

There were a number of learning points for Trish Butler from her first quick search. First, it was going to be considerably more difficult than she had expected to retrieve values-relevant literature. The number of false positives was considerably greater than she had anticipated, far more than she could easily skim through, and this in turn meant that, even with more time at her disposal, it would be difficult to cover the field adequately.

On the other hand, there were upsides: for very little time investment, Trish had already found some useful ideas to follow up – the "teachable moments" paper, for example, and the reminders about positive values and, importantly for her clinical problem, of the links

between COPD and depression. Furthermore, the large number of returns was encouraging in that there clearly had been a great deal of relevant work in this area. This could be helpful, she realized, in planning both her PLT training session and her research dissertation (including, in relation to the latter, the two researchers working on smoking in older people whom she might be able to contact for advice and ideas).

Overall then, Trish Butler had not got the result she started out looking for, namely research-based information on values that might shed light on Sandy Fraser's motivations, but she had gained a number of broader insights into smoking values and related research that could help her with all three of her initial problems – not a bad result for an informal quick "search and skim" that took her in all about 20 minutes.

Values PUNs and DENs

Trish Butler's initial experience of exploring the Internet to find relevant material on the values dimension was thus positive enough to set her off on further explorations. She had found some pointers: some partial answers that had taken her further along the path. Now she wanted to go further and deeper in her exploration of the values knowledge base. Her research inclinations played a part in this, but just as many working clinicians decide to explore scientific evidence-bases, so the way is open for them to explore values-bases as well. The NHS provides access to research data free of charge (by means of Athens Internet passwords) in the hope that many clinicians will want to develop their knowledge and thereby improve their service to patients.

Subsequent exploration of a wider variety of sources of knowledge would give Trish a deeper understanding of the diversity of values – positive and negative – attached to smoking. This would support her both in managing the clinical problems presented by Sandy Fraser and other persistent smokers for the practice, and in training and feedback sessions with her colleagues. An additional personal gain would be the ideas she got that would help her complete the first outline of the proposal for a research project that she had to submit as part of her MSc in Health Sciences.

Taking her knowledge of values further, however, as we will see, turned out to be less straightforward than Trish had found when using the Internet to research other areas. Before following the next stage of her story, it will be worth looking briefly at why this should be so.

Searching for evidence on values versus science

One reason why searching for research on values is difficult is because scientific knowledge in areas like diagnosis and treatment is more easily aggregated by the nature of the studies contributing evidence: generalized knowledge is meta-analyzed, meta-synthesized and distilled into summaries and overviews. Favorite sites will correspondingly yield digests and distillates of immediate clinical value, and in daily practice, it is rarely necessary to read original papers to stay sufficiently up to date on clinical knowledge.

The knowledge base for values is different. Values are about people: each one of us is different, each situation is different and each research project on values has to take account of this "N of 1" context – even more so than in some other social sciences. Summarizing data through meta-analyses is thus considerably more problematic and, indeed, original papers contain much of the richness of the values that underpins the very need for values-based practice. This is one reason why this book about the *essentials* of values-based practice is built around the stories of individuals rather than focusing on general theory and research findings.

These difficulties are inherent in the nature of values, but there is a further reason for the difficulty in retrieving knowledge of values, which is to do with the way the research databases themselves are set up. Trish Butler, as we will see, runs straight into this difficulty when she goes beyond her initial Google searches. But, to anticipate a little, the essential problem here is that the databases themselves are insensitive to the search terms we would naturally use when searching for values. We will return to this point later and to early attempts to overcome the difficulty. But one obvious example is the very term "values" – as Trish found, the many meanings of this term means that using for example a scientific database like PubMed produces a large number of false positives along the lines of "the value of the hemoglobin"!

Accessing discipline-specific databases

Now having made an explicit decision to explore her questions further, Trish Butler returned to her search that evening when she had more time and with the benefit of the research handbook that had been among the supporting materials for her MSc. Signing up for an MSc also gave her electronic access to a number of discipline-specific databases via a university library. (As someone working in the NHS in the UK, she could have got access to a similar range of resources with an Athens code – see websites at the end of this chapter.)

PubMed

Looking through the wealth of databases available, she decided to start with the most obvious discipline for work on smoking and disease, medicine. PubMed, her handbook told her, was the industry standard for medical research and she accordingly tried her two search strings. The result was not encouraging: zero returns for "qualitative, smoking, persistent, reasons, values," and when she tried "understanding why people keep smoking," the program asked her if she was looking for "gene information"!

"Oh well," she thought, "perhaps I'm doing it wrong." Rather than getting stuck, she decided to switch to the most obvious discipline for the other side of her search, values, and look in the social sciences.

Social science databases

Here, there was no obvious front-runner database. Indeed, Scopus (a bibliographic database containing abstracts and citations for scholarly journal articles), although one of the best (so her handbook told her), was considered too expensive by her university and like many others they did not have a subscription. Instead, they recommended the Web of Science database (an online academic citation index) – but this too proved unhelpful, with her two word strings between them producing only two returns, neither of which looked interesting.

Returning to her friendly Google, she searched for social science databases and found the initially promising Social Science Research Network, or SSRN. But once more she had no luck. Searching on "understanding why people keep smoking" produced just one return – but it was about economic theory. When she tried "qualitative, smoking, persistent, reasons, values," she did get a large number of returns (12,883), but, scanning the first page, they were again all about economics with titles like *Value Maximization, Stakeholder Theory, and the Corporate Objective Function* and *Performance of Private Equity Funds.* "Not really my cup of tea!" she thought, wryly.

PsycINFO

Finally, with counseling in mind, she turned to the psychological sciences. For this, her handbook recommended PsycINFO (an abstract database providing systematic coverage of the psychological literature from the 1800s to the present day), noting that the "Scholars Tab" function was useful for finding not only published literature but also researchers working in particular fields.

Here she struck if not gold at least silver. Both word strings produced sizeable but manageable returns (between 200 and 250). So she went on to scan the first 50 of each: "understanding why people keep smoking" produced little of direct interest, but "qualitative, smoking, persistent, reasons, values" looked more promising. There were still many false positives, but the majority of papers were about smoking, and of these, one was explicitly about values (cultural values), while a further eight were implicitly so (i.e. including terms such as quality of life (QoL), perceptions, attitudes, concerns, reasons and desires). The majority of the returns reflected work that was broadly in the same areas as her earlier Google search had signaled, but there were three that added a distinctly new angle to her thinking.

> **Reflection point**
>
> Fig. 6.2 reproduces the three returns that caught Trish Butler's eye in particular from the first 50 returns of her PsycINFO search.
>
> Why do you think she found these particular returns of interest?

The key word linking these three returns is depression, something that had been connected with COPD in her early Google Scholar searches. The recent emphasis on looking for comorbidity in general practice, underlined by changes in the NHS Quality Outcome Framework (QOF), meant that Trish was well aware of depression in chronic disease. But, somewhat uncomfortably, she reflected that she could not actually recall doing a depression scoring with Sandy Fraser. Maybe depression could explain his reluctance to "open up"?

Added value from Trish Butler's further search

In order to get more "in-depth" material on values than she had found on Google Scholar, Trish had had to adopt a flexible approach. Follow-up would also be important. The Internet had been helpful in a general way in showing her the extent and richness of established research from which she might learn – and

4. Name: Bonnie Spring

Affiliation: Professor, Behavioral Medicine, Northwestern University, 2005 – Current

From Publication Abstracts: Despite the strong co-occurrence between lifetime prevalence of depression and *smoking*, a history of major depressive disorder (MDD history) does not reliably predict *smoking* cessation outcomes . . . history smokers most at risk for *smoking* relapse. Anhedonia, in particular, is a core feature

25. Name: Jane Wardle

Affiliation: Professor/Director, Epidemiology and Public Health, University College London

From Publication Abstracts: their intentions to have the HPV vaccine and *reasons* for this decision. Most intended to have the vaccine . . . of *smoking*, alcohol consumption and physical activity was compared in cancer survivors and those . . . with better QoL and lower depressive symptoms, and *smoking* with poorer QoL and higher depressive

36. Name: Wayne J. Katon

Affiliation: Adjunct Professor, Department of Health Services, University of Washington

From Publication Abstracts: depression with the Patient Health Questionnaire-9. We controlled for baseline demographics, *smoking* . . . with a higher risk of obesity, sedentary lifestyle, *smoking*, and poor adherence to medical regimens

Fig. 6.2. Returns of interest to Trish Butler from her search in the PsycINFO Scholars Tab using "qualitative, smoking, persistent, reasons, values" (edited).

she would talk with her supervisor about contacting one or more of the researchers she had come across.

Furthermore, the reminder about depression that she had now had from PsycINFO prompted a number of specific ideas for follow-up with each of her three problems.

The clinical problem

She would explore the possibility that Sandy Fraser might be depressed or at any rate suffering depressive thoughts that were blocking his motivation: helplessness, guilt and indifference were among the obvious possibilities.

The training problem

Trish Butler's problem here was what to do for the PLT session that would ameliorate rather than aggravate the growing disagreements within the practice about how to manage patients like Sandy Fraser. Again, it would be counterproductive to tackle this directly: she was well aware of the dangers of foisting one's enthusiasms (for motivational approaches) on others; and merely challenging her colleagues would push everyone into even more polarized and defensive positions.

Whilst her computer was on and whilst her brain was in search mode, Trish had a quick look on Google Scholar for references that might help her with the values-based training problem. She found three quite quickly. The first was a nursing journal columnist (Castledine, 2004) writing about how nurses can deal with doctors they find difficult. The other two were both entitled "How doctors learn," one of them being an old Royal College of General Practitioners Occasional Paper from 1990, and the other being Hank Slotnick's aforementioned paper (Slotnick, 1999).

The key to doctor learning was not that different to nurse learning, or for that matter anyone else's learning, Trish realized. It depended on there being a problem that the learner wants to address. She realized straight away that depression and its links to COPD could be a common starting point, a place of shared values from which they could move forward together, if not to wider agreement, then at least to better mutual understanding. Everyone in the practice, Tom Peters included, recognized the need for a patient-centered approach in managing mental health problems. So, as Tom had offered to help with the PLT session, she would ask him to have a look at the latest literature on depression and other common psychiatric comorbidities for COPD with a view to presenting this in the session. This might trigger in Tom Peters' mind a different and more supportive way of understanding patients like Sandy Fraser; and presenting this literature in the PLT session would lead naturally to a discussion of the need to find a common approach to managing this aspect of smoking cessation. The wider problem of "challenging versus supportive" approaches would remain. But at least the session would strengthen their ability as a practice to work together in a well-coordinated way.

The research problem

Trish's interest had been well and truly caught by the challenge of masked depression in older people with COPD. She had as yet no very clear idea about what she would do for her research. But she recognized that depression and other affective disorders profoundly affected people's values and hence motivation; and she was drawn to the idea of doing something qualitative as a way of exploring individual narratives. She could perhaps compare the health beliefs and values of people with COPD with and without depressive thinking and look at how this affected their engagement with motivational approaches to smoking cessation. "Yes," she thought with growing enthusiasm, "this looks interesting ..."

Encouraged by this flood of new ideas, she put out a call to her supervisor. Her supervisor was encouraging, saying that the broad area sounded just right for a dissertation – "and great that it will tie in so closely with your day job."

"You'll need to narrow it down quite a lot in due course" she added. "... but a more careful look at the literature is the next step." And she put Trish on to two more specialized sources, the Healthtalkonline (formerly DIPEx) program at Oxford University, which collects narrative evidence of patients' experiences in different areas of healthcare, and the website for values-based practice at Warwick Medical School (i.e. the website supporting this series).

Emerging resources for knowledge of health-related values

We do not have space here to follow through in detail with Trish Butler as she moved to the next step in developing her research. The two specialized sites she accessed are available either directly or via the website supporting this series (web addresses are given at the end of the chapter).

Both sites extended her knowledge of values and smoking, although neither proved to be a panacea. Indeed, perhaps the most important overall learning point for Trish Butler from her experience of searching for values-related literature was that, as with values themselves, diversity is the key. There is no gold standard in searching for values. The "gold standard," such as it is, is to use a diversity of methods in a flexible and creative way within the constraints (of time and access) of a given search.

Healthtalkonline

Although there was no database as yet on smoking cessation, Healthtalkonline had a large database of narrative materials on patients' experiences of illness ranging across a wide variety of conditions. Much of this was available in various formats on the website, indexed by conditions but searchable by perspectives that readily exposed values dimensions in patients' thinking. What came across was the huge variety of world views, affecting the way in which patients tackle their illness and make their choices. Taking the time to read more of these would surely be rewarded by some reflections from people who had some traits in common with Sandy Fraser, she thought.

As to her research, an initial call to the friendly Healthtalkonline contact number confirmed that, although there was no database as yet on smoking cessation, they had just such a study underway. Thus, she realized that staying in touch could be very valuable for her research, and the Healthtalkonline team was interested in her ideas for looking at clinicians' experiences, as well as those of patients.

The values-based practice website

The values-based practice website supporting this series proved helpful to Trish Butler at a number of levels. First, despite her interest in motivational interviewing, she had been unaware of the wide range of disciplines now offering tools of different kinds for working with values: these are the tools in what we called in Part 1 of this book the clinical values toolbox. She was encouraged that there was a growing interest in this aspect of healthcare, not least among those working in evidence-based medicine.

When it came to her research, the values-based practice website gave examples of a range of research methods that had been used successfully in exploring values. Again, she found the variety fascinating: besides the familiar quantitative and qualitative empirical protocols, she found examples of philosophical methods, including both analytical (for example Sadler, 2005, on values in diagnosis) and phenomenological studies (for example Stanghellini, 2004, on schizophrenia; also, and importantly, Carel, 2008, and Toombs, 1993, both of whom used phenomenological methods to explore their own experiences of lymphangioleiomyomatosis and multiple sclerosis, respectively). Colombo *et al.*'s study (2003) of multidisciplinary teams using a combined empirical–philosophical approach looked particularly relevant to her research interests. (Details of these are given on the series website and we return to Colombo's study in Chapter 9.)

Reviewing the range and variety of studies was helpful to Trish Butler in providing context for her research. But it was clear from the examples given that most were beyond the scope of what she could achieve with the time and resources (including specialized research skills and supervision) available to her for her dissertation project. Again therefore, she wisely decided to stick with her plan for a qualitative/narrative study of some kind.

VaST: a search tool for everyone interested in values

Moving on from these examples of research, she found her way to the values search manual that her supervisor had mentioned. Called VaST (Values Search Tool), the manual set out clearly many of the difficulties and limitations she had already encountered in her search for values-related literature. Helpfully, though, it also included a brief search method for those who, like her, needed to get a reasonable idea of the research available without aiming for anything approaching a comprehensive review of the literature.

At the heart of this brief VaST search was a string of search terms called a "values filter," shown in Fig. 6.3. This had been derived from a much longer list as providing the best hit rate (technically, precision and sensitivity, see website) for relevant values literature (Petrova *et al.*, 2011). (The search string can be downloaded from the series website.)

The manual emphasized that the VaST string had been validated only for a handful of conditions that did not include COPD, and the brief values filter had been validated only for PubMed. Nonetheless, Trish spent a few minutes following the instructions in the manual and ran her own brief values search for COPD in PubMed. We have summarized the results of Trish Butler's search in Fig. 6.4.

> **Reflection point**
>
> Running a VaST search in PubMed clearly produced a very different result from Trish Butler's earlier nil return. But had this helped her? And if so, how had it helped?
>
> We look in a moment at what Trish Butler learned from her further search of PubMed. But what do *you* think?
>
> Look at the search terms (Fig. 6.3) as well as at the returns she got (Fig. 6.4).

1. attitude* [tw]
2. perceptions [tw]
3. qualitative [tw]
4. coping [tw]
5. counseling [tw]
6. cultural [tw]
7. ethics [tw]
8. experiences [tw]
9. interviews [tw]
10. perceived [tw]
11. personal [tw]
12. professionals [tw]
13. QOL [tw] OR Quality of Life [mh]
14. relations [tw]
15. respondents [tw]
16. satisfaction [tw]
17. staff [tw]
18. well-being [tw]
19. Adaptation, Psychological [mh]
20. Nurse's Role [mh]
21. Social Support [mh]
22. OR/1–21

Fig. 6.3. A brief values filter for PubMed from the VaST manual. Note: [mh] indicates "Medical Subject Headings" (i.e. search terms listed in PubMed) and [tw] indicates "Text Words" (i.e. free text words). (From Petrova et al., 2011.)

Learning points from the search terms

Trish Butler learned a good deal just from the terms that made up the VaST brief values filter. In the first place, she was surprised that, as we noted earlier, many of these validated terms were far from being intuitive: "ethics, "quality of life," "satisfaction" and "well-being" certainly made intuitive sense as being about values. But what about, say, "coping"? Certainly, she could see the connection with values when she thought about it: coping is a concept with connections to recovery, for example. But she would *not* have thought about it, she now realized, unprompted. Indeed, there was only one word on the list ("qualitative") that she had included in her two original intuitive word search strings ("understanding why people keep smoking" and "qualitative, smoking, persistent, reasons, values"). No wonder her original PubMed search had been unproductive.

The largely non-intuitive nature of the brief search filter showed Trish Butler the limitations of relying only on intuition in searching for values. Intuitive searching could certainly be helpful in its own right, particularly when doing a quick search in real time for clinical purposes. But intuition alone was clearly not enough for training and research purposes. In relation to her own research, she was encouraged to see "Nurse's Role" as a term on the VaST list that was effective in retrieving research on health-related values (clearly this was an area where her profession was

"research active"); and no less than three terms that tied in with the research project that was now coming together in her mind: "counseling," "experiences" and "interviews." This was important as her supervisor had pointed out: it suggested she would find like-minded colleagues with whom to share and develop ideas; and when it came to dissemination, she should be able to find both conference and journal outlets for her work.

Learning points from what Trish Butler found

As to the return itself, the main result from this was to consolidate what she had learned already from her more intuitive searches:

* Clinically, there were papers about patients' and families' understanding and experiences (e.g. paper 1 on patients' and families' experiences of COPD and paper 19 on the language of breathlessness).
* For her training session, the link with depression came up again, and now with additional references on other comorbidities such as panic attacks, which she could pass on to Tom. There was also paper 5 on a new Helplessness Index and patient self-management.
* For her research project, there were helpful pointers to possible methodologies for her own research: one of these (paper 46, by Kessler et al., 2006) used an "observational, interview-based" methodology for exploring patients' experiences (in this case of exacerbations), which looked right up her street.

Using the brief search filter had been a little more complicated than any of her intuitive searches, but it had still taken only a few minutes (including downloading the filter for future use), and this had produced a shorter and better focused selection of the literature. This meant that she could effectively scan the complete list of 47 references in a few minutes rather than having to wade through much longer lists. True, there were still many false positives but now at a lower rate than in her earlier searches: all the papers were about respiratory diseases, and all but two were about COPD; and of these, 14 out of 45 were either directly (e.g. paper 1 on perspectives, and paper 41 on quality of life) or indirectly (e.g. paper 5 on self-management and paper 36 on person-centered care) about values. The rate of true positives was thus about 30%, and as the VaST filter used validated search terms, she could be reasonably confident that the return was representative of the literature she might access in a wider and more comprehensive search.

1. Living and dying with severe chronic obstructive pulmonary disease: multi-perspective longitudinal qualitative study.

4. The impact of disability on depression among individuals with COPD.

5. The COPD Helplessness Index: a new tool to measure factors affecting patient self-management.

8. Depression and health-related quality of life in chronic obstructive pulmonary disease.

10. Cognitive decline among patients with chronic obstructive pulmonary disease.

11. Comorbidities, patient knowledge, and disease management in a national sample of patients with COPD.

16. COPD as a systemic disease: impact on physical functional limitations.

19. The language of breathlessness differentiates between patients with COPD and age-matched adults.

20. Panic attacks and perception of inspiratory resistive loads in chronic obstructive pulmonary disease.

23. Impact of cough across different chronic respiratory diseases: comparison of two cough-specific health-related quality of life questionnaires.

31. Sex differences in the prevalence of psychiatric disorders and psychological distress in patients with COPD.

36. Impact of COPD exacerbations on patient-centered outcomes.

37. Summaries for patients. Combination inhaler therapy for chronic obstructive pulmonary disease.

39. Summaries for patients. Interval versus continuous high-intensity exercise for patients with chronic obstructive pulmonary disease.

41. Does quality of life of COPD patients as measured by the generic EuroQol five-dimension questionnaire differentiate between COPD severity stages?

44. Effect of rollator use on health-related quality of life in individuals with COPD.

45. Nurse-conducted smoking cessation in patients with COPD using nicotine sublingual tablets and behavioral support.

46. Patient understanding, detection, and experience of COPD exacerbations: an observational, interview-based study.

Fig. 6.4. Sample results from Trish Butler's VaST search for health-related values and COPD (titles only, total return 47).

Learning points from what Trish Butler did *not* find

> **Reflection point**
>
> Taken together, Trish Butler had learned a good deal from what she had found in literature searches. But what did she learn from what she did *not* find, i.e. from what was noticeable by its absence?
>
> Think about this question for a moment, particularly with the values aspects of smoking cessation in mind.

In her initial review of the returns from her literature searches, Trish Butler had focused, as most of us would have, on what was there rather than on what was not there. But reflecting on all of her searches later, she realized that what was *missing from the returns* was, from the point of view of values, at least as interesting as what was included. In particular:

- First, there was nothing about patients' experiences *of smoking-cessation interventions*. There were papers aplenty on different kinds of intervention and their effectiveness (including a nurse-led program). But surprisingly, given the acknowledged importance of motivation in smoking cessation, there was nothing about how different interventions came across from patients' perspectives. The study underway by Healthtalkonline in Oxford aimed to fill this gap, but it was a surprising gap all the same, given the widespread adoption of motivational interviewing in this area.

- A second absence was anything on *clinicians' experiences* of smoking-cessation interventions. This, although perhaps more understandable, was clearly relevant to her second problem (the growing disagreements within the practice about how to manage resistant patients like Sandy Fraser). Moreover, her experience of motivational interviewing had taught her the importance of understanding motivation as arising from relationships *between* people rather than from within an individual. Again, this was a surprising gap, and Healthtalkonline were interested in her ideas for looking at this in her research.

- Thirdly, there was nothing about *the positives*. Recall here that Trish Butler, despite her generally positive approach to life, had realized from her first Google search that she had slipped into the clinician's negative bias (see Chapter 4 where we illustrated just such an unintended negative bias by some members of the mental health team – it was the support worker who was able to start work on the StAR qualities of strengths, resiliencies, and aspirations of Fig. 4.3). This bias towards looking at the negatives while neglecting the positives was evident again in the literature returned by VaST from PubMed.

There could well be studies out there that she had not yet identified. But the fact that the VaST values search filter used validated search terms suggested that such studies were not finding their way, in any numbers at least, into PubMed. Clearly, there was all to play for in clinically relevant research on values in this area.

Sandy Fraser and stage 4 of Slotnick's learning cycle

Although not the focus of this chapter, you will recall that the fourth element of Hank Slotnick's learning cycle was crucial to how new learning becomes embedded. So how did things go for Trish Butler from here?

The PLT session was a success: Tom Peters came away from his reading of the depression and COPD literature with a more reflective approach to the challenges of smoking cessation; and as Trish Butler had anticipated, the shared focus within the session on identifying comorbid conditions side-stepped a polarized debate about the rights and wrongs of smoking and persistent smokers. As for her dissertation proposal, her tutor was pleased with her first draft. She encouraged Trish to slim her plans down still further but also complimented her on the way she had followed through on her initial leads – the mark of a natural researcher, she had said.

An *n* of 1

Sandy Fraser, however, remained an enigma. They found no evidence of depression. Trish Butler had been planning to ask him if he would take part in her research, but while she was waiting to hear from the Research Ethics Committee, he suddenly stopped coming to her clinic. She thought at first that he had just given up, but then she heard from the District Nursing Service that Ivy had died suddenly and that Sandy had moved away. Three months later, Trish Butler had a letter from Sandy Fraser thanking her for all her support and wanting to let her know that he had not had a cigarette since Ivy died. Why, he didn't say, and they never found out.

Sandy Fraser, the puzzle of whose persistent smoking had brought Trish Butler to the stuck point from which all her new learning was to flow, thus taught her what is perhaps the most important lesson of all about research on values: however much we may learn from research about the values likely to be in play in a given situation, each of us as a unique individual remains in the language of research an *n* of 1.

Chapter summary

This chapter has shown that, like most things values-related, retrieval of relevant literature from electronic databases is a lot trickier than we might imagine. There are a number of relatively simple innovations in the categorizing of research that would help here. But we hope that Trish Butler's experience has indicated that, even in the current relatively undeveloped state of the field, with a little flexibility and follow-up there is a good deal that we can learn about values from the Internet. We might summarize what Trish Butler learned as prompts and points to pursue:

- *Prompts* – reminders of things she knew but had for the moment overlooked (a key reminder was about the link between depression and other comorbidities and COPD).

Type of search	Advantages	Disadvantages
Google Scholar	Time – immediate: ideal for quick clinical query Can be done without learning specific search methods or obtaining passwords Easy to follow links to free online source documents Very easy to re-word and research May include "lay" perspectives neglected by researchers	May be hard to convince research colleagues or librarians that it is a legitimate method or to use it in formal research (although many academics do use it)
Established databases	Once learned, gives useful skills in formal searches Can save searches More "acceptable" methodology for formal research	Time to learn methods is significant Time to actually run a search is greater Access to sites requires passwords Harder to find open access versions of source documents from search results
VaST search	Improves on intuitive database searches by using validated values-related search terms, which may increase results (higher proportion of true positives) A short search word filter (Fig. 6.3) can be downloaded and "saved" for repeat use in PubMed Makes using databases easier in this context As per databases, may be more acceptable for formal research	Requires the same database access and learning of methods as formal database searches Need to download and install the VaST filter from the series website Only validated for PubMed

Fig. 6.5. Advantages and disadvantages of three main ways of searching for values.

- *Points to pursue* – ideas to build on from published research (a key idea for Trish Butler to pursue in her research was to look at clinicians' as well as patients' experiences of smoking cessation; and she had found a useful paradigm for her study).

We draw together the advantages and disadvantages of the various search methods used by Trish Butler in Fig. 6.5. There are two key messages from this figure. The first is about getting the knowledge. The message is that, when it comes to values, there is no one method of searching that is suited to all topics and all contexts: there is, as we said, no "gold standard." What is needed, rather, is a flexible approach, like that adopted by Trish Butler, in which different searches are "test driven" and leads followed up.

The second key message from Fig. 6.5 is about *not* getting the knowledge. This message is that none of these methods, separately or together, can tell us about the values in play between *particular individuals* in

particular situations. The generalized evidence from research on values is helpful, as Trish Butler found, in suggesting the *kind of values* likely to be in play (hence the importance of the prompts and points to pursue summarized above). But each individual is always, as we put it, an *n* of 1. Thus it was that in this story the *n* of 1, Sandy Fraser, the patient who brought Trish Butler to her initial stuck point, lived and died a smoking enigma.

References

Butler, C. C., Pill, R. and Stott, N. C. H. (1998). Qualitative study of patients' perceptions of doctors' advice to quit smoking. Implications for opportunistic health promotion. *British Medical Journal* **316**, 1878–81.

Carel, H. (2008). *Illness*. UK: Acumen Publishing.

Castledine, G. (2004). Nurses must learn methods to deal with difficult doctors. *British Journal of Nursing* **13**, 479.

Colombo, A., Bendelow, G., Fulford, K. W. M. and Williams, S. (2003). Evaluating the influence of implicit models of mental disorder on processes of shared decision making within community-based multidisciplinary teams. *Social Science & Medicine* **56**, 1557–70.

Edwards, R. (2004). ABC of smoking cessation. The problem of tobacco smoking. *British Medical Journal* **328**, 217–19.

Eve. R (2003). *PUNs and DENs: Discovering Learning Needs in General Practice*. Oxford: Radcliffe Publications.

Kessler, R., Ståhl, E., Vogelmeier, C. *et al.* (2006). Patient understanding, detection, and experience of COPD exacerbations: an observational, interview-based study. *Chest* **130**, 133–42.

Maudsley, G. and Strivens, J. (2000). Promoting professional knowledge, experiential learning, and critical thinking for medical students. *Medical Education* **34**, 535–44.

Miller, W. R. and Rollnick, S. (2002). *Motivational Interviewing: Preparing People for Change*. New York/London: Guildford Press.

Monden, C. W., de Graaf, N. D. and Kraaykamp, G. (2003). How important are parents and partners for smoking cessation in adulthood? An event history analysis. *Preventative Medicine* **36**, 197–203.

Petrova, M., Sutcliffe, P., Fulford, K. W. M. and Dale, J. (2011). Search terms and a validated brief search filter to retrieve publications on health-related values in MEDLINE: a word frequency analysis study. *Journal of the American Medical Informatics Association* [16 August; Epub ahead of print].

Polanyi, M. (1967). *The Tacit Dimension*. London: Routledge and K. Paul.

Richards, H. (2003). Victim-blaming revisited: a qualitative study of beliefs about illness causation, and responses to chest pain. *Family Practice* **20**, 711–16.

Ritchie, D., Amos, A. and Martin, C. (2010). Public places after smoke-free – a qualitative exploration of smoking behavior. *Health and Place* **16**, 461–9.

Royal College of General Practitioners (1990). *How Doctors Learn*. Occasional Paper No. 44. London: Royal College of General Practitioners.

Sadler, J. Z. (2005). *Values and Psychiatric Diagnosis*. Oxford: Oxford University Press.

Slotnick, H. (1999). How doctors learn: physicians' self-directed learning episodes. *Academic Medicine* **74**, 1106–17.

Stanghellini, G. (2004). *Deanimated Bodies and Disembodied Spirits. Essays on the Psychopathology of Common Sense*. Oxford: Oxford University Press.

Thornton, T. (2006). Tacit Knowledge as the unifying factor in EBM and clinical judgement. *Philosophy, Ethics, and Humanities of Medicine*, 1:2doi:10.1186/1747-5341-1-2 at http://www.peh-med.com/content/1/1/2.

Toombs, S. Kay. (1993). *The Meaning of Illness: a Phenomenological Account of the Different Perspectives of Physician and Patient*. Dordrecht, The Netherlands: Kluwer Academic Publishers.

Websites

- http://www.library.nhs.uk offers access to databases (including PubMed and PsycINFO), librarian support and, in the case of clinicians in England, a query answering service, which can find information to answer clinical queries. NHS workers can get an NHS Athens password giving them access to most health-related journals. Those in Scotland get valuable library resources through the website http://www.knowledge.scot.nhs.uk/home.aspx.
- The resources of the Oxford DIPEx program can be accessed through http://www.healthtalkonline.org.
- VaST, the search manual for values, can be found on the website supporting this series.

CHAPTER 7 begins on following page

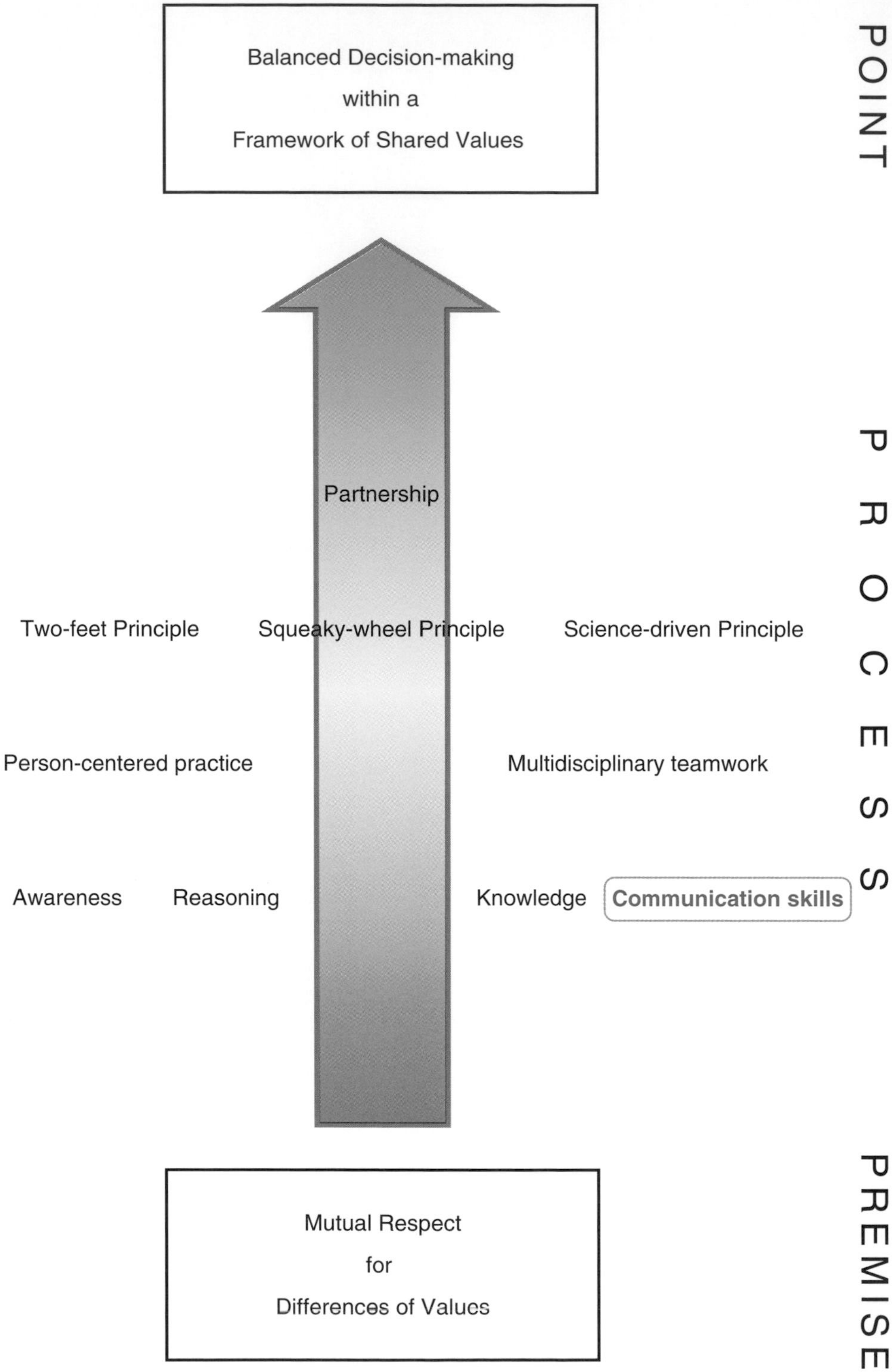

POINT

Balanced Decision-making
within a
Framework of Shared Values

PROCESS

Partnership

Two-feet Principle   Squeaky-wheel Principle   Science-driven Principle

Person-centered practice   Multidisciplinary teamwork

Awareness   Reasoning   Knowledge   **Communication skills**

PREMISE

Mutual Respect
for
Differences of Values

Map of values-based practice – communicatin skills.

Chapter

7

Diabetic control and controllers: nothing without communication
Values-based practice element 4: communication skills

Topics covered in this chapter

The rich two-way interplay between traditional communication skills and values-based practice is illustrated by the way a GP, Dr. Mellon, manages a challenging problem of diabetes control presented by one of his teenage patients, Vicky Bartlett, and her mother.
    Other topics include:

- ICE and ICE StAR
- Eliciting values
- Clinical leadership and conflict resolution
- Management theory and clinical leadership
- Self-management and diabetes
- Adolescent health and parental involvement
- Team work.

Take-away message for practice

*Values-based practice can enhance our communication skills in particular by **adding strengths** to the traditional focus on needs and difficulties.*

At the most elementary level in communication skills training, students are taught to elicit ideas, concerns and expectations. Suggested originally by David Pendleton *et al.* (1984) and developed further by Roger Neighbour (1987) and others, the familiar acronym is ICE. We will use the acronym throughout this chapter but we do so respectfully, aware that all too often citing "ICE" has become some sort of substitute for really engaging with the ideas, concerns and expectations that are really about values. Indeed, linking ICE explicitly with values, as we will see in this chapter, is an important counterbalance to the tendency to "tick-box" reduction. This in turn is an aspect of the rich two-way relationship that, as we outlined in

Chapter 2, exists between communication skills and values-based practice:

- Communication skills support values-based practice particularly with (i) skills for *eliciting values* (of self and others) and (ii) skills of *conflict resolution*.
- Values-based practice in turn supports communication skills by helping us to go behind the mantra and to really explore the values attached (by ourselves as well as our patients) to a condition, to the patient's lifestyle and to their significant relationships.

Values-based practice, as we saw in Chapter 3, emphasizes the importance of exploring, in particular, strengths, aspirations and resources (StAR values) as well as (negative) needs and difficulties. Values-based practice plus communication skills thus takes us from ICE to ICE StAR.

From ICE to ICE StAR

In this chapter, we explore the two-way relationship between communication skills and values-based practice through a story of diabetes control involving 16-year-old Vicky Bartlett, her mother and their long-standing GP, Dr. Stuart Mellon. Working with others in the practice and in the hospital clinic, Dr. Mellon exhibits well-developed communication skills in coming to an understanding of the ideas, concerns and expectations at play in the situation (his own as well as those of Vicky and her mother) and in the clinical leadership he shows in resolving the developing conflicts between Vicky Bartlett, her mother and the many others concerned with and for her.
    Key to Dr. Mellon's success in all this, as we will see, is a balanced values-based approach: in tacitly recognizing the many positive values in play behind the ideas, concerns and expectations of those involved, as well as the more obvious negatives, he

felt he had let down; his fear that he will not be able to live up to Vicky and her mum's expectations of him; and Dr. Patel's QOF point reminder), and he fully expects (from what Trish and Achila have told him) that this is going to be a tricky interview in an area (diabetes management) that, even at the best of times, he finds difficult.

Small wonder then that, although Dr. Mellon is courteous and welcoming, he is a little heavy-handed at first with Mrs. Bartlett, Vicky's mum, and then with Vicky herself. Clearly, he needs to talk to Vicky on her own and his intention is that he will then be giving her mum a proper opportunity to talk about how she feels about what has happened, either with Vicky there or (depending on how things go and if Vicky agrees) on her own. But he gives Mrs. Bartlett no indication of this. She is effectively just dismissed. This is the opposite of what she had expected from a doctor who had, over the years, "been more like an uncle" and she is understandably taken aback and doesn't understand Dr. Mellon's attitude. However, she acquiesces, albeit feeling hurt and indeed offended.

Again, when Dr. Mellon has Vicky on his own, he reopens the consultation appropriately with an open question (these being more effective than closed questions for eliciting feelings and values) but qualifies it unhelpfully with a directly critical comment ("I didn't expect all this from you"). He is, as we have seen, disappointed. But the risk here is that Vicky will take his comment as an indication that he is just another adult with no real idea what it is like to be hag-ridden by diabetes and who is simply "siding" with everyone else lining up to tell her how to run her life.

Vicky responds

Vicky Bartlett, though, for all her bravado, is frightened by what has happened. She wants help, and the support and care that Dr. Mellon has given her and her mum over the years is still there as a basis on which to build. So with her mum now out of the room, she is ready to talk and she does so freely, expressing many of the concerns that so many young people in her situation feel (Bryden *et al.*, 2001; Dickinson and O'Reilly, 2004). Here are some of the things that, with an occasional nod of encouragement and brief clarification from a carefully attentive Dr. Mellon, she said:

- "I just feel that I've had enough of diabetes ruling my life. I can't get away from it, or from you lot. I can't forget it just for one day."

- "I just want to be normal, for a change. I'm sick of people treating me differently. How do you think it feels that everyone saw me dragged off in an ambulance after a night out?"
- "I know you always harp on about problems later on in life, but that's not what bothers me at the moment."
- "I'm not going to have another hypo in public. It's so humiliating. I don't care if I run a bit high. Better that than ending up with a hypo. My friends thought I was bonkers when I didn't know where I was, and my boyfriend thought I was dying when I passed out. It's all too much."
- "Having the HbA1c you want me to would mean being half a stone heavier and being totally miserable through hypos and testing every two minutes. No thank you."

Eliciting skills

Before looking at how the consultation went from this point, it will be worth reflecting for a moment on how Dr. Mellon's skills of eliciting information compare with one of the lists in a book on communication skills by a GP and medical educator, Peter Tate, *The Doctor's Communication Handbook* (Tate, 1994). Published originally some time ago, Peter Tate's book, which has gone through many subsequent editions, remains an invaluable resource of down-to-earth detailed practical tips for improving communication skills in a number of key areas, one of which is eliciting information. We summarize Tate's checklist of eliciting skills and how Dr. Mellon performed against it in Fig. 7.1.

Peter Tate's checklist should, of course, not be read as encouraging a tick-box approach to communication skills. But using it here as a quick audit of Dr. Mellon's abilities shows just how many eliciting skills he has shown already in this brief exchange with Vicky Bartlett and her mother. The two exceptions (the two "No" answers in Fig. 7.1) both involve the implicitly critical comment that, as we noted earlier, slipped into Dr. Mellon's opening gambit with Vicky after her mum had left the room ("I didn't expect this of you . . .").

In the consultation then, as much as in giving feedback, Pendleton's golden rule "good things first" applies (Pendleton *et al.*, 1984). We come back to the significance of the two exceptions to Dr. Mellon's otherwise exemplary eliciting skills for how he manages the situation shortly.

Eliciting skill	Dr. Mellon
Speak the patient's language, do not talk down to them, and avoid jargon	Yes
Remember that, at the beginning, the patient is always right	No (his opening negative comment suggests Vicky Bartlett is wrong)
Let the patient go first	Yes
Make statements that make good questions, for example, "I was wondering whether . . .?"	Not applicable
Ask open questions; they are good for finding out about patients' beliefs, for example, "Would you tell me about . . .?"	No (his opening question was largely open, but his negative comment gave it a negative "steer" – see text)
Ask closed questions, which are good for obtaining facts	Not applicable
Give encouragement, such as, "Go on." Eye contact and nodding encourage patients to continue . . .	Yes
Check what they have said	Not applicable
Explain why you are asking a question	Not applicable
Use silence – allow pauses. The patient will invariably fill them if you wait long enough	Yes

Fig. 7.1. Checklist of Dr. Mellon's eliciting skills (based on Tate, 1994, pp. 67–68).

Vicky Bartlett's ICE

Small wonder then, given the skills Dr. Mellon has shown, and the secure therapeutic relationship that he had already established with Vicky Bartlett and her mum, that Vicky's ICE comes through loud and clear in the above extracts from what she said: she wants to be a normal young woman with normal friends in normal relationships and with a normal social life – and let the future go hang. Again, we will come back to what this implies in terms of practical agendas for management in a moment. First, we need to ask two questions: what is missing from what Vicky Bartlett has said, and why?

> **Reflection point**
>
> Think about these two questions as questions about values.
>
> In terms of communication skills, Dr. Mellon has very effectively ticked the "Vicky Bartlett ICE" box. But in terms of values, what information is he still lacking and why is he missing it?

In terms of values then, what is missing from what Vicky Bartlett has said is that Dr. Mellon knows the negatives but not the positives: he knows as he put it in his opening question "what's wrong" with Vicky Bartlett but nothing about "what's right."

Negative ICE

As to "why?" this is again, in terms of values, a matter of the negatives, although in this case the negative values not of Vicky Bartlett but of Dr. Mellon. To be clear, Dr. Mellon's positive values were essential to the effectiveness of the way he was able to use his well-developed communication skills in getting Vicky Bartlett to open up as she did where others (including her friends as well as other skilled professionals) had failed. His success here, as we have seen, built directly on the excellent therapeutic relationship that he had built up over the years with Vicky Bartlett and her mum, which in turn reflected the value he placed on providing long-term continuity of care. But his failure nonetheless to elicit "what's right" about Vicky Bartlett as well as "what's wrong" reflected his negative values, both background professional negative values and foreground personal negative values:

- *Background professional negative values.*
  Dr. Mellon is a health professional, and health professionals, as we noted in Chapter 3, have a natural tendency to focus on the negatives simply because our patients and clients come to us *as* professionals with *problems* of one kind or another with which they want help. This (natural) negative bias is reflected even in Peter Tate's book: there are many and detailed sections dealing with different

87

aspects of clarifying and managing patients' problems but nothing about clarifying and building on their strengths.

- *Foreground personal negative values.* Dr. Mellon's natural tendency as a health professional and as a doctor to focus on the negatives was further enhanced in this instance by the negative personal values that he brought to the consultation: his disappointment that his hitherto-successful patient had "let him down," his lack of confidence (in dealing both with diabetes and with adolescents), his performance anxiety (the expectations of success inadvertently loaded on him by Trish Gore as well as by Vicky Bartlett and her mother) and the pressures from his practice to "up" their diabetes data for QOF point prizes.

- All these factors are in the background to the negative loading he gives to his opening question to Vicky Bartlett ("I didn't expect all this from you – you've always done so well with your diabetes . . . What's the problem? What's wrong?"), and the same factors are reflected again in her correspondingly close focus on the negatives in what she says in reply.

Dr. Mellon was, of course, aware of Vicky Bartlett's potential strengths. The child Vicky Bartlett he knew in the back of his mind had indeed had a number of distinct strengths to her credit: she was intelligent and competent in her own right (he had found her at times as a child slightly formidable), she had the support of a caring and sensible mother (with whom he had always got on well) and she had exhibited a settled determination not to let her diabetes get in the way of her future. But in his present uneasy state of mind, Dr. Mellon's background memories of Vicky Bartlett served only to underscore his negative bias towards the apparently very different young woman in front of him now.

Again, it was important that Dr. Mellon was able to elicit all the information he did about Vicky Bartlett's take on the problem. This will be important for him when, as he will shortly have to do, he moves in the consultation from information-gathering to problem-solving. But while he now has a fair idea of what the problem is that has to be solved, he has no idea at all (at least from what he has just heard) what strengths and other assets Vicky Bartlett might bring to the task of problem-solving. Moving forward, therefore, from information-gathering to problem-solving on the basis only of negative information will mean that

Dr. Mellon is working in effect with one arm (his positive arm) tied behind his back.

From ICE to ICE StAR

In the next section, we will follow Dr. Mellon as the consultation develops, first with Vicky Bartlett and then when he sees her mother, Mrs. Bartlett. Again, Dr. Mellon's communication skills will be evident. The difference, however, is that, with Dr. Mellon's now growing confidence, a number of Vicky Bartlett's strengths become evident for the first time. Dr. Mellon thus moves in effect from ICE to ICE StAR. In the final section of the chapter, in which Dr. Mellon sees Vicky Bartlett and her mother together, Vicky Bartlett's strengths will prove important as the basis for a way forward that promises to defuse the growing conflict between her and her mum, and thus open up a path for both of them towards independence.

Eliciting ICE StAR

We are now about five minutes into the consultation (including the period when Mrs. Bartlett was also in the room), and although Dr. Mellon had allowed a double session for Vicky, he is aware that he needs to start moving the agenda on from problems to problem-solving. Vicky, having now found her voice, is showing no signs of running out of steam. So instead of trying to shift her focus directly, he picks up in an encouraging way on her stream of concerns and redirects it by saying, ". . . yes, there's obviously a lot going on for you at the moment, Vicky, and we'll get a chance to go through everything in more detail later on. Shall we start by thinking about that hypo?"

Vicky stops talking and looks towards him attentively but without either agreeing or disagreeing. Dr. Mellon takes this as a "yes" and sets the agenda with, "This is really difficult, Vicky. I've known you so long and I feel responsible for your diabetes; and I don't need to tell you how dangerous a hypo is . . . but then there's so much of it that's really only down to you."

Reflection point

Before reading it will be worth taking a moment or two to think about how Dr. Mellon has moved the consultation on at this point.

What agendas has he set? What communication skills has he shown in setting them? And how does all this relate to the values of those concerned?

The agendas

In this brief intervention, Dr. Mellon has set at least three key agendas:

1. *The hypo.* Dealing with the hypo is the explicit clinical agenda item number 1; but tied in here implicitly are also points 2 and 3.
2. *Who is involved?* Vicky's diabetes is a matter of legitimate concern to others besides Vicky: "It"s *my* life," if this means "It's my life and *no one else's*," is nearly always disingenuous but recognizing this is an achievement that many, not least in adolescence, find peculiarly hard.
3. *Responsibility.* Vicky has reached an age and maturity where the balance of responsibility for managing her diabetes is shifting fast from others (her mum and various professionals) towards herself.

The skills

Dr. Mellon's well-developed communication skills, shown in the extreme economy with which he has set these three important agendas, are now working on full power as he begins to settle into the consultation and gain confidence in his ability to manage the situation and find a way forward.

There is no inappropriate use of "exploring feelings" (powerful as this may be in the right setting). Instead, Dr. Mellon takes control. He does this of course not by domineering but by engaging with Vicky Bartlett's own agenda in an encouraging way. He makes it clear that everything she has said is important (all her adolescent angst): he does this partly by saying something positive about what she has been telling him (his ". . . a lot going on for you . . ." says that he has heard and understood) and partly by signaling that he will be coming back to all this (his ". . . we'll get a chance to go through everything in more detail later on . . ."); and only then does he set up the agendas for the rest of the consultation by suggesting they focus first on the hypo.

The precise wording he adopts here is important. Again, reflecting his well-developed communication skills, his choice of words is instinctive and is the more effective for that. Thus, he uses a *permissive* ("shall") and combines this with the first person *plural* ("we") in a *rhetorical* question ("Shall we start by thinking about that hypo?"), which neatly avoids the equal and opposite errors of either prescribing or leaving wholly up to Vicky the agendas on which

they will focus. These three aspects of Dr. Mellon's wording here thus work together to bring the two of them to the nub of the matter (the hypo, agenda 1) but working together (agenda 2), and with Vicky already having in effect taken a (manageable) degree of responsibility (agenda item 3).

The values

The values driving this stage of the consultation are very much in the foreground for each of the three agendas. First, Dr. Mellon's focus on Vicky Bartlett's hypo (agenda 1) neatly takes them to a point of intersection of the values of everyone concerned. There is much else over which Vicky Bartlett, Dr. Mellon, the other professionals concerned and Mrs. Bartlett will disagree. But all of them (picking up agenda 2) are worried about the hypo.

Vicky Bartlett, in particular, despite her professed "sufficient unto the day" attitude to long-term harms from poorly controlled diabetes, has, as we noted earlier, had a bad scare. Moreover, her scare was not just that she had had a hypo: she had had similar episodes before. Her scare was that this hypo was (addressing agenda 3) down to her. She had started to move from doing what others told her to relying on her own judgment and it had all gone (nearly disastrously) wrong.

Similar values play out again in what follows, as Dr. Mellon uses a moment of self-disclosure to head Vicky Bartlett towards ownership of her problems (agenda 3). Self-disclosure, as discussed originally by Balint (1957), is an advanced communication skill that used judiciously can help to avoid defensive patterns in the consultation (Salinsky and Sackin, 2000). It is used here by the skilled Dr. Mellon judiciously. Each element of what Dr. Mellon says is well judged:

- "This is really difficult, Vicky," as his opening phrase leaves the two of them neatly poised in ambiguity between his and her responsibilities for managing Vicky's diabetes. We might translate Dr. Mellon's "This is really difficult, Vicky, *for X*," where "X" stands for *everyone* involved, not just (as it is) Dr. Mellon and certainly not just Vicky Bartlett, the aggrieved teenager.
- Dr. Mellon has thus effectively located their relationship appropriately as being (as it should be in working with a mature 16-year-old; see Department for Constitutional Affairs, 2006,

Chapter 12) at the tipping point between paternal care and adult autonomy. He has also left Vicky Bartlett potentially open to recognizing that she is at a similar tipping point in her relationship with her mother.

- Vicky is thus able to hear what follows, "I've known you so long and I feel responsible for your diabetes," not as an abnegation of her doctor's care for her but as an affirmation of her potential for self-care. This is an important message, given the knock to her self-confidence that she has suffered from allowing herself to end up with a hypo, especially in front of her friends.
- Dr. Mellon's affirming message is then further reinforced with his "I don't need to tell you how dangerous a hypo is": and he doesn't, for he knows from her intelligent and competent approach as a child that Vicky Bartlett fully understands the danger in which she placed herself.
- Dr. Mellon has thus paved the way for handing her an appropriate degree of responsibility for managing her diabetes based on a realistic, affirming acknowledgment of her ability to take on that responsibility. Vicky Bartlett is thus ready to accept the responsibility finally made explicit in Dr. Mellon's concluding, "... but then there's so much of it that's really only down to you."

To anticipate a little, it is worth noting how important all this will be when they move from information-gathering to problem-solving and in particular to resolving the conflicts between Vicky Bartlett, her mum and others. Dr. Mellon is showing what we will describe later as effective clinical leadership. There is no attempt to bludgeon or manipulate Vicky Bartlett. Instead, there is a clear effort to negotiate and to find compromise, a strategy that is indeed explicitly supported by the guidelines from the National Institute for Health and Clinical Excellence (NICE, 2004).

First steps towards a plan for Vicky Bartlett

With the consultation now on a secure footing, the first steps towards Vicky Bartlett taking control of her diabetes follow readily enough. Dr. Mellon asks Vicky how much she knows about alcohol-induced hypos. As he suspects, she proves to be well aware that she should prime herself with carbohydrates and then "top up" before going to bed. But this is where Vicky's concern about her weight has got in the way.

"What about exercise?" Dr. Mellon asks. Vicky has been studying for her GCSE exams, she explains, and working mainly from home, and now she thinks about it, she has had relatively little exercise for some months. Dr. Mellon explains that regular exercise will help with blood sugar control and at the same time allow her to eat properly without gaining undue weight. Vicky likes this idea. She had been a good swimmer as a child and says she had been thinking of taking this up again, adding, "My boyfriend likes swimming."

This gives Dr. Mellon an opening to ask, "What about your mum?"

Vicky had forgotten about her mum for the last few minutes. She looks surprised and after a moment replies rather defensively, "What about her?"

"Well, mums don't always like boyfriends!" Dr. Mellon says.

"Oh, no," Vicky replies, now smiling, "She's fine about my friends . . ." (and then with her smile slipping, continues) ". . . it's just the diabetes – she's on about it all the time . . ."

But before Vicky can get back into her stride on the subject of her mum and diabetes, Dr. Mellon, relying now on their re-established relationship, chips in with, "Well she's worried about you, you know, any mum would be." And then he adds (with his fingers mentally crossed), "Why don't I have a chat with your mum on her own for a few minutes and then we can agree a plan together." And Vicky, who is at her wits end with her mum, readily agrees.

Mum's the word

In reply to Mrs. Bartlett's natural opening question about what they have been talking about, Dr. Mellon says, "I think we're getting somewhere but can I ask you a bit more about what's been happening to Vicky recently and then, if you agree," (he knows she will) "the three of us can put our heads together to work out a plan."

Notice again that, with Dr. Mellon now feeling increasingly on top of the situation, he gives a clear signal of acknowledging what is important to Mrs. Bartlett as Vicky's mum, that they are "getting somewhere" with her daughter's diabetic control, and that (with his ". . . can I ask you a bit more about what's been happening to Vicky recently?") she is being firmly included in, rather than excluded from, whatever is agreed. In what follows, he builds on this, as again he had done a couple of minutes earlier with

Vicky, by using a small dose of self-disclosure. But on this occasion he gets some unexpected results.

"I have to admit," Dr. Mellon continues, "to being very worried when I heard what happened to Vicky last weekend. I spent long enough working in A&E to hate seeing what binge drinking does to young people."

But at this mention of binge drinking, Mrs. Bartlett switches suddenly from critic to defender of her daughter. "But it's not that, Doctor, she's never been much of a drinker. That's why I can't understand what's happened. Things *have* got more difficult recently, but I put it down to her exams. She wants to be a forensic scientist you know, but she needs to get really good results and she's been studying too hard. I thought I was doing the right thing encouraging her to go out more, and then . . ." (now suddenly in tears) ". . . this happens, and she might have died if it hadn't been for her boyfriend realizing what was happening . . ."

> **Reflection point**
>
> Clearly, this gives a very different picture of the events of the weekend. But in terms of values, what new information does Dr. Mellon now have about Vicky? And how will this contribute to resolving the growing conflict between Vicky and her mum as a step towards helping them establish mutual independence?

Vicky Bartlett's ICE StAR

In the early stages of the consultation, it was mainly negative values that were in play, "negative ICE" as we called them. True, the positive values of Dr. Mellon's commitment to long-term relationships and continuity of care avoided the consultation foundering and allowed him to find out a good deal about, as he put it in his opening question to Vicky, "What's wrong?"

But what he has now learned from Vicky's mum is a great deal also about "what's right" with Vicky Bartlett. Recall here that Dr. Mellon was well aware of the child Vicky Bartlett's ICE StAR. Now, in this short response from her mother, the many aspects of the adolescent Vicky Bartlett's ICE StAR come through loud and clear:

- Her *strengths* – she works hard; far from being a binge-drinking teenage alcoholic, she errs on the side of "all work and no play"; and she has good social skills (having built up a good group of

friends and found a boyfriend in whom she had felt able to confide).
- Her *aspirations* – her plan to become a forensic scientist is both realistic (she is good at science, especially the "practicals") and well directed (at the time there was a shortage in this area).
- Her *resources* – her boyfriend, to name but one, who had proved to be well up to the mark when it came to dealing with an acute situation (he was in fact two years older than her and had a place at medical school).

It is worth noting here that, even on the issue of "what's wrong," Dr. Mellon had been misled, by the predominantly negative values he brought to the consultation, into assuming that Vicky Bartlett made a habit of binge drinking whereas in fact it was out of character – it seems an obvious question with hindsight, but he never thought to ask her whether this had happened before.

However, Vicky Bartlett's positive values will be even more significant when, towards the end of the interview, he gets her to join himself and her mother to agree a shared management plan. Building on what Dr. Mellon knew before (Vicky Bartlett's negative ICE, her problems), he had been able to take a number of important steps in partnership with her towards managing the risks presented by her alcohol-induced hypo. Now he has a much enriched ICE StAR on which to build a more secure and comprehensive plan to help Vicky move towards responsible adult self-management of her diabetes.

First steps towards a plan for Mrs. Bartlett

Before he can get to this, however, he has to engage Mrs. Bartlett in moving towards Vicky's independence. Here, he is acutely aware he has to be very careful. Vicky's mum is clearly blaming herself for what happened. It was, as she has just pointed out, she who had encouraged Vicky to go out when she had her hypo.

In this, ironically, she was taking her own first steps towards letting go: she was trying to support Vicky in, as she saw it, "having fun" as a normal teenager. She understood the risks: she knew well enough that adolescence was a danger time for diabetes control; and she was very much aware that her daughter had been "slipping" from the meticulous control she had maintained as a child. But she also knew the risks of a parent "hanging on too long": at some point, as she put it to herself, they have to cross the road on their own. Yet for all this, rationalize what had happened as she might, there was no escaping the fact that, deep down, she felt responsible – it was her fault; she had failed her daughter when her best endeavors to let go a little had ended up in near catastrophe.

So Dr. Mellon has to find a way of getting Mrs. Bartlett to take the heat off Vicky without making her feel even more fearful and demoralized and thus increasing rather than decreasing the level of conflict between them. Reassurances won't do: they will read as insincere to Mrs. Bartlett in her present state of mind and anyway she won't believe him. Nor will asking her about how she feels help. This is not a situation that calls for exploration of feelings, however helpful this may sometimes be: they both know how she feels, and "exploring feelings" will simply stir up emotions that he will not have time to work through.

Mrs. Bartlett's ICE StAR

What Dr. Mellon does is simple but effective. He switches the focus away from Vicky and onto her mother. He does this by first sharing a memory, reminding her how, even when Vicky was only five, she had wanted to do something medical, so he wasn't surprised at her choice of career. "But," he added, "what about you? Do you have any plans now?"

"Oh, me? Well, I was planning to get back into nursing ..." Mrs. Bartlett, it transpired, had been a nurse before she gave up work to look after Vicky and (as a further indication of her awareness of the need to let go) she had already started to explore retraining options.

"How does Vicky feel about that?" Dr. Mellon asks.

"Vicky's fine about it. She has been really encouraging to me, in fact ... but obviously I'll have to put all that on hold."

Dr. Mellon doesn't push her on this (he knows that she would be unable to take on a challenging retraining program until her daughter is living independently), but he asks her if she would be interested in helping one of the other practices in the group who is looking for volunteers, and is much encouraged when she says she will follow this up.

"Let's get Vicky back in then," Dr. Mellon says, "and put our heads together."

Getting it together

From this point, with Vicky Bartlett and her mother now both feeling listened to and understood, and

with Dr. Mellon armed with all his new positive information about Vicky, the consultation runs well. Dr. Mellon starts by inviting Vicky to talk about what they had discussed earlier, but she defers to him. So starting with, "OK, but tell me if I get anything wrong," he notes that Vicky is going to, (i) be more careful about carbohydrate intake before and after having a drink with her friends, (ii) eat better, but also (iii) look into going swimming regularly, perhaps with her boyfriend, and (iv) check her blood glucose more often (and she nods agreement when he adds ". . . and will that include keeping your diary up to date?").

This is all, of course, what he and Vicky had agreed earlier, but his confidence that she is likely to manage it all is much improved by his new picture of the ambitious and capable young woman that he now understands her to be. His confidence in Vicky combined with his understanding of her mother's strengths (notably her insight into and practical steps towards "letting go") further allow him to bring Mrs. Bartlett in with a direct, "How does that sound to you?"

"Fine," she says, "but I'm still worried what happens if Vicky has another hypo and her boyfriend isn't there?"

"What do you think, Vicky?" Dr. Mellon asks her. "How do you feel about talking to one or two of your friends about things in advance, so they know how to help you? Would you be able to do that?"

She answers that she would.

Bringing in the rest of the team

"Looking ahead," Dr. Mellon continues, "we need to think how best to help you manage things during your exams. It's bound to be a difficult time and I do feel a bit out of my depth when it comes to working out how to best juggle your insulin round your lifestyle. But there are people like Trish Gore at the hospital who you know, and Achila here, who we can work with. Trish would you be happy to see you in the adult clinic if you would like me to send her a letter?" This gets a nod of acceptance from Vicky and a silent "thank you" from her mum. "And Achila is starting a group for young people with diabetes if you would be interested in talking to her?"

This one gets only a "Let me think about that one."

Follow-up

Dr. Mellon concludes the consultation with a question about a follow-up appointment. "Shall we see how things are going in a couple of weeks?" he asks, deliberately directing his question at the room in general rather than at either mother or daughter in particular.

Somewhat to his surprise but also to his clinical gratification, Mrs. Bartlett instead of insisting that she comes along, asks Vicky if she would like her to; and Mrs. Bartlett looks positively proud of her daughter when Vicky says, "No, that's fine Mum, I can handle it."

It is worth noting finally, as a mark of the growing confidence that Dr. Mellon's handling of the situation had already given Vicky, that in the event she did not take up the offer of joining Achila's group. Instead, the offer prompted her to go online to find a community of peers with whom she could relate on equal terms. Among the sites she found were a number of extreme groups advocating a "devil may care" approach to their diabetic control. These groups, as she later described to Dr. Mellon, gave her a shock in that she recognized in them something of the direction in which she had been in danger of traveling. There has been much interest in the role of peers in general (Greco *et al.*, 2001; Coleman *et al.*, 2011) and in particular as mediated through mobile phones and other web-connected technologies (Sutcliffe *et al.*, 2011). But in Vicky's case at least, her experience helped her to engage fully with the shared agenda between herself, her mother and her GP of achieving a mature self-management of her diabetes.

Resolving conflicts and clinical leadership

Dr. Mellon had thus, at least to this point, effectively defused the conflicts brewing over control of her diabetes between the teenage Vicky Bartlett, her mother and the other professionals involved in her care. This was an important clinical outcome in the short term: it is the paradox of adolescent diabetes that just when a young person most needs help with blood sugar control, they are least able to accept it. There was a clear risk here of the strong-minded Vicky Bartlett and her equally strong-minded mother getting drawn into a vicious cycle of mutual opposition and distress, with further loss of blood sugar control and potentially dangerous hypos the inevitable outcome.

Holistic skills of conflict resolution

So how had Dr. Mellon avoided this? We have noted at a number of points his considerable skills of eliciting information and the interplay between these and the

values in play (his own and others). Here we were able to draw on a considerable body of well-established medical communication skills literature: as we saw from our quick audit of Dr. Mellon's skills (Fig. 7.1), he measured up well against recognized standards.

With conflict resolution, there is – perhaps surprisingly – no corresponding well-defined canon of medical communication skills literature on which to draw. This is in part because conflict resolution, unlike eliciting skills, is not a well-defined aspect of any particular part of the consultation but rather is a product of the way the consultation as a whole is managed. We saw this holistic aspect of conflict resolution for example in Chapter 1 when Dr. Gulati defused the potential conflict with Roy Walker over his clinically inappropriate demand for an off-work certificate by arranging for him to come back for a longer session at the end of the week. We will come to other elements of values-based practice that support conflict resolution in later chapters, for example dissensus in Chapter 13, and the use of frameworks of shared values in Chapter 14.

For the moment, though, the point is that the holistic nature of conflict resolution means that, while conflict resolution as such is not as widely discussed as other aspects of communication skills in the medical literature, there is much in this literature that is relevant in principle. The skills shown by Dr. Mellon correspond for example with some of the "tasks" in the consultation listed by Pendleton *et al.* (1984):

1. *To choose with the patient an appropriate action for each problem.* Dr. Mellon and Vicky Bartlett chose to focus on her hypo, which was also central to Mrs. Bartlett's concerns and this led to a number of practical actions.
2. *To achieve a shared understanding of the problems with the patient.* By the end of the consultation, all three of them recognized the importance of finding a way to balance Vicky Bartlett's need for normal adolescent freedoms against the constraints of blood sugar control.
3. *To involve the patient in the management and encourage him or her to accept an appropriate level of responsibility.* Again, the balanced way Dr. Mellon handed an appropriate level of responsibility to the 16-year-old Vicky Bartlett was central to his management of the situation, both with Vicky and with her mother.

Almost any consultation model can be used to map what was going on in this consultation. For example, in the terms of Heron's six category intervention analysis, Dr. Mellon is avoiding being prescriptive and the main interventions are informative, confronting and supportive (Heron, 1975). There are also powerful models in particular areas of healthcare: Dr. Mellon's approach, for example, once he had got past his initial inadvertent dismissal of Mrs. Bartlett, showed many of the essential features of an approach to shared decision-making in mental health called "trialogue" (Amering *et al.*, 2002). But that said, where the medical communication skills literature on eliciting skills is detailed and practical, the corresponding literature on conflict resolution in the consultation is relatively high level and general.

Communication skills in the management literature

This is in marked contrast to the communication skills literature in the area of management and leadership. Managers and clinicians are often set at odds by their inherently very different priorities and other values: we explore some of the tensions here in a later chapter (Chapter 11). The management and leadership literature nonetheless offers a rich and largely untapped resource for understanding how communication and the skills for working with values together support conflict resolution through the skills of effective leadership.

We can get a sense of the potential of this resource for medical communication skills in the area of conflict resolution by carrying out a further quick audit of Dr. Mellon's consultation, this time focusing on his skills of clinical leadership, and by reference to a model of leadership from the management literature called "adaptive work" (Heifetz, 1994).

Adaptive work and clinical leadership

"Adaptive work" is especially helpful for understanding the conflict resolution aspects of Dr. Mellon's consultation with Vicky Bartlett and her mum. It was developed at the Harvard Business School as a model of leadership for use primarily in commercial and political contexts. But its author, Ronald Heifetz, was a doctor; thus, many of his examples are from medicine, and Heifetz indeed argued that as a model of leadership "adaptive work" is equally applicable in health care as in any other context.

Adaptive work, moreover, consistent with the themes of this chapter, puts values and conflicts of values at the heart of leadership (Heifetz, 1994, p. 23). It also shares with values-based practice a clear recognition that differences of values are a resource for, not an impediment to, effective decision-making (Fulford and Benington, 2004). Adaptive work also shares with values-based practice the key insight that, although values are always there, we tend to notice them only when they cause trouble (as paradigmatically they do in conflict situations). Thus, Principle 2 of adaptive work (Heifetz's "pressure cooker" principle, see Fig. 7.2 below) corresponds with the "squeaky-wheel" principle of values-based practice. Moreover, these two principles provide a clear link with medical communication skills through Roger Neighbour's concept of "values under pressure": it is when values are under pressure, Neighbour points out, that they reveal themselves – hence the importance of conflict situations in bringing important issues to the surface where they can be understood and dealt with (Neighbour, personal communication).

How then do Dr. Mellon's skills of clinical leadership measure up against the principles of adaptive work? Fig. 7.2 summarizes five elements of adaptive work as set out by Heifetz in a chapter on the use of authority in resolving conflict and how these elements relate to Dr. Mellon's work with Vicky Bartlett and her mother.

As with our audit of Dr. Mellon's eliciting skills (Fig. 7.1), it is clear that he ticks the requisite boxes. What was required for him to do this was anything but a tick-box approach, however. Yes, he had well-developed communication skills. But as Fig. 7.2 indicates, the effective way in which he *used* those skills in resolving the conflict between Vicky Bartlett and her mother was crucially driven by the *values*, his own values as well as their values, at play in the consultation. With ICE then, they could have gone a long way. With ICE StAR they went a lot further.

Chapter summary

This chapter has illustrated the two-way relationship between values-based practice and communication skills:

- Values-based practice depends critically on good communication skills – values-based practice as we said in Chapter 3 is nothing without communication skills. Dr. Mellon's management of Vicky Bartlett's diabetes in this chapter depended critically first on his skills of eliciting the values of those concerned (Vicky herself, but also her mum's values and Dr. Mellon's self-understanding of his own values), and secondly on the clinical leadership he showed in his skills of conflict resolution.

Five principles of adaptive work as skills for clinical leadership	Dr. Mellon
Principle 1: Diagnose the situation in light of the values at stake and unbundle the issues that come with it.	**Yes** – especially positive values: Dr. Mellon's values of long-term relationships and continuity of care were essential to the successful start of the interview; Vicky's StAR values (and those also of her mother) were essential to its successful outcomes.
Principle 2: Keep the level of distress within a tolerable range for doing adaptive work. Like a pressure cooker, keep the heat up without blowing the vessel.	**Yes** – with a partial exception at the start of the interview (when he summarily dismissed Mrs. Bartlett), Dr. Mellon maintained at each stage of the interview a balance between challenge and support, again. This was effective because the balance reflected the values (positive and negative) of those concerned.
Principle 3: Focus on the tractable issues, counteracting avoidance mechanisms like: • Denial • Scape-goating • Externalizing the enemy • Pretending the problem is technical • Attacking individuals, not issues (blaming someone else).	**Yes** – in concentrating on Vicky's hypo as a central and shared value of all those concerned, Dr. Mellon firmly countered the various avoidance mechanisms listed by Heifetz: there was no scope for example for anyone, least of all Vicky, to continue denying the gravity of what had happened to her at the weekend.
Principle 4: Give the work back to the people with the problem (but at a rate they can stand) (i.e. patient active not passive).	**Yes** – at the heart of Dr. Mellon's management was a process of resolving the conflict between Vicky Bartlett and her mum by making them both active agents rather than merely passive recipients of "advice": and his scope for doing this directly reflected the many strengths that both brought to the situation.
Principle 5: Protecting voices of leadership without authority (no more unauthorized voices than those of children).	**Yes** – at 16, Vicky Bartlett was moving towards assuming an adult authority for self-leadership but still needing the support of her mother and others. She had the strength to do this but it took Dr. Mellon's skills of clinical leadership to find a way forward that protected her growing voice of authority as she moved from childhood dependence to adult independence.

Fig. 7.2. Heifitz's five principles of leadership as adaptive work and Dr. Mellon's skills of clinical leadership (conflict resolution) (based on Heifetz, 1994; adapted from Fulford and Benington, 2004).

• Communication skills are in turn enhanced and extended by values-based practice. Values-based practice, as we put it at the start of this chapter, helps us to "get behind the mantra." The mantra on which we focused here was the helpful mnemonic acronym ICE. Each of these ideas, concerns and expectations is deeply value-laden. So each of the elements of values-based practice can all in principle enhance the way ICE is used. Again, we have focused here in particular on values-based skills of raising awareness of values with a particular emphasis on the importance of eliciting positive strengths (the StAR values of Chapter 3), as well as (negative) needs and difficulties. Hence our mantra for this chapter that adding values-based practice to traditional communication skills takes us from ICE to ICE StAR.

In the next part of the book, we will see how similar two-way relationships support clinical decision-making in the areas of person-centered practice and multidisciplinary teamwork, respectively.

References

Amering, M., Hofer, H. and Rath, I. (2002). The "First Vienna Trialogue": Experiences with a new form of communication between users, relatives and mental health professionals. In H. P. Lefley, D. L. Johnson, eds, *Family Interventions in Mental Illness: International Perspectives*. Westport, CT/London: Praeger.

Balint, M. (1957). *The Doctor, His Patient, and the Illness*. London: Pitman. [Millenium Edition (2000). Edinburgh: Churchill Livingstone,]

Bryden, K. S., Peveler, R. C., Stein, A., Neil, A., Mayou, R. A. and Dunger, D. B. (2001). Clinical and psychological course of diabetes from adolescence to young adulthood. *Diabetes Care* **24**, 1536–40.

Coleman, K. J., Clark, A. Y., Shordon, M., et al. (2011). Teen peer educators and diabetes knowledge of low-income fifth grade students. *Journal of Community Health* **36**, 23–6.

Department for Constitutional Affairs (2006). *Mental Capacity Act Code of Practice*. Code Number CP 05/06. London: HMSO.

Dickinson, J. K. and O'Reilly, M. M. (2004). The lived experience of adolescent females with type 1 diabetes. *The Diabetes Educator* **30**, 99–107.

Fulford, K. W. M. and Benington, J. (2004). VBM²: a collaborative values-based model of healthcare decision-making combining medical and management perspectives. In R. Williams and M. Kerfoot, eds., *Child and Adolescent Mental Health Services: Strategy, Planning, Delivery, and Evaluation*. Oxford: Oxford University Press, pp. 89–102.

Greco, P., Shroff Pendley, J., McDonell, K. and Reeves, G. (2001). A peer group intervention for adolescents with type 1 diabetes and their best friends. *Journal of Pediatric Psychology* **26**, 485–90.

Heifetz, R. (1994). *Leadership Without Easy Answers*. Cambridge, MA: Harvard University Press.

Heron, J. (1975). *A Six Category Intervention Analysis*. Human Potential Research Project, University of Surrey, Guildford, UK.

Larme, A. C. and Pugh, J. A. (1998). Attitudes of primary care providers toward diabetes: barriers to guideline implementation. *Diabetes Care* **21**, 1391–6.

Neighbour, R. (1987). *The Inner Consultation*. Lancaster: MTOPress.

NICE (2004). *Type 1 Diabetes: Diagnosis and Management of Type 1 Diabetes in Children, Young People and Adults* (updated April 2010). London: National Institute for Health and Clinical Excellence.

Pendleton, D., Schofield, T., Tate, P. and Havelock, P. (1984). *The Consultation: an Approach to Learning and Teaching*. Oxford: Oxford University Press.

Salinsky, J. and Sackin, P. (2000). *What are you Feeling, Doctor?* Oxford: Radcliffe Medical Press.

Sutcliffe, P., Martin, S., Sturt, J. et al. (2011). Systematic review of communication technologies to promote access and engagement of young people with diabetes into healthcare. *BMC Endocrine Disorders* **11**, 1.

Tate, P. (1994). *The Doctor's Communication Handbook*. Oxford/New York: Radcliffe Medical Press.

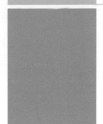

Introduction to Part 3

This part is concerned with the relationships, respectively, between professionals and patients, and between professionals of different kinds working together in multidisciplinary teams.

- "Person-centered practice" means different things in different contexts. Chapter 8, through the story of a woman, Brenda Forest, with early breast cancer, shows that in all its various meanings person-centered practice must include attention to the values – the needs, preferences, strengths and above all aspirations – of the particular person concerned. Person-centered practice, the chapter concludes, is nothing if it is not person-*values*-centered practice.
- Multidisciplinary team work has become increasingly the norm in many contexts in the ever more complex environment of modern healthcare. In part, this is because team members from different professions bring with them different skills and experience. In values-based practice, the concept of the multidisciplinary team is extended to include different team *values*. In Chapter 9, we illustrate the importance of team values in supporting balanced decision-making in a child safeguarding case.

"Person-centered practice" and "multidisciplinary teamwork" are both very much among today's buzz words in health care. There are good reasons for this. Like any buzz word, they can become misused as empty mantras. But person-centered practice represents an important shift of focus away from the priorities of providers and back to the needs of individual patients and their families, while multidisciplinary teamwork is essential for the effective delivery of care that is genuinely person-centered. Values-based practice, as we will see in this part, both draws on and in turn contributes to the multidisciplinary delivery of person-centered care.

Balanced Decision-making
within a
Framework of Shared Values

POINT

Partnership

PROCESS

Two-feet Principle   Squeaky-wheel Principle   Science-driven Principle

Person-centered practice

Multidisciplinary teamwork

Awareness   Reasoning   Knowledge   Communication skills

Mutual Respect
for
Differences of Values

PREMISE

Map of values-based practice – person-centred practice.

8

"Best" in breast cancer: clinician values and person-centered care

Values-based practice element 5: person-*values*-centred practice

Topics covered in this chapter

The story of Brenda Forest described in this chapter shows the importance of values (alongside evidence) in tackling two kinds of problem presented by person-centered practice: problems of *mutual understanding* and problems of *conflicting values*.

Other topics include:

- The many varieties of person-centered medicine
- Body image, sexuality and (desired) outcomes in women with breast cancer
- NICE guidelines on the management of early breast cancer
- Jainism and Gujarati culture.

Take-away message for practice

*Genuinely person-centered practice means person-**values**-centered practice.*

Values-based practice is very far from being alone in promoting a person-centered approach to clinical decision-making in medicine. Indeed, although there is a sense in which medicine has always been centered on people (what else could medicine be about but people), person-centered has become one of the buzz words of current clinical practice, following the work of McWhinney's group (Stewart *et al.*, 2003).

Like many such buzz words, however, as we saw in Chapter 1, exactly what it means to be "person-centered" varies widely with context. In therapeutics, "personalized medicine" means tailoring drugs and other treatments to the individual, including, in principle at least, the individual's unique genetic profile. With breast cancer, which is the focus of this chapter, there have been major developments in recent years towards more personalized approaches in this sense. Again, terms like "patient-led" and "expert patient" are scattered liberally in current policy and service developments, not to mention research. And in medical law and ethics, correspondingly, it is the individual who is the primary holder of rights: in this chapter, the right to individual autonomy will play an important role in a person-centered approach to the management of breast cancer.

Values and person-centered practice

Values are clearly important in each of these varieties of person-centered practice. The role of values is perhaps most self-evident in person-centered ethics and law: the language of rights and autonomy just *is* the language of values. But values are also the driving factor in recent policy, service development and research initiatives: the aim of patient-led and expert patient programs in each of these areas is, precisely, to bring what really *matters* to patients more fully to the fore.

Values are no less important, too, in the therapeutics of personalized medicine. The potential ability to tailor drugs to an individual's genetic profile makes it more rather than less important that such drugs are used in the *interests* of the individual concerned. With further developments in personalized medicine, then, it will become more important than ever to remember from Chapter 1 David Sackett and colleagues' definition of evidence-based medicine as combining best research evidence with each individual patient's unique "values," the "unique preferences, concerns and expectations each patient brings to the clinical encounter."

With values, however, in person-centered as in other areas of medicine, goes the challenge of complexity; and with complexity, as we outlined in Chapter 2, goes the need for values-based alongside evidence-based practice.

The clinical context

For once, Mr. Satish Shah was at a loss for words. A consultant surgeon specializing in breast cancer at a large local hospital in the East End of London, Mr. Shah was used to dealing with women who knew their minds and were not afraid to make their wishes known. But Brenda Forest had him stumped. The referral letter from her GP had noted her concern about her appearance and he had anticipated some "discussion" about reconstruction rather than a simple mastectomy. But Brenda Forest seemed determined to limit any surgical intervention to removal of the primary tumor.

Foreground values

Brenda Forest, aged 42, was described in the referral letter as a single mother who worked as a hairdresser. The story was that she had noticed an area of puckering skin near her left nipple and had immediately telephoned for an appointment. Her GP, Dr. David Anderson, had in turn referred her for an urgent appointment with Mr. Shah in the local "breast clinic." Cancer services were well developed in the area and she had been seen within a few days.

Keen to make a good impression, Brenda Forest had "dressed down" for her hospital appointment. She knew well enough that a mastectomy was on the cards and had rehearsed carefully what she would say. But somewhat to her surprise, she had found herself in the event uncharacteristically tongue-tied. Mr. Shah had been courteous and professional. But she could see that he had little understanding of what the prospect of losing a breast meant for a woman in her situation; and she felt that he had given her little encouragement to explain.

Mr. Shah, also in his 40s, was a Gujarati Indian. He had come to the UK with his parents as a young child and had followed his father into medicine. As a family, they had worked hard to integrate with the local community but at the same time had kept up their cultural and family ties with their country of origin. Mr. Shah in particular had maintained the traditional Jainist religious beliefs and practices that the family brought with them from India. The modest ethic and disciplines of Jainism had suited Mr. Shah's personality and had helped him to cope with what he saw as the excesses of Western individualism. In addition, Gujarati culture is strong on diversity and inclusion. Between his religion and his culture, therefore, Mr. Shah had considerable resources on which to draw in approaching each

of his highly heterogeneous group of patients in what he hoped was a fully person-centered way.

But this patient, Brenda Forest, was proving a challenge. Yes, her skirt was perhaps a little short and her heels a little high, but she was obviously intelligent and had come prepared with a better knowledge of breast cancer than the majority of his patients at the same stage. Yet she seemed unaccountably resistant to his evidence-based suggestions about the best way to proceed.

Two problems in person-centered practice

> **Reflection point**
>
> Before reading on you, may want to try thinking for a moment about why in the clinical scenario above Brenda Forest and Mr. Shah appear to be heading for a standoff over what to do about her breast lump.
>
> We will be giving you more information about Brenda Forest and Mr. Shah shortly. But from what you have read thus far, it is clear that both of them are thoughtful and mature people. Mr. Shah, moreover, is by temperament and training very much committed to a person-centered approach.
>
> So what do you think could be the problem or problems here?

This exercise takes us to the heart of the values-related problems presented by person-centered medicine. We will be looking at these problems and how values-based practice can help to tackle them in detail in this chapter as we follow the story of Mr. Shah and Brenda Forest. But to anticipate a little, the problems we will encounter with person-centered medicine here are of two main kinds, namely problems of *mutual understanding* and problems of *conflicting values.*

- *Problems of mutual understanding.* The presenting problem for Mr. Shah is that, for the moment at least, he simply cannot understand why this particular individual, Brenda Forest, should be so peculiarly insistent on limiting the surgical options as he saw it so drastically. Importantly, however, Brenda Forest for her part is finding Mr. Shah's difficulties of understanding equally incomprehensible.
- *Problems of conflicting values.* Problems of mutual understanding in person-centered medicine are challenging enough. Mr Shah will have to dig deep

into his commitment to person-centered medicine to get any understanding of where Brenda Forest is coming from. But this, as we will see, leads him straight into problems of the second kind, problems of conflicting values, that turn out to be even more challenging: for Brenda Forest is coming from a very different set of values from where he, Satish Shah, as a person-centered clinician working within evidence-based principles is coming from.

In the rest of this chapter, we will be exploring these two kinds of problem presented by person-centered practice – problems of mutual understanding and problems of conflicting values – and indicating some of the ways in which values-based practice, working (as always) alongside and in partnership with evidence-based practice, can help to tackle them. We will start by taking a closer look at the consultation between Mr. Shah and Brenda Forest.

A person-centered consultation

In this section, we set out how Mr. Shah's consultation with Brenda Forest went up to the point where, as in the clinical scenario at the start of this chapter, he found himself stumped.

Mr. Shah, as we have seen, is fully committed to a person-centered approach. As such, he manages problems of the first kind outlined above, problems of mutual understanding, up to a point. But even as he comes to understand (in part) Brenda Forest's concerns about mastectomy, he runs straight into problems of the second kind, problems of conflicting values, and it is here that, as a person-centered clinician, he finds himself stumped.

Reflection point

As you read through the consultation that follows, you may find it helpful to keep in mind the two kinds of problem with person-centered practice outlined above:

- Problems of mutual understanding
- Problems of conflicting values.

In the course of this and later sections, we will be looking at where in the consultation these two kinds of problem arise and the extent to which the resources of values-based practice (in particular the clinical skills outlined in Chapters 3–6 of this book) can help us to tackle them.

After the usual introductions, Mr. Shah opened the consultation by indicating that he had had a detailed letter from Brenda Forest's GP, Dr. Anderson, but would like to hear from her exactly what had brought her to see him. Brenda Forest knew from her own work as a hairdresser how important it is to give people a chance to talk about what they want rather than rushing in with "solutions" and she was impressed that, like Dr. Anderson, Mr. Shah was a "listening doctor."

Accordingly, she described how she had noticed an area of dimpled skin on her left breast and that Dr. Anderson had confirmed she needed urgent assessment for possible breast cancer. No, she had no family history (her mother died suddenly from a stroke in her 80s); yes, her general health was good; she had lost no weight; and she had given up smoking in her late 20s (at the time because she had seen how it "aged" people). Mr. Shah then examined her confirming a 1 cm area of firm puckered skin in her left breast close to but clearly separate from the nipple. Underlying this, he found a 4 cm diameter hard lump. "Oh," he thought as he continued his examination, "at least there are no clinical pointers to locoregional spread, and the other breast seems OK."

"Well," he said when Brenda Forest had got dressed and was sitting down again, "Dr. Anderson was quite right that you did well to pick this up so promptly."

"So, what is it?" Brenda Forest had asked, emphasizing that she wanted to "know the worst."

"Well, we can't be absolutely sure until we undertake some further tests: you'll need a mammogram, an ultrasound of the breast and your armpit, and a needle biopsy of the lump," Mr. Shah said. He went on, "As Dr. Anderson suspected, this is very likely to be an early breast cancer. But if it really is very early, with modern treatments you have an excellent chance of being completely cured."

"Yes," Brenda Forest said, "one of my stylists was diagnosed with breast cancer a few years ago and apart from an annual check up she seems absolutely fine. But she had to have a mastectomy," she added, looking Mr. Shah firmly in the eye.

It was at this point that this hitherto standard consultation started to get difficult. Forewarned by Dr. Anderson's letter, Mr. Shah thought he understood what Brenda Forest meant – no simple mastectomy for her if she could possibly avoid it – and he expected the consultation to go on to a discussion of reconstructive options. He was right but, as we will see in a moment, only up to a point. He started with his usual reassurances

101

about "modern" treatments – mastectomies were less extensive nowadays, chemotherapy did not have to involve hair loss and his team were experts at helping with really effective prostheses. But he could see that he was not hitting the spot; and he was considerably surprised when Brenda Forest, instead of asking about breast reconstruction, said "And what about breast-conserving surgery?"

This was the first indication to Mr. Shah that he was dealing with an unusually well-informed patient. Being unaware that Brenda's son was a medical student, he assumed she could only have got this phrase from a careful reading of the NICE or some similar website and he took her question fully seriously. He explained straightforwardly that, although breast-conserving surgery was now used for some cases, with a cancer of this kind the evidence was that the chances of successful treatment were better with a mastectomy.

"How much better?" she asked.

"Impossible to be exact," he had replied, "but certainly better."

"So how much smaller would this thing need to be for me to avoid losing a breast?"

"Well, not much smaller, certainly, but our guidelines are very firm about this, so I really couldn't advise . . ."

And then Brenda Forest asked the question that finally brought Mr. Shah up short. As just noted, he was expecting her to plead the usual "cosmetic concerns." But Brenda Forest had looked up breast cancer in one of her son's medical textbooks. Here she read about the move over recent years to ever more conservative options in surgery for breast cancer and away from mastectomy as the standard treatment, other than in very advanced cases. Mastectomy was presented to students as an area of active debate and research. Thus, being well informed, she asked, "But does everyone agree with the guidelines?" Mr. Shah was well and truly stumped.

Background values

To understand exactly why Mr. Shah as a person-centered clinician was so stumped by Brenda Forest's question, we need to look at what we called in Chapter 1 the background values in play between Brenda Forest and Mr. Shah. We need to look in more detail at the beliefs and values with which both of them came to the consultation and how these had brought them into their now opposed positions in the consultation. In order to

appreciate their significance for the problems Mr. Shah had run into as a person-centered clinician, we need to set them in context briefly by reference, respectively, to his and to Brenda Forest's biographies.

Mr. Satish Shah

Mr. Shah was proud of his deservedly good reputation for breast surgery, both locally and nationally among his peers. Two of his colleagues had been off sick in the past year so there had been considerable pressure from management to keep within the guideline times for seeing new referrals and also to offer definitive surgical treatment.

This had meant some "gentle persuasion" to offer more mastectomies and wide local excisions rather than reconstruction mammoplasties, which take more time in surgery and may require a series of operations to achieve optimal results. Mr. Shah and his team had found the pressure of extra work difficult to keep up with at times. But they shared the management's objectives of early treatment. And they had no problem of principle with recommending simple mastectomy as the treatment of choice. Their clinical experience as a team was consistent with early research suggesting that reconstructive surgery offers no long-term advantages in relation to overall psychological or psychosexual outcomes (see for example Schover, 1994).

To be clear, Mr. Shah and his team never coerced anyone into accepting a simple mastectomy. Aside from issues of consent, they were well aware of and followed NICE guidelines about discussing options for breast-conserving procedures where appropriate with early and non-invasive cases (NICE, 2009). Mr. Shah, committed to person-centered medicine, made a point of trying to understand where his patients were "coming from." But he believed, again with the backing of research evidence (see Johnson et al., 1998), that, although most women faced with breast cancer welcome discussion of the options for treatment, at the end of the day a large majority find the choices confusing and difficult and are actually looking for him to say what he as "the expert" believes the best option to be.

Saving lives

Mr. Shah was also concerned that raising issues of appearance could lead to too much importance being placed on what was after all an unattainable cosmetic result rather than focusing on what he regarded as the bottom line, life-saving surgery.

Like all clinicians, Mr. Shah regarded saving lives as an important priority. This also fitted well with his respect as a Jain for the sanctity of life – Jainists are vegetarians and are careful to avoid unnecessary killing of any living thing. So for Mr. Shah, a Jain and a clinician, it was natural that saving lives should figure strongly in his scale of values, personal as well as professional.

Team values

The clinic nursing team broadly supported Mr. Shah's approach of tending to recommend mastectomy. Most of the team had worked together for many years and they enjoyed their shared success. They knew little about Jainism (very few of them even knew that this was Mr. Shah's religion), but they all respected him as a "fantastic surgeon" who really cared about his patients. They had found that his sometimes rather down-to-earth style could come across as blunt, but they saw it as part of their role to give their patients a chance to talk through their concerns "woman to woman" (the nursing team were in fact all women); and they had many opportunities for this while they were carrying through all the preparatory tests and procedures.

Mr. Shah for his part valued the nursing team's caring and supportive approach with their patients. He was well aware that this had been a major factor in achieving their excellent psychological outcomes: a large majority of their patients found their initial concerns about body image allayed as treatment progressed and they were helped to "put things in perspective."

Brenda Forest

Brenda Forest's first thought when her GP, David Anderson, confirmed that she probably had breast cancer was that this could mean a mastectomy. Dr. Anderson had focused (reasonably enough) on her (relatively speaking) good prognosis. He had reassured her that she had done well to catch it at a very early stage and that statistically she was very likely to be completely cured. He told her that they had an excellent surgeon locally, Mr. Shah, who would see her within a few days.

"What about chemotherapy?" Brenda Forest asked, thinking that this could be an alternative to surgery.

"Yes," Dr. Anderson had explained, missing the point of Brenda's question, "but this usually comes after surgery." Mr. Shah and his team would want to do some tests and would then discuss everything with her in detail.

That first full acknowledgment of the reality of her situation – an urgent appointment with a surgeon specializing in breast cancer – gave Brenda Forest a lot to think about. She was, of course, not alone in being concerned about the cosmetic effects of breast surgery. But at 42, she was unusual in the nature and extent of her concerns. Had she been 22, with a 22-year-old's psychosexual drives and ambitions, Dr. Anderson might have anticipated that breast conservation could be a prime concern, but his experience suggested that most of his middle-aged patients were focused almost exclusively on survival at this stage. Research findings in this area (see for example Schover, 1994) confirm that, for the younger woman, cosmetic concerns would be likely to weigh against the fear of death.

But Brenda Forest – this particular Brenda Forest – was different. At 42, Brenda Forest was psychosexually closer to a 22-year-old and with the added urgency of a life that had been in this respect largely on hold for the last 15 years.

Girl deferred

Thus it was that, as the implications of her (probable) diagnosis sank in, Brenda grew increasingly angry at a fate that appeared to be conspiring to cheat her of the life she had worked so hard to build up following her divorce. In the best traditions of her kind, she had taken that early disappointment on the chin. Not for her the gratifications of regret. She picked herself up, dusted herself down and got on with life. Using her divorce settlement for a downpayment on a small house, she had set out to earn her living as a hairdresser and to ensure a secure home for her son, John. There were difficult periods financially. But as property values rose in the late 1990s, she used the security of her house to negotiate a bank loan to start her own salon. With her warm personality and shrewd business sense, the salon had prospered. She now employed six stylists and had recently paid off both bank loan and mortgage.

Throughout the time she was building the business, John had been Brenda Forest's priority. It was perhaps for this reason, as much as from the disaster of her first marriage, that she had avoided getting too deeply involved in any new relationship over this period. She was an attractive woman who, despite that unhappy early experience, liked men and she had not been short of opportunities. But she had thus far firmly deflected all offers of anything permanent.

First love

Then, out of the blue, a few weeks earlier, Brenda had been contacted by her very first love, Brian Davies, through the website Friends Reunited. They had exchanged emails. There had been no talk of romance, but hearing from Brian had made Brenda realize that since turning 40 she had become increasingly aware of a gap in her life. Her business continued to prosper – even in times of recession people wanted to look good – and John was doing well at medical school. But for all her success as a parent and as a business woman, she realized now that her life was very far from complete. Where would she be in another 15 years?

"Where indeed?" she now thought ruefully. But if she was going to survive, she was not going to end up alone. And losing a breast (whatever they said about reconstruction) was about as good a way as she could imagine of doing just that.

Sex versus survival?

Mr. Shah and Brenda Forest thus brought partly shared but also importantly different values and beliefs to the consultation. The differences of values between them could be summed up aphoristically as "sex versus survival." For the Jain and clinician Mr. Shah, survival was an important priority. Brenda Forest had shown herself over the last 15 years to be nothing if not a survivor. But in the new situation in which she now found herself, she wanted to survive, certainly, but not on any terms. Survival with the partner she had never had, yes. Survival alone, and with, as she saw it, even the prospect of finding a partner (literally) cut away, no thank you.

Matters were not so starkly drawn between them, of course. Nor indeed was there anything at this stage remotely approaching a standoff. With other characters, there might have been. Faced with such a conflict of values, and a conflict the true extent of which neither of them still fully understood, the consultation with other characters involved might well have broken down altogether, at least as an exercise in person-centered medicine. A different Mr. Shah might have ridden roughshod over a different Brenda Forest's concerns: a different Brenda Forest might have given up, accepting against her true wishes the "inevitable" mastectomy. That theirs was by contrast a moderated standoff directly reflected what these two particular if very different characters brought to their respective sides of the consultation.

From problems to (partial) solutions

In the next two sections, we are going to move from the problems presented by person-centered medicine to the role of values-based practice as a resource for dealing with them. We will consider first the importance of the values-based clinical skills set out in Chapters 4–7 above, and then, in a subsequent section, the contributions to person-centered medicine of other elements of values-based practice.

Two preliminary points

Two points about values-based practice and person-centered care are worth bearing in mind:

- *Order of presentation*. As we noted in our initial overview (Chapter 3 above), the skills for values-based practice – awareness, reasoning, knowledge and communication skills – although described and illustrated separately in the four chapters of Part 2, have to be used in practice in a seamlessly joined-up and fully integrated way. Hence, in what follows in this section, they are described in the order in which they emerge from and drive the consultation.
- *Theory and practice*. In reflecting on the consultation, we will be setting out what went on in rather more detail than would have been apparent to either Mr. Shah or Brenda Forest at the time. We will also be drawing on all the additional information we now have about both characters, much of which would, of course, not have been available to them at the time.

This section and the section that follows should thus be understood as an exercise in reflective thinking. What this will show is the role of values-based skills (their strengths but also, as we will see, their limitations) in meeting the problems presented by person-centered medicine in practice.

Values-based skills in person-centered medicine

In this section, then, we are going to look at the contributions to person-centered medicine of the skills for values-based practice by reviewing the ways and extent to which these skills were operative in the consultation between Mr. Shah and Brenda Forest.

As just noted, it was their respective skills in this area that allowed the consultation as an exercise in person-centered medicine to get as far as it did.

Patient and doctor, in terms of the first of the two problems with person-centered medicine outlined above, had achieved a degree of mutual understanding. Yet at the point of standoff they had now reached, they had come close to foundering on a problem of the second kind, a problem of conflicting values. It is at this point, therefore, with problems of conflicting values that, as we will see in the next section, the further resources of values-based practice for person-centered medicine come in to play.

Reflection point

Before reading on you may want to go back briefly to the consultation described above between Mr. Shah and Brenda Forest.

Try running through the consultation briefly looking for *where* and *to what extent* Mr. Shah is (explicitly or implicitly) exercising the skills for values-based practice. Look out for examples (not necessarily in this order) of:

- Awareness (of values and of differences of values)
- Knowledge
- Reasoning skills
- Communication skills.

Look out also for the extent to which Brenda Forest is exercising the same skills. Values-based skills are, of course, not the preserve of clinicians and, as we will see in a later chapter (Chapter 12), partnership between those directly concerned as clinicians and as patients in a given decision is of the essence of a values-based approach.

Nothing without communication

Values-based practice, like evidence-based practice, is, as we saw in Chapter 7, dependent on good communication skills to achieve a positive influence on clinical decision-making. Values-based practice is, as we said, nothing without good communication skills, and this certainly applies in the devastating situation of breast cancer (Lerman *et al.*, 2006).

Mr. Shah is exemplary in this respect. He will have heard stories like Brenda Forest's hundreds of times, and as a busy surgeon working against challenging targets, he might have been forgiven for cutting straight to the quick. But he takes time to put Brenda at her ease as far as possible. He opens with a positive reference to Dr. Anderson's referral letter: Brenda is thus reassured by their mutual respect (Dr. Anderson

having remarked to her what a good surgeon they had locally). Mr. Shah builds on this reassurance for Brenda that the system on which her life depends is working well, by listening carefully to her own account of her story.

An example from mental health

Mr. Shah's person-centered communication skills should not be taken for granted. It is not at all uncommon for clinicians to believe that they are working in a person-centered way while in fact paying little attention to the values of the actual persons concerned.

A clear example of this comes from the early work of Kim Woodbridge in developing values-based skills training in mental health for a Community Mental Health Team in East London. The team in question was a well-functioning multidisciplinary team with an explicit commitment to person-centered practice and they had asked for training in values-based practice to support them with their very challenging work load. Much to the team's surprise, an early learning point for the team from the training was that their practice had been anything but person-centered!

This became apparent from a preparatory stage in which Kim Woodbridge sat in on one of the team's case review meetings and with their permission recorded the content of the comments made. What she found, as Fig. 8.1 shows, was that, despite the team's commitment to person-centered practice, a large majority of the comments reflected their own priorities rather than those of their patients. Thus, it has been known since the pioneering survey work of the sociologists Anne Rogers, David Pilgrim and Richard Lacey in the 1990s that what matters to people with long-term mental disorders are issues like housing, employment and a social friendship group (Rogers *et al.*, 1993). But the case review meeting was almost entirely taken up with clinician priorities such as medication and risk management. The team's surprise at the extent of the disjunction between their person-centered intentions and their person-centered practice provided a strong basis for the training that followed.

Awareness up to a point

Mr. Shah with his person-centered approach ensured that, as we saw, the consultation got off to a good start with Brenda Forest appreciating, as she put it to herself, a "listening doctor." Brenda Forest was a good communicator herself. She would not have lasted long

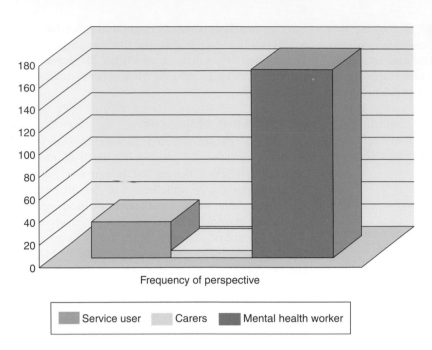

Fig. 8.1. Perspectives expressed in a mental health team meeting. (Fulford and Woodbridge, 2007).

as a hairdresser if she had not been a good listener, and her wider communication skills in areas such as negotiation and conflict resolution had stood her in good stead in building up her business in a highly competitive field. She had indeed dealt with many difficult interviews in her time and, as we have seen, had prepared carefully for the consultation.

Yet in the event, Brenda Forest found that she was unable to explain her real concerns about a mastectomy to Mr. Shah in the clear and straightforward way she had rehearsed. She recognized that this was no fault of Mr. Shah's. He was much as she had expected from what Dr. Anderson had told her and from what she had learned about him and his team from the Internet: caring, quietly competent and highly professional in his approach. He was also, as she had now found, a good listener. But she had been considerably more thrown than she had anticipated by the fact that Mr. Shah was a man and (as she assumed) a Muslim man, and she just could not bring herself to talk with him openly about her real feelings. Hence, as the consultation progressed, Brenda Forest became in her unaccustomed frustration more challenging and Mr. Shah correspondingly more defensive.

In fact, Mr. Shah was closer to understanding Brenda Forest's concerns than she realized. He had had of course no difficulty in picking up that Brenda Forest was worried about the cosmetic effects of a mastectomy: Dr. Anderson had indicated as much in his referral letter and it was understandably a common concern among women in her situation. But there was clearly, he saw, something different about the way Brenda Forest was reacting. In the first place, she had apparently read up on the options (that phrase "breast-conserving" was a giveaway), and then as the consultation progressed she had seemed unimpressed not to say indifferent to his usually well-received arguments about relative survival rates. All this wrong-footed Mr. Shah. He found himself in unfamiliar territory. He was not sure what that territory was but he certainly did not feel comfortable in it.

Again, it is important to recognize the extent to which Mr. Shah was ahead of the communications game here. As a genuinely person-centered practitioner, he had avoided what we called in Chapter 3 the "delusion of sameness": he picked up straight away that whatever Brenda Forest's values were they were not the same as his. As a genuinely person-centered practitioner, similarly, he avoided stereotyping: he was immediately aware that whatever Brenda Forest's concerns about the cosmetic effects of mastectomy might be, they were different from those of most of his patients.

In Chapter 4, we introduced the acronym of StAR values, to remind us of a person's strengths, aspirations and resources. Mr. Shah picked up readily on Brenda Forest's many strengths where many consulters only consider their patient's needs and difficulties.

Crucially, however, in terms of these StAR values, Mr. Shah missed Brenda Forest's aspirations (the A in StAR). Indeed, she had deliberately held back from telling him about her hopes of finding a belated life partner. On the plus side, he had recognized some of Brenda's resources. Although unaware at this stage of her successes as an entrepreneur and as a parent, he was nonetheless very much aware of her competencies: her clear and practical account of how she had found her breast lump and what she had done about it, her command (as he saw it) of the consultation and her obvious knowledge of breast cancer.

A degree of mutual understanding

Brenda Forest and Mr. Shah thus both had a better understanding of each other than many would have achieved after the first few minutes of an initial consultation on a potentially life-threatening condition. Their mutual respect, too – their recognition of each other's strengths – was important in sustaining the consultation. Yet for all this, the consultation clearly *was* in difficulties.

> **Reflection point**
>
> Think for a moment here about the level of mutual understanding Brenda Forest and Mr. Shah have achieved.
>
> Would still greater mutual understanding help or hinder the problem of conflicting values that is emerging between them?

It is important for understanding the way values-based practice supports person-centered medicine to recognize that, in this instance at least, greater mutual understanding between Mr. Shah and Brenda Forest would certainly not have resolved, and might actually have made more acute, their conflict of values.

Thus, Mr. Shah, had he understood the real basis of Brenda Forest's resistance to a mastectomy, in her hopes for finding a new life partner, might have felt more sympathetic – in his scale of values, her aspirations in this respect would have rated considerably higher than as he saw it "mere cosmetics." But greater sympathy in this instance would have made the conflict between Brenda Forest's priorities and his personal and professional commitment to saving lives sharper and more difficult for him to deal with: it was easier for him within his scale of values to discount cosmetics as a concern than relationships.

Brenda Forest, similarly, had she understood that Mr. Shah was a Jainist and not a Muslim might well have felt less inhibited in talking about her divorce and current ambitions. There would have been no shadows in her mind of the treatment of women under Shariah Law in some Muslim countries. But given the resistance she was picking up, she might nonetheless have associated this with the (mistaken) stereotype of Jainism as protecting life at all costs. As an experienced negotiator, she might thus have decided that this was a battle she was not going to win and that she had better look to alternatives (she had the resources to "go private").

Either way then, greater awareness of each other's values supported by excellent communication skills, important as both of these two skills areas are for values-based practice, would not have been sufficient to sustain the consultation between Mr. Shah and Brenda Forest. One way or another, the consultation as an exercise in person-centered medicine would have broken down. So, how far would the other skills outlined in Part 2, knowledge of values and reasoning skills, bridge the gap?

Getting (and not getting) the knowledge

In Chapter 6, we illustrated the importance of having a strong evidence base for values-based practice as for any other area of medical practice through the story of Sandy Fraser as an "unreformed" smoker with COPD. A key message from Chapter 6, however, was that, helpful as the evidence from research may be in indicating the *kind* of values that might be in play in a given situation, research can never tell us the *actual* values in play between particular individuals concerned. Everyone is, as we put it, an "*n* of 1," and indeed Sandy Fraser remained at the end of Chapter 6 a smoking enigma.

Breast cancer is an area where there is a relatively well-developed values evidence base. Dr. Anderson and Mr. Shah were both aware of this evidence and drew on it in their respective consultations with Brenda Forest. But here the story lines, about Sandy Fraser with COPD and about Brenda Forest with breast cancer, separate. For where the research findings in Sandy Fraser's case were helpful in a general way in deciding how to manage his situation, although again without actually getting to the bottom of what was motivating him, in Brenda Forest's case, the corresponding research findings were actually misleading.

Thus, Mr. Shah and Dr. Anderson were aware of the research noted above suggesting that a majority of

107

women of Brenda Forest's age will be less concerned about the cosmetic effects of mastectomy than women in their 20s. But Brenda Forest's values were in this respect closer to those of a woman in her 20s. Similarly, as doctors they were aware that this research also suggested that overall psychological and sexual outcomes are for a majority of women no different between simple mastectomies and reconstructive mammoplasties. This was indeed consistent with the clinical experience of Mr. Shah and his team in their clinic. But for all that there were clear indications that, for Brenda Forest, losing a breast would have put her at significant risk of long term psychological and sexual difficulties. Being the person she was, she would no doubt have coped with these difficulties as effectively as she had with other challenges in her life. But that would hardly be a successful person-centered outcome.

"Use with care," then, is the message of Chapter 6. Research evidence, more so in values-based even than in other areas of clinical decision-making, has to be drawn on with full awareness that the individual concerned in a given decision may well be relevantly different from the norms of the research in question.

Reasoning for and against

If (unmediated) knowledge of values was unhelpful in Mr. Shah and Brenda Forest's case, what about reasoning? Here the skills "boot" ends up on the other foot. Up to this point, although both our leading characters have shown considerable values-based skills, it has been Mr. Shah as the expert on breast cancer who has had the greater influence on the course of the consultation. When it comes to reasoning skills, however, their roles are reversed.

This is how things go. Faced with an increasingly intransigent Brenda Forest, Mr. Shah, like Dr. Gulati in Chapter 2, falls back on the "guidelines." Recall Mr. Shah's reference to "... our guidelines are very firm about this ..." He has in mind locally agreed treatment protocols that in turn are based on NICE guidance. Further back in his mind but still important in what he says are ethical guidelines about acting in his patient's best interests. The "best interests principle" is implicit in his further comment "... so I really couldn't advise ...." But this is where Mr. Shah is so effectively stymied by Brenda Forest's question, "But does everyone agree with the guidelines?"

At first glance, it may not seem obvious why Mr. Shah should feel so stumped by this question.

Could he not, you may think, simply acknowledge that, as in so many other areas of medicine, there are competing views, but that the majority view was that, on best current evidence, as he had already said, a mastectomy offered the highest chance of a successful outcome.

The Bolam principle

This, however, would be to miss the (implicit) point of Brenda Forest's question and hence the force of its impact on Mr. Shah as a clinician committed to a person-centered approach. Brenda Forest did not think of her question this way, of course. But what she had in effect done was to use a principle of medical ethics and law, the Bolam principle (a principle that normally operates to protect doctors) against Mr. Shah.

The Bolam principle was introduced into English law in 1957 following a case in which a patient tried to sue a doctor for negligence for failing to warn her of a rare but serious side effect of a treatment she had received from him (*Bolam* v. *Friern*, 1957). The defense was that, although some doctors, possibly even the majority of doctors, might have warned of this side effect, at least *some* doctors would not have done so – that is to say, some doctors would have considered the side effect in question to be so unusual that it would not have been in patients' best interests to worry them unnecessarily about it and thus perhaps to wrongly bias their decision about whether or not to go ahead with the treatment. This defense succeeded and the Bolam principle was accordingly established: that a doctor could not be sued in negligence under English law if he or she acted in accordance with a recognized body of medical opinion.

With the current move towards ever greater patient autonomy, the Bolam principle has been progressively undermined. As a so-called "prudent doctor" test of non-negligent practice, the Bolam principle has been increasingly replaced by a "prudent patient" test (Samanta and Samanta, 2003). In other words, the onus is now on the doctor to spell out all the pros and cons of a proposed treatment so that the patient, being fully informed, is in a position to make up their own mind about whether or not to accept it.

The Bolam principle, case-based reasoning and person-centered medicine

A prudent patient test of negligence certainly suits many patients (it would have suited the independent-minded Brenda Forest), though whether the very long and detailed lists of side effects with which patients are nowadays so often presented really amount to being "fully informed" is, we believe, an open question. Such lists are an aspect of the increasingly defensive practice that we argued in Chapter 2 is among the adverse consequences of an overly legalistic development of ethics in medicine.

Indeed, the thinking behind the Bolam principle was precisely to avoid this. The Bolam principle sought to ensure that doctors would have the freedom to exercise their clinical judgment within proper professional limits rather than being obliged for fear of being sued to follow the majority view.

Although described as a principle then, the effect of "Bolam" was to leave room in clinical decision-making for reasoning processes that are closer to what we called in Chapter 5 case-based (or casuistic) reasoning. And case-based reasoning is essential to person-centered decision-making. For case-based reasoning, as we described in Chapter 5, contrasts with principles reasoning precisely in that, instead of being "top down" from general principles (ethical or legal), it is "bottom up," driven by the particular circumstances of individual cases.

Person-centered guidelines

Case-based or bottom-up reasoning, therefore, is essential to person-centered practice. This is why Mr. Shah was so stumped by Brenda Forest's question about differences of views among experts on the role of mastectomy in the treatment of early breast cancer. For clinical judgment, and hence reasoning based on individual cases, is a requirement of the very guidelines on which he was relying in his attempt to reason with Brenda Forest.

NICE guidelines always include a direction (reproduced in Fig. 8.2) that they are not to be read as a substitute for clinical judgment in individual cases. The introduction to the NICE guidelines for the treatment of early breast cancer, moreover, on which Mr. Shah's local protocols were in turn based, includes an explicitly person-centered requirement (also given in full in Fig. 8.2) that "Treatment and care should take into account patients' individual needs and preferences."

The reverse Bolam maneuver

Brenda Forest, then, had in effect and without realizing it, reversed the normal effect of the Bolam principle. Bolam was introduced as a defense for doctors

Extract from General Statement of NICE's Remit, p. 2
This guidance represents the view of NICE, which was arrived at after careful consideration of the evidence available. Healthcare professionals are expected to take it fully into account when exercising their clinical judgement. However, the guidance does not override the individual responsibility of healthcare professionals to make decisions appropriate to the circumstances of the individual patient, in consultation with the patient and/or guardian or carer, and informed by the summary of product characteristics of any drugs they are considering.

Extract from Opening Section of the Guidance, p. 4
Patient-centered care
Treatment and care should take into account patients' individual needs and preferences. Good communication is essential, supported by evidence-based information, to allow patients to reach informed decisions about their care. Follow Department of Health advice on seeking consent if needed. If the patient agrees, families and carers should have the opportunity to be involved in decisions about treatment and care.

Fig. 8.2. Person-centered practice – two extracts from NICE Clinical Guideline 80 (underlining added).

against negligence where in exercising their clinical judgment they went against majority opinion, albeit remaining within the bounds of current thinking among their peers. Brenda Forest had used the same principle to put pressure on Mr. Shah to do just that, to *exercise his freedom of clinical judgment* to depart from the majority view as expressed in the guidelines. And as Mr. Shah was all too uncomfortably aware, the guidelines themselves made explicit provision for this as an aspect of person-centered care.

If Mr. Shah had not been so fully and genuinely committed to a person-centered approach, he could have fudged the issues. He could have said to himself that he had, in the words of the guidelines, "taken account" of Brenda Forest's "needs and preferences" while in fact paying them merely token regard. Or he could have fallen back on a more paternalistic understanding of "best interests." True, Brenda Forest was right that at worst she was trading only a small but unquantified, increased risk of relapse in return for the chance of saving her breast. But the surgeon is usually better placed than the newly diagnosed patient to understand through experience the realities of the late stages of breast cancer. Surely he, with all his experience, knew better than Brenda Forest what would be truly in her best interests.

None of these specious arguments would do for the highly professional and genuinely person-centered Mr. Shah, however. Brenda had him stumped. If he went with her "needs and preferences" by agreeing to removing merely the primary tumor, he would be acting consistently with his professional values of

109

person-centered care as supported by current guidelines, but, by the same token, he would be going against his personal and professional principles. If, on the other hand, he insisted on her having a mastectomy (even assuming he could eventually get anything resembling her genuine consent to this), he would be acting consistent with his principles but by the same token going flatly against his commitment to person-centered care.

An interim person-centered audit

At the start of this chapter, we noted two kinds of problem raised by person-centered practice: problems of mutual understanding and problems of conflicting values. To the point that Mr. Shah and Brenda Forest had now reached in the consultation, they had achieved, as we said earlier, a rather better degree of mutual understanding than many would have done in similar circumstances. This reflected their excellent skills in two areas important to values-based practice, *communication skills* and the consequent *awareness* of each other's values that this gave them.

Yet their relative success in understanding each other left them at risk of becoming impaled on a particularly acute problem of the second kind, namely a direct conflict between their respective values: we might summarize this as "sex before survival" (Brenda Forest) versus "survival before sex" (Mr. Shah). Here the further skills of values-based practice, *knowledge of values* and *reasoning skills*, have brought a degree of further mutual understanding but without resolution:

- Knowledge of the values of women undergoing treatment for breast cancer, based on the research literature and the surgical team's clinical experience, proved to be positively misleading: this was because Brenda Forest's perspective was very different from that of most women of her age in her situation.
- Reasoning skills, far from resolving the conflict, were the basis of what we called Brenda Forest's reverse Bolam maneuver that left Mr. Shah stumped.

The exercise of values-based skills has thus allowed patient and clinician to identify and in part to understand the problem between them. This in itself is important for person-centered medicine. The mutual understanding that Mr. Shah and Brenda Forest had reached was a step towards a person-centered

resolution of the issue. As often as not, this may be enough. As often as not, conflicts of values in person-centered medicine arise from misperceptions and misunderstandings the resolution of which is the resolution of conflict – to understand all is to forgive all, as they say. But in this case Mr. Shah and Brenda Forest's skills were not sufficient in themselves to resolve the differences between them. Indeed, any further clarification of the full extent of the conflict of values between Brenda Forest and Mr. Shah, far from resolving their difficulties, could actually have sharpened them.

From understanding to conflict resolution in person-centered medicine

Values-based skills, then, are necessary for person-centered practice but not always sufficient. So how can Brenda Forest and Mr. Shah move forward? What else is needed to go from understanding (mutual if still incomplete understanding of their conflict of values) to resolution?

> **Reflection point**
>
> In a final reflection in this chapter, you may find it helpful to think about this question briefly before reading on.
>
> Try looking back for a moment at the summary of the elements of values-based practice from Chapter 3 (Fig. 3.1), which is reproduced at the start of this chapter.
>
> Which of these elements (besides the skills areas described above) might be helpful in allowing Brenda Forest and Mr. Shah to reach resolution?

As we have indicated several times, the elements of values-based practice, although described separately in this book, have to come together in an integrated way to support practice. We do not have space here to follow in detail how the story between Brenda Forest and Mr. Shah went forward from their point of stand-off to resolution. We will be looking at conflict resolution again in the next chapter in relation to the very different issues raised by child protection. But there are three elements of values-based practice (in addition to its skills base) that together support resolution of conflicts of values, whether in person-centered or in any other area of clinical decision-making:

- Its premise of mutual respect.
- Its aim of balanced decision-making (through dissensus-based partnership).
- Multidisciplinary team work.

In the remainder of this chapter, we will look briefly at how each of these elements might have been important in how Brenda Forest and Mr. Shah's story eventually worked out.

The premise of mutual respect

Without mutual respect, Brenda Forest and Mr. Shah would not have got as far as they did towards mutual understanding. As we noted earlier, Brenda Forest was immediately impressed with Mr. Shah as a "listening doctor," and Mr. Shah in his turn was impressed with Brenda Forest's evident strength of character and her grasp of the issues involved in the management of breast cancer.

Gujarati culture, you will recall, is strong on inclusion and diversity, and it thus came naturally to Mr. Shah to adopt an open and reflective approach to his work with his diverse group of patients. Nonetheless, whether Mr. Shah with his "survival before sex" values would be able to accommodate Brenda Forest's "sex before survival" values remained to be seen. Not that he should compromise or give up his values any more than Brenda Forest should compromise or give up her values. Mutual respect means *mutual*. Hence, the need as we noted in Chapter 3 for dissensual decision-making (described fully in Chapter 13).

The premise of *mutual* respect marks one of the differences between values-based practice and some of the more regulatory moves in medical ethics, as reflected in the principle of autonomy of patient choice. As noted in Chapter 2, autonomy is an important principle of current medical ethics and law replacing earlier "doctor knows best" approaches. But the recent emphasis on autonomy has in some contexts had the (unintended) effect of replacing "doctor knows best" with an equally unbalanced principle of "patient knows best." This drift towards a consumerist model of clinical decision-making is evident in the shift noted earlier in this chapter from the "prudent doctor" Bolam test of negligence to a "prudent patient" test. The principle of mutual respect by contrast leads to partnership in decision-making based on a balance of both clinician and patient perspectives.

Balanced decision-making, partnership and dissensus

Mutual respect in values-based practice thus means respecting the values of staff as well as patients. Person-centered medicine, correspondingly, understood in terms of values-based practice, means *person-*centered and not just patient-centered. This carries with it, of course, the need outlined in Chapter 3 for a shift from pre-set "right outcomes" to a reliance on "good process" in clinical decision-making, a move that we characterized there as paralleling the shift from a totalitarian to a democratic model of political decision-making.

This is why good clinical skills are so fundamental to values-based practice. In the present case, Mr. Shah and Brenda Forest knew enough about conflict resolution to pull back from their standoff. In what followed between them, instead of pressing for resolution either way, they "gave each other space," as we put it in Chapter 7. Mr. Shah suggested and Brenda Forest readily accepted that they should get on with the various pre-operative assessment tests that had to be done and then come back for a further discussion about which surgical option to go for.

This further exercise of good communication skills would not, however, have led ultimately to a values-based resolution if this had meant either Mr. Shah or Brenda Forest simply acceding to the other. Coming to a consensus view in this way is, as we indicated in Chapter 2, an appropriate basis for partnership in decision-making in many contexts. In values-based practice, by contrast, the basis of partnership in decision-making is a dissensual process in which differences of values, instead of being subsumed one to another, are balanced according to the particular circumstances of a particular situation.

We look further at dissensus and its relationship with consensus in Chapter 13. Whether Mr. Shah and Brenda Forest would have been able to come to a dissensus is an open question. But as we indicated in Chapter 3, multidisciplinary team work can often make a vital contribution to the balance of values on which genuine partnership in decision-making critically depends.

Multidisciplinary team work

In values-based practice, as we will see in the next chapter, multidisciplinary team work is important not just for the diversity of *skills* that it represents but also for the diversity of team *values*. And one way in which the diversity of team values is important is in providing the balance of perspectives that is essential to dissensual decision-making.

We have not explored in any detail in this chapter the importance of the breast clinic nursing team in the story of Brenda Forest and Mr. Shah. It will be evident, though, from the little that has been said how important they, and others involved in the modern multidisciplinary approach to cancer care, are likely to have been in the further development of this story of person-centered medicine.

Sister Clare Moody, for instance, who headed up the nursing team, had wide experience of helping women faced with mastectomy to work through their concerns and fears. Brenda Forest would have had little hesitation in confiding her aspirations to Sister Moody. In her turn, Sister Moody, who had given her life to nursing and was now in her mid-50s and facing the bleak prospect of a lonely retirement, would have understood exactly where Brenda Forest with her "sex before survival" values was coming from.

Then again, in the multidisciplinary review of Brenda Forest's case, the oncologist, Dr. Brendon Roley, who had wider experience even than Mr. Shah of late-stage cancer but whose values were closer to the "good death" values of modern palliative care (see Chapter 13), would bring an important balance to the decision-making process.

These different balancing perspectives would have had little effect if Mr. Shah and his colleagues had not all been equally committed to a multidisciplinary approach. This is why values-based practice, as we noted in Chapter 3, contributes to, as well as draws on, multidisciplinary team work. Managing the diversity of professional and personal values of different team members is essential for effective multidisciplinary team work. Without this, there is a risk of failures of communication and of joined-up practice (Colombo *et al.*, 2003). Well managed, however, that same diversity of values becomes, as we will see in the next chapter, a positive and powerful resource for balanced values-based decision-making.

Chapter summary

In this chapter, the opening moves in a consultation between Mr. Shah and his patient Brenda Forest about the management of her early breast cancer have illustrated the role of values-based practice in relation to two kinds of values-related problem arising in person-centered medicine:

1. *Problems of mutual understanding.* Here the clinical skills for values-based practice were important, notably communication skills and awareness of values.
2. *Problems of conflicting values.* In moving towards conflict resolution other elements of values-based practice (besides clinical skills) were needed as well: its premise of mutual respect, its aim of balanced decision-making based on dissensus and its reliance for balanced decision-making on the diverse values (as well as skills) of the multidisciplinary team.

We hope that looking in detail at these two particular kinds of problem has helped to illustrate just how deeply the diversity of individual human values, of clinician as well as patient, are involved in any genuinely person-centered approach to clinical decision-making. Given this diversity, there can be no single right answer to what is "best," even in such a well researched area as breast cancer. Guidelines based on current research evidence and the experience of clinicians and patients indeed provide vital guidance. But in person-centered medicine, the final decision *is* personal. "Best" then, means "personal best." This is why, as we put it epigrammatically in the summary box at the start of this chapter, genuinely person-centered practice means person-*values*-centered practice.

References

Bolam v. Friern HMC [1957] 2 All ER 118.

Colombo, A., Bendelow, G., Fulford, K. W. M. and Williams, S. (2003). Evaluating the influence of implicit models of mental disorder on processes of shared decision making within community-based multidisciplinary teams. *Social Science & Medicine* **56**, 1557–70.

Fulford, K. W. M. and Woodbridge, K. (2007). Values-based Practice in Teaching and Learning. Ch 12 in Stickley, T. and Basset, T. (eds) *Teaching Mental Health*. London: JohnWiley & Sons, pp. 145–160.

Johnson, J., Roberts, C., Cox, C, *et al.* (1998). Breast cancer patients' personality style, age and treatment decision making. *Journal of Surgical Oncology* **3**, 183–6.

Lerman, C., Daly, M. and Walsh, W. (2006). Communication between patients with breast cancer and healthcare providers: determinants and implications. *Cancer* **72**, 2612–20.

NICE (2009) *Early and Locally Advanced Breast Cancer. Diagnosis and Treatment*. NICE Clinical Guideline 80. London: National Institute for Health and Clinical Excellence.

Rogers, A., Pilgrim D. and Lacey, R. (1993). *Experiencing Psychiatry: Users' Views of Services*. London: Macmillan Press.

Samanta, A. and Samanta, J. (2003). Legal standard of care: a shift from the traditional *Bolam* test. *Clinical Medicine* **3**, 443–6.

Schover, L. (1994). Sexuality and body image in younger women with breast cancer. *Journal of the National Cancer Institute* **16**, 177–82.

Stewart, M., Brown, J. B., Weston, J. W., McWhinney, I. R., McWilliam, C. L. and Freeman, T. R. (2003). *Patient-Centred Medicine: Transforming the Clinical Method*, 2nd edn. Oxford: Radcliffe Press.

Website

- Guidelines for counseling in infertility: http://ec.digaden.edu.mx/moodle/moodledata/99/03ginobs/101epi2tf3lbm/333a1301.pdf.

POINT

PROCESS

PREMISE

Balanced Decision-making
within a
Framework of Shared Values

Partnership

Two-feet Principle   Squeaky-wheel Principle   Science-driven Principle

Person-centered practice   Multidisciplinary teamwork

Awareness   Reasoning   Knowledge   Communication skills

Mutual Respect
for
Differences of Values

Map of values-based practice – multidisciplinary teamwork.

Risks in safeguarding children: team values as well as skills

9

Values-based practice element 6: the extended multidisciplinary team

Topics covered in this chapter

The importance of diverse team values (as well as knowledge and skills) in values-based practice is illustrated by the issues of risk and safety in a child protection case.

Other topics include:

- Risk assessment and values
- Strengths and limitations of protocols and procedural guidelines
- Balanced clinical judgment
- Diverse team values and person-values-centered care
- The "extended" multidisciplinary team.

Take-away message for practice

*Working in teams opens up a resource of **diverse value perspectives** that can support you in making balanced decisions in areas like risk assessment that require difficult judgment calls.*

Like person-centered care in the last chapter, values-based practice brings an extra dimension to multidisciplinary teamwork. Teamwork is important in modern health care in part because no single profession, let alone individual, can hope to encompass all the diverse knowledge and skills required for effective evidence-based practice in the increasingly complex environment of modern health care. But the complexity of modern health care, as we saw in Part 1, is a complexity as much of the *values*-base of practice as of its evidence-base. Correspondingly, teamwork is important in values-based practice as much for the diverse values that different team members bring to the decision-making process as for their diverse knowledge and skills.

In this chapter, we illustrate the importance of the diverse value perspectives of team members through the story of how a GP, Dr. Lee Chew, manages the child protection issues raised when a young mother, Jade Spence, arrives in an "Extras" clinic on a Friday evening concerned that her four-month-old baby, Brit, has become sore "down below." Although experience shows the innocent nature of most perineal complaints in childhood, Dr. Chew has alarm bells ringing on this occasion. He is faced with the possibility that there could have been abuse. Available protocols and guidelines make clear that the responsibility for safeguarding baby Brit rests firmly with Dr. Chew but offer him at best limited help with exactly how he should do this. There is no "perfect solution" here. By working collaboratively initially with an experienced practice nurse, Lyndsey Carlton, on the Friday evening and then with a wider circle of colleagues early the following week, Dr. Chew finds a way forward that:

- *balances* the risks of the various courses of action available to him in a way that proves acceptable to all those concerned (including Jade Spence);
- gives Dr. Chew as the interim "buck stopper" the *support and security* of multiple ownership; and
- allows the team as a whole to offer Jade Spence and her family *the help she was really seeking*.

The knowledge and skills that different team members brought to each stage of the decision-making process were important here. But so too were their different value perspectives.

Who's who?

As there are rather more people involved in this than in earlier stories, we have summarized the cast of characters in the order in which they appear in Fig. 9.1.

115

Characters in the Friday evening consultation
- **Patient:** baby Brit Spence, aged 4 months.
- **Family:** mother Jade Spence, with Griff, Jade's first child, now aged two and a half, in tow. Jade's current partner, Wayne Ball, is at home.
- **Responsible clinician:** Dr. Lee Chew, the GP who sees Brit and thus becomes responsible for safeguarding.
- **Liz Robson:** receptionist.
- **Lyndsey Carlton:** practice nurse who took the triage call and joins Dr. Chew in the consultation.
- **Dr. Steve Fawcett:** GP partner.

Other characters in the story:
- **Beth Stokes:** health visitor.
- **Dr. Dev Chowdhury:** consultant pediatrician.
- **Dr. Fauzia Hussein:** consortium lead for safeguarding.
- **Obioma Abiola:** case worker for Social Services.

Fig. 9.1 The characters involved in Brit's story.

The clinical context

It is Friday evening surgery and Dr. Lee Chew, a family doctor of many years' standing in the practice, sees that Brit Spence (aged just four months) is on the list to be seen as an extra following a triage call taken by the practice nurse, Lyndsey Carlton, earlier in the day for "sore bits down below." Although Dr. Chew has not seen Brit before (he checks that Brit is a girl), he knows her mother, Jade Spence, well. He reflects on what he knows about Jade while he takes a sip of his coffee before buzzing for her to be shown in. Jade Spence, he recalls, is 19 and unemployed, as is her current partner, Wayne Ball. She does occasional bar jobs and he believes Wayne works for cash to supplement their benefits.

Reflection point

To get a sense of the problem Dr. Chew faced here, you may find it helpful to try filling out the likely backgrounds of Jade Spence and her partner, Wayne Ball, a little for yourself before reading on.

Jade is 19 and, in addition to baby Brit, she already has a two-and-a-half-year-old child, Griff, possibly by another man. Neither she nor Wayne (her current partner and Brit's presumptive father) is in regular employment. The referral is for "sore bits down below."

What kind of narratives about Jade and Wayne do you think are likely to be running through Dr. Chew's mind as he readies himself for this triage referral on a Friday night?

What Dr. Chew knew

Shortly after Dr. Chew came to the practice, Jade Spence was excluded from school for glue sniffing, and he managed to establish quite a good working relationship with her by helping her to assert herself in a very troubled and somewhat violent home. He did not see much of her for a couple of years when she went off to live with a boyfriend, but she had returned to the area two years ago as a single parent to Griff who was now two and a half years old. Dr. Chew wrote a very strong letter of support for Jade and Griff to get a council flat when he learnt that she was expecting another baby last year. The family home was overcrowded, Jade's mum had developed a serious alcohol problem and, with her father often still violent towards her, it seemed all-in-all an unhealthy place in which to bring up children.

Wayne Ball he knew was not a local man. He came with Jade to some of her antenatal appointments, where Dr. Chew noted that he had "HATE" tattooed rather clumsily on his knuckles. This looked the sort of tattoo that might have been done by a bored prisoner and a two-year gap in Wayne Ball's medical records suggested that he could well have been "inside." There were a number of entries about drug dependency in Wayne's notes, although he had never consulted about drug issues in their practice.

Consultation on a Friday evening

With this background running through his mind, Dr. Chew presses the buzzer and in comes Jade Spence with baby Brit cradled in her left arm and Griff holding on tightly to her other hand. Griff, quickly summing up the situation, lets go of Jade's hand and makes a beeline for the toys in the children's corner. Asked what the problem is, Jade explains that she is worried about Brit having trouble "down below," and taking off the baby's nappy she reveals a sore perineum. Dr. Chew notes a lot of nappy rash generally but around the vulva there is definite swelling and he finds a little dried blood on the nappy.

"How did she get this sore, Jade?" Dr. Chew asks.

"I don't know, Doctor" Jade replies, "but she's that sore that she keeps scratching herself."

"Scratching inside her nappy?" Dr. Chew is now starting to get a little alarmed at the credibility gap opening up in the story and Jade's proffered explanation does nothing to reassure him.

"She don't have her nappy on all the time, Doctor, and Griff might have taken it off her – he could have fiddled with her a bit – you know what kids are like."

Alarm bells are by now ringing loud and clear in Dr. Chew's head, and he is thinking, "Why does this always happen on a Friday evening?"

Reflection point

You may like to think what you would do next in this situation. Irrespective of whether or not you are a clinician, or have any experience in this area, think about the interpersonal communication. What would you like to say to Jade at this point?

Cards on the table

Thinking rapidly how to play this, Dr. Chew decides to rely on his good relationship with Jade and adopt a straightforward approach.

"Look, Jade" he says kindly, "we have got a problem here. We really have to be very careful to understand what is happening with Brit. It may be that she has just got a little skin soreness. This can happen to any baby in nappies. But we do also have to think about the possibility that someone could be abusing her, and that can be very harmful to a little baby."

He lets the words sink in. Jade does not look shocked, but her face is worried. "I guess that's why I brought her, Doctor, but I don't want anything to happen to her."

With this answer, Dr. Chew perceives a gleam of light. He believes Jade and thinks she could become an ally in the formidable task of safeguarding a vulnerable baby. But he realizes he will have to be very careful not to frighten her into a defensive shell. He knows from his previous contact with her that she is nothing if not strong-minded and he is in no doubt that now as a mother she will fight like the proverbial tiger not to lose her children. So he needs to find a way of getting her to fight with him rather than against him while at the same time ensuring baby Brit's safety.

"You did the right thing, Jade," he says, ignoring a crash as Griff is happily demolishing a tractor in the corner. "Let's have a think about this together."

Alternative strategies here

Some of you might have wanted to ask Jade about her other concerns first. This might have been a more effective step than the one taken by Dr. Chew himself bringing up the possibility of abuse. We will see later that this would indeed have been productive. But this is with hindsight. With the pressures of a Friday night and with what Dr. Chew knew of the background to Jade's presentation, it is easy to see why he (as any of us might easily have done) moved so directly to what he saw as the crunch issue.

What Dr. Chew actually does is to involve a second clinician at this stage, the nurse practitioner, Lyndsey Carlton. And to anticipate a little, the bottom line of the chapter will be that it was by bringing together their different values as well as skills that they were able to find a balanced way forward between them in these difficult circumstances.

Building partnerships

Explaining that he needs to check who else is waiting to see him, Dr. Chew then rings Liz Robson, on reception. He tells Liz that he will not be able to see any more Friday evening "extras" as it is now 5.45 p.m. and he asks that the remaining two patients be diverted to Dr. Steve Fawcett, the other partner on duty. In reply to his question, Liz says that Beth Stokes, the health visitor, has gone home. This is a disappointment to Dr. Chew, as a health visitor, being a trained children's nurse who focuses on preventative medicine and family support, could bring valuable skills to bear here. Lyndsey Carlton, the nurse practitioner who took the call originally from Jade, is still around, tidying up the treatment room before she leaves for the weekend.

"Could you ask her to hold on a minute?" Dr. Chew asks, mentally thanking his lucky stars that Lyndsey is still in the practice. He is well aware from safeguarding protocols that it is important to widen the circle of people involved in making the decisions which are facing him, and he and Lyndsey had worked successfully together before on other difficult cases. In fact, Lyndsey Carlton had asked Liz Robson (the receptionist) to let her know when Jade Spence was coming. She suspected from her talk with Jade on the telephone that whoever saw her might need someone else with them and she had deliberately stayed on with the excuse of tidying up just in case.

Turning back to Jade, Dr. Chew asks, "You know you talked to nurse Lyndsey on the phone earlier? Would you mind if she joined us?" Jade readily agrees to this and Lyndsey comes in, perching herself on the examination couch under which Griff is now playing with his tractor.

It takes two

Between them, Lyndsey Carlton and Dr. Chew establish that Jade first noticed Brit's sore perineum the previous day when changing her nappy. It had got neither worse nor better since then. The only other time she had seen any blood was when Brit was about ten days old, and that was "round the back," where she had got very sore after a dirty nappy had been left on too long. On that occasion, Beth Stokes, the health visitor, had helped Jade sort out the problem with creams and advice about managing nappies. Dr. Chew then asks Jade about Wayne.

"And how's Wayne?" Dr. Chew asks. "Is he still around?"

"Yeah, he's at home now."

"What's he up to these days?"

"Not a lot. There's no work around, so he hangs around home most of the time. But he's quite useful with these two. We take them out together. And he can do anything with his hands."

"Does he help with nappy changing?"

"Sometimes he does. But" (suddenly looking defensive) ". . . he wouldn't hurt her, if that's what you're thinking."

"We aren't thinking *anything*, Jade." Dr. Chew's riposte comes back perhaps just a shade too quickly; and then, continuing after a pause but now palpably holding himself in check, "We are just trying to think *with you* about all the possibilities, so that between us we can make sure Brit is safe and well cared for. That's what you want too, isn't it?"

But Jade, now openly challenging as the full implications of what is going on start to sink in, persists, "You're not thinking about taking her away or anything, are you?"

Catching Dr. Chew's eye, Lyndsey Carlton picks up the interview.

"What we are trying to do," she says, "is to work with you, Jade, to help you look after Brit together, like the health visitor helped you before. You were a bit worried, which is why you were right to bring her here. When I had my babies, I was always at the doctor's! Dr. Chew is trying to understand what could have happened and then we can work out together how to help you look after Brit."

Reflection point

The interview has now clearly reached a critical point. Before reading on, you may want to think for a moment about what Lyndsey Carlton has just said and how Jade Spence is likely to react and why.

There is a key difference between what Dr. Chew and Lyndsey Carlton, respectively, bring to the interview at this point. What is it?

Jade Spence's reaction to Lyndsey Carlton's intervention is that she relaxes a little and, although still looking decidedly wary, a feeling of trust comes back into the interview.

So, what made the difference? Why was Jade Spence starting to bristle with Dr. Chew but then calms down when Lyndsey Carlton comes into the interview saying almost the same as Dr. Chew? Lyndsey Carlton and Dr. Chew both endorsed Jade's initiative in bringing her baby to the clinic and both talked in terms of working together to make sure she was well looked after; moreover, both drew on essentially the same knowledge and skills in approaching the interview with Jade Spence in this inclusive way. The difference, however – and it was a crucial difference at this critical stage in the interview – was that Lyndsey Carlton as a "mum" was able to bring a perspective to the interview with Jade Spence that Dr. Chew could not. Implicit in the mum's perspective is *a shared set of values* that Lyndsey could claim to share with Jade where Dr. Chew could not. Additionally, Lyndsey is on the same side of the male/female gender divide, which may for some people be value-laden in child rearing. Perhaps more importantly, she is closer to Jade in terms of power balance.

Values in the interview

In talking about values here, we need to be careful on two points. First, the difference between Dr. Chew and Lyndsey Carlton really was a difference in the way their respective values affected their perspective on the situation more than the way it affected their empathic understanding for Jade. The difference was one of degree of course, but it was critical nonetheless in driving how each of them reacted as they approached the "crunch" issue of whether baby Brit was safe to remain at home over the weekend.

- Dr. Chew's reaction as the GP responsible was, as we have seen, to become more anxious and then defensive – the buck, after all, stopped with him if he failed to take Brit away from the family home and things "went wrong" over the weekend.
- Lyndsey Carlton, on the other hand, who was not under the pressure of direct responsibility for safeguarding, was able to build on her shared values with Jade as a mother fighting for her child.

Jade Spence no doubt picked all this up partly from what was actually said, notably Lyndsey Carlton's reference to her own children ("When I had my babies I was always at the doctor's!") and perhaps even more strongly from their respective body languages. Either way, with Jade Spence partially reassured through Lyndsey Carlton's intervention, the interview got back on to a more collaborative footing.

But that brings us to the second point about which we need to be careful when talking about values, namely that what was important in the interview was, simply, *different* values and *not* right or wrong values. This becomes immediately clear when we look at how the interview progressed from this point. Lyndsey Carlton's "family over safeguarding" values (if we can summarize it this way) may have got the interview back on track. But now Dr. Chew's "safeguarding over family" values ensured that they were not sidetracked from the main issue but pressed on with the hard questions.

Back to the interview

"Who else visits the house, Jade?" Dr. Chew (his equanimity restored) asks kindly. There is a pause as Jade looks at the floor.

"I guess you know Wayne has a bit of a habit, Doctor. I don't do more than the odd spliff myself but Wayne, he's into baseballing – coke, you know. He does a bit of dealing – they all do these days, and so there's quite a lot of people come to the house, some of them right weirdoes."

"Are there any that you are particularly worried about?"

"Yeah, one or two. There's this creep, Whizzer, who stinks, and he's always trying to grab at me. Wayne says he'll kill him if he catches him after me."

"Could Whizzer or anyone get alone with the baby?"

"I don't think so, but I don't know. I have to pop out sometimes, like when I take Griff to nursery, and sometimes I leave Brit with Wayne indoors."

Decision time deferred

With Griff tugging at his knee and trying to show him his tractor, Dr. Chew realizes that he needs to draw some threads out of his by now tangled thoughts and come to a decision about how to manage the situation over the weekend. Still far from sure what to do, he is nonetheless about to turn the interview in the direction of perhaps Brit being "safer away from Wayne and his friends" until we have got things sorted out, when Brit herself (who up to this point has been lying

contentedly in Jade's arms) reminds them of her presence by starting to cry rather loudly.

"Sorry, Doctor," Jade explains. "The receptionist was just going to find me somewhere where I could feed her when your buzzer went. I'm still breast-feeding . . . would it be OK?" she adds hesitantly.

Dr. Chew, inwardly breathing a sigh of relief for a decision deferred, says immediately that of course that would be fine. Lyndsey Carlton, however, offers instead to go with them round to the next-door consulting room (which would by now be free) so that Jade can give Brit her feed in peace while she and Griff see if they "can make that tractor work."

Lyndsey Carlton accordingly takes Griff in tow and, as the family troop out, Dr. Chew sits back in his chair and tries to sort out his ideas . . .

Protocols and guidelines

In this section, we will be following Dr. Chew as he tries to decide what to do. As with other situations of this kind, we will be making his thought processes rather more explicit than they would have been to a tired and troubled Dr. Chew late on a Friday evening. But drawing out his thoughts in this way will illustrate both the strengths and limitations of protocols and guidelines in supporting difficult judgment calls in demanding situations of the kind in which Dr. Chew was now placed.

Tangled thoughts

We will start with a brief reflection on what was likely to have been in Dr. Chew's mind as he watched Lyndsey Carlton usher Jade and her children out of his room.

Reflection point

What do you think is likely to be going through Dr. Chew's mind at this point?

Don't try to organize Dr. Chew's thoughts here or to come to a decision in your own mind about what he should do. The idea here is simply to do a "brainstorming" exercise to get a sense of the competing considerations that are likely to be in Dr. Chew's mind as he struggles with this difficult Friday night decision.

We give our own brainstorm in Fig. 9.2 in the form of a "cloud diagram." The various "clouds" are not in any particular order but instead offer a visual representation of Dr. Chew's own tangled state of mind.

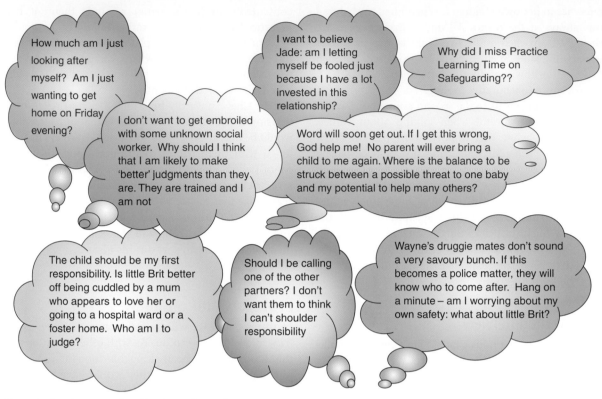

Fig. 9.2. Cloud diagram of Dr. Chew's initial thoughts.

Again, as with previous similar exercises, we imagine our brainstorm will be similar in some respects to yours and different in others. One shared thought is likely to be Dr. Chew's dilemma about what to do (represented by the bottom left cloud): he has a direct safeguarding responsibility towards Brit, however the evidence of possible abuse is circumstantial and there is a risk of serious long-term harm if the children end up being taken away for no good reason from a mother who shows every sign of warmth and care. But there is a good deal more going on in Dr. Chew's mind than just this central dilemma.

We return to the significance of the full range of Dr. Chew's tangled thoughts in a moment. First, we need to follow him a little further as he tries to bring order out of chaos by looking at one of the many published protocols and guidelines on safeguarding.

The PCT protocol

"Let's see what our local guidelines have to say," Dr. Chew says to himself as he reaches up to the shelves over his desk – a repository of countless guidelines and protocols. Between a pamphlet on disfigurement and last year's pediatric BNF (British National Formulary) he finds what he is looking for: the local Primary Care Trust (PCT) *General Practice Protocol for Safeguarding Children* dated three years previously. Making a mental note to spend some time updating his guidelines, he turns to the relevant page. We give an extract of what he found in Fig. 9.3.

> **Reflection point**
>
> What do you think of this protocol? Does it help Dr. Chew? What do you think Dr. Chew himself thought about it?

A muttered "Thanks a lot" is what Dr. Chew thinks about this protocol. He was broadly familiar with the protocol already, of course, but had hoped he had forgotten some "gem" that might have resolved his dilemma. Clearly written by a lawyer (with its embedded cross-references), the main thrust of the protocol

In the event of a GP becoming aware of, or suspecting that a child has suffered significant harm, he/she should consult the Trust Child Protection guidelines 2.1–2.42, and take the following actions:

- Share concerns with other clinical staff (GP, Health Visitor, and School Nurse) in order to build up a fuller picture and clarify if other concerns have been identified
- If a GP is concerned that significant harm may have occurred, or is occurring, the suspicion should be discussed and a referral made to Social Care using the Inter-Agency Referral Form
- Record, date, and sign all actions
- It is the GP's responsibility to pass on details of the referral to:
  - The patient/parent unless doing so increases risk of harm to the child
  - Named Health Visitor and/or School Nurse
  - Members of the Primary Health Care Team, Safeguarding Children and Families Team as appropriate.

Please Note

GPs are accountable for their own actions under General Medical Council Guidelines. Guidance for GPs relating to Safeguarding Children is available within Good Medical Practice 24–28. (GMC 2006)

Fig. 9.3. Extract from the PCT safeguarding protocol.

1. Morally and legally we must place Brit's best interests first. Our responsibility is to her and her safety and well-being are paramount.
2. We don't *know* that any harm at all has happened to her. She may be sore for perfectly innocent reasons. But it could also be that she has been molested, and if so she is in danger of it happening again.
3. There are lots of people we need to consult including Beth Stokes and some of the children's experts in the practice and at the hospital.
4. Jade, I am sure, has Brit's interests at heart; otherwise she would not have brought her here tonight.
5. Although ideally we would get Brit to the hospital for some tests straight away, I am not sure that Friday night is the ideal time for that either . . .
6. . . . and once we have raised concerns with the duty team, there is no going back.
7 If we end up with Brit (and probably Griff into the bargain) being torn away from Jade, who is clearly a caring and affectionate mother, is that really in anyone's best interests – especially if it turns out that there has been no abuse?

Fig. 9.4. Dr. Chew's checklist of issues.

was to remind him (if reminder were needed) that the buck stopped with him.

Needless to say, he has no copy of the said "Inter-Agency Referral Form" to hand. But he decides to start organizing his thoughts by making a checklist of the issues that he thinks he will have to cover when he writes his referral. We give a tidied up version of his checklist in Fig. 9.4.

> **Reflection point**
>
> What do you think of Dr. Chew's checklist? How does it compare with his thoughts in the cloud diagram in Fig. 9.2?

Perhaps the most striking thing about Dr. Chew's checklist is that, at first glance, it bears little relation to the cloud diagram of thoughts going through his mind just a few minutes earlier. The only obvious overlap is the primacy of baby Brit's best interests (point 1 on Dr. Chew's list of issues and bottom left in the cloud diagram). Closer inspection, however, shows that the two lists are in fact deeply related and in ways that illustrate both the strengths and limitations of protocols of the kind prepared by the PCT's lawyers.

- *Strengths*: the protocol has focused Dr. Chew's mind firmly on his prime responsibility to ensure Brit's best interests. This, as we have seen, has now

been made explicit in point 1 (i.e. right at the top of Dr. Chew's list) and the protocol has also reminded him of some of the key steps he should consider taking in this respect: wide consultation (point 3), including a hospital referral for further tests (point 5).

- The protocol has further helped Dr. Chew to draw out and highlight some of the hazards of precipitous action: the harm to the children of being separated from a loving mother (point 7) who clearly has their best interests at heart (point 4), especially if after all it turns out there has been no abuse (point 2). He is acutely aware that experienced staff may be thin on the ground at this time on a Friday night (point 5) and that there will be no "going back" once he has raised his concerns with the "duty team" (point 6).
- *Limitations*: so far so good, and yet the protocol had taken him no further towards an actual decision about what to do. There were indeed two limitations of the protocol in this respect, one of which Dr. Chew was aware and one of which he was not. The limitation of which Dr. Chew was aware was that, as his muttered "Thanks a lot" testified, the protocol, although indeed clarifying the horns of his dilemma, left him as the buck stopper firmly impaled thereon.
- The limitation of which Dr. Chew was not aware was that the protocol in focusing his mind firmly on Brit's best interests had by the same token deflected him from all the competing interests that,

121

as we put it above, were also tangled up in his thinking about what to do. In terms of the distinction we introduced in Chapter 1 then, the protocol had effectively highlighted the foreground interests (Brit's best interests in this case) but at the expense of a number of background interests.

From a narrowly legal point of view, the effectiveness of the protocol in focusing Dr. Chew on the foreground (Brit's best interests) at the expense of the background (all the other elements in Dr. Chew's thinking) may seem like a "good thing": the central concern in this case as we have emphasized several times is indeed Brit's best interests. But as we saw in Chapter 1 (and again when we looked at awareness of values in Chapter 4), background values, too, may critically influence decisions and actions.

We will return shortly to exactly how critically Dr. Chew's background thoughts (although he was largely unaware of them) were influencing him at this point. But that they were *likely* to be influencing him is evident from the extent to which Dr. Chew's background thoughts were thoughts about his *own interests*.

Thus, one cloud (bottom left), as we have noted, was concerned with the central dilemma facing Dr. Chew about Brit's best interests. But the remaining seven clouds (which have now largely disappeared from the foreground of Dr. Chew's thinking) are all in one way or another not about Brit's interests but about the interests of Dr. Chew: his need to get home on a Friday night; his "investment" in his relationship with Jade; his wish to be thought by his partners capable of standing on his own feet; his plain fear of Wayne's "druggy mates"; and above all (in his "God help me if I get this wrong!" cloud) a worry about his reputation as a doctor. He wraps this worry up in a (utilitarian) justification about ensuring that he remains in a position to help other children in the future. But this is mere sophistry. Dr. Chew's real fear (and it is a fear with which many of us will readily identify) is that he will find himself at the center of the next high-profile child protection scandal.

For the moment, then, much that was available to Dr. Chew in self-understanding from his original (tangled) thinking has now been lost to view in his post-protocol-reading checklist of issues. None of his self-interested thoughts is a matter for criticism, it is important to emphasize. We have surely all "been there" with Dr. Chew. The point is rather that, in displacing these thoughts from his awareness while leaving them still very much in play in the background, the PCT protocol (although helpful in other respects)

had (in this respect) actually impaired Dr. Chew's ability to come a balanced judgment about Brit's best interests.

The BMA toolkit

Aware that Jade Spence and her family ware likely to reappear with Lyndsey Charlton at any moment, Dr. Chew starts a final quick search for further guidance.

Googling "Safeguarding Children England" on his computer brings up "Child Protection – a toolkit for doctors" by the British Medical Association (BMA) and this seems more promising. Skimming the different "cards" into which the toolkit is helpfully organized, he picks up much that reassures him that he is at least not wholly out of line in hesitating before leaping in with both feet on the full safeguarding procedures. This is broadly how his thoughts ran as he scanned through the toolkit:

- *The primary responsibility is to the child's "best interests"* (p. 3, and again on p. 6). "No problem there," he says to himself, "but the issue is *what* exactly is Brit's best interests here?"
- *This has to be judged on its merits* (p. 4). "Again, fine, but back to me as the buck stopper!"
- *We should seek to work with parents (p. 6/7)*. "Very much what Lyndsey and I are doing then, and good to see this emphasized – it's undoubtedly in Brit's best interests that we build on our good relationship with Jade, and indeed try to build up Jade's confidence in us and in herself as a mother."
- "Interesting that there's nothing much here about the actual signs of sexual abuse . . . although signs of physical and social/emotional abuse are covered in detail. It's clearly a difficult area then."
- *Write everything down.* "Yes, we're good at record keeping in our practice."
- "Ah! A whole card about what to do when you have initial concerns" (card 7) . . . *important to involve others* ("Yes, doing that") and you . . . *may consider the evidence too uncertain to warrant the immediate commencement of child care proceedings* (p. 17).

So, Dr. Chew reflects, sitting back again in his chair as he takes in this last proviso, it's clear that there is no absolute obligation to launch in with the full safeguarding process in this case and perhaps good grounds not to. "So, *why am I still so reluctant to let Jade take Brit home?*"

The (unwelcome) crunch

And then Lee Chew had a quick look at the site of the Royal College of General Practitioners (RCGP). Much of what was said in the *Keep Me Safe* document (developed in 2009 by the RCGP and National Society for the Prevention of Cruelty to Children (NSPCC)) was similar to the BMA guidance, but one particular section caught his eye. We have reproduced what he found of relevance about "barriers to implementation" in Fig. 9.5.

Reflection point

At this point, you may find it helpful to reflect for a moment on Fig. 9.5 before reading on.

Dr. Chew has found broad endorsement in the BMA toolkit for his hesitation over simply calling up the duty social worker and starting a full-scale safeguarding process. Clinically, it would be entirely consistent with the guidelines to proceed cautiously. And yet he finds himself very reluctant not to "press the button."

The "Barriers" section seems intended to encourage practitioners to move in the direction of "pressing the button," but an aspect of the focus here helps to clarify the issues for Dr. Chew and brings him to the crunch. Where do you think the focus helped him, and what do you think he decides to do?

What struck Dr. Chew as he read this section was that his reluctance not to involve the duty safeguarding team arose primarily not from a concern about Brit's best interests but from his own concern for "relationships" and "trust." In that moment of unwelcome self-awareness, everything fell into place. There was no ducking the fact that, while of course he could not be certain, it was on the evidence to date unlikely, perhaps very unlikely, that Brit was being sexually abused. Whether other people would see it like that next week with 20:20 hindsight if things went wrong over the weekend was an entirely different matter. That, he now realized, was exactly what he was really worried about. But with this realization went the further and more painful (to him) realization of the harms that were likely to have accrued to this little family if he had (as he had so nearly done) started a course of action that had ended up with Brit and quite possibly Griff too being dragged away from a distraught and demoralized Jade. It was clear then on balance where Brit's best interests lay . . .

And then with a sudden retreat . . .

Normalising the problem:
We should not be more tolerant of neglectful behaviour where there is material deprivation. Neglect is more common where there is deprivation, but deprivation does not cause neglect.

Not seeing the child:
We must put the needs of the child above all others (*The Children Act 1989 Paramountcy Principle 48*) and see the child, not just the parents. The needs of the child can easily be overshadowed by those of the parents.

Not looking:
There is no doubt that child abuse is upsetting. It is easier to ignore the problem or seek other, more comfortable explanations for our observations.

Doing nothing:
Acknowledging that there is a problem can cause a lot of work and strife. It is less trouble, at least in the short term, to do nothing.

Relationships:
We are often concerned for our relationship with the family; they will be angry and upset and we may fear for our safety if we raise the issue of child abuse. The family may feel betrayed by us if we express our concerns. Relationships may be fragile anyway or we may feel that the family is doing their best under very difficult circumstances.

Trust:
Our relationship with our patients is founded on trust and mutual respect. Where there are suspicions of child abuse, we have to adopt a much more assertive and forensic approach that cuts across this relationship of trust.

© **Royal College of General Practitioners & National Society for the Prevention of Cruelty to Children**

Fig. 9.5. Some of the barriers for healthcare professionals in recognizing and responding to child abuse, identified in these extracts from *Keep Me Safe*, the RCGP strategy for Child Protection.

"That's all very well," his mind threw back at him, "but I'm not a saint. Can I take the risk?"

But before he could answer his own rhetorical question, the door opened and Jade, Brit and Griff, with a smiling Lyndsey Carlton beside them, were coming back into the room.

Decision time

Still uncertain of his final decision, Dr. Chew, looking Jade straight in the eye, asks, "Jade, do you think you can make sure that Brit is never out of your sight, even for five minutes, over the whole weekend? We *have* to accept that it is possible that someone, we don't know who, could have harmed her, and if we are going to keep her in the family over the weekend, we have to know that you are keeping her safe. Can you do that?"

"Yes, Doctor, I can do that," Jade replies. "She won't ever be out of my sight and she sleeps beside me at night."

Turning to Lyndsey Carlton, Dr. Chew says, "Lyndsey, what do you think? Can Jade really manage this OK, given everything that is going on at home?"

"Jade has been telling me a lot more about how Wayne looks after them all," Lyndsey replies. "I'm sure they can manage over the weekend."

Dr. Chew now makes up his mind. "Right, Jade, so this is what we will do. I am going to give you some cream for Brit, called Cetraben, and you can dab that on the sore spots gently at every nappy change. You must do *all* the changes yourself and never ever let her out of your sight at any stage. That means you are going to have to be quite clever with Griff, having him sorted out with toys every time you have to change Brit. You must be ever so careful to stay sharp and on the ball all weekend, so that means you must not have a drink or do spliffs, and if they ask you out to the pub, you will have to say no. Is that clear?"

"Yes, Doctor."

"Here is my mobile phone number – it will be switched on all weekend and if you have any concerns whatsoever, I want you to call me day or night. I need to trust you to do that. If you can't get hold of me, then just dial 999 and tell them the doctor said the baby needs safeguarding and they will know what to do. I want you to bring Brit back at ten o'clock on Monday morning to see Beth Stokes, the health visitor who helped you before. You may be here for quite a while as we work out what to do for her. Will Griff be in nursery?"

"Yes Doctor."

"Very well, we'll see you then – and Jade," he adds, "you did the right thing bringing Brit to see us." Jade smiles at them both. "And get here on time on Monday or we'll be worrying about you!"

Jade, gathering up her things, takes the prescription and leaves with her chin up.

De-brief

After the door had closed, Lyndsey Carlton described to Dr. Chew how Jade had opened up to her while she was breast-feeding. And what Jade had told Lyndsey in the very different context of talking mother to mother in an informal way had revealed the situation at home in a very different and more positive light.

Wayne Ball, it turned out, was father to both Jade's children. But as Dr. Chew had suspected, he had been in prison for a period after Griff was born and it was at this time that Jade had come home. She had, however, visited Wayne regularly while he was inside and they had done their best to set up home together when he came out (they both knew that Dr. Chew's letter of support had made this possible). Wayne had tried hard to find a job (he had done a woodworking course in prison), but his record had been against him and he had gradually slipped back

into his old habits. But there was a whole other side to Wayne Ball when it came to his family. Wayne had been brought up mainly in care, and from what Jade said (and the way she had said it), it was clear to Lyndsey that whatever Wayne's faults, Jade, Griff and Brit now meant everything to him.

None of this guaranteed that Wayne (or more likely one of his drug-dealing contacts) was not abusing Brit, but it clearly showed that, as parents, Wayne as well as Jade had actual and potential strengths on which to build. The balance of benefits and harms had thus seemed to the experienced Lyndsey Carlton to have come down firmly in favor of keeping the family together over the weekend with appropriate support and with a view to pulling together a robust care plan for them with a wider team of colleagues the following week. Hence her smiling demeanor when she brought Jade and her children back into Dr. Chew's consulting room and her subsequent confident support for Jade in reply to Dr. Chew's direct question about her ability to keep Brit safe over the weekend.

Roles and values

Before we finish this chapter, we will be giving you a brief progress report on how things worked out for Jade, Wayne and their children. We will see that a much wider team was needed to take things forward successfully from this point. But to understand the importance of different team values (alongside their respective knowledge and skills) in multidisciplinary teamwork, it will be worth looking first in a little more detail at the precise roles played by Dr. Chew and Lyndsey Carlton in coming to this critical Friday evening decision. There are three key questions to consider here:

1. Who made the decision? Dr. Chew had clinical responsibility. Did he exercise that responsibility?
2. How did Lyndsey Carlton contribute to the decision?
3. Who else besides Dr. Chew and Lyndsey Carlton contributed to the decision?

> **Reflection point**
>
> What would your own answers be to these questions?
>
> As we will see, they take us to the heart of the extended multidisciplinary team of values-based practice. So you may find it helpful to think what your own answers would be before reading on.

Dr. Chew's decision

The answer to the first question is "yes," the decision was indeed made by Dr. Chew. A common misunderstanding about multidisciplinary teamwork is that it ends up with no one being responsible. That was clearly not the case here. Dr. Chew was throughout acutely aware that the safeguarding responsibility rested firmly with him and that this meant acting in Brit's best interests.

It was (Dr. Chew felt at the time) bad luck that he had got landed with this responsibility, particularly at this time on a Friday evening – "particularly" because in normal working hours he could have passed on the case to various safeguarding experts with a fair degree of confidence that they would not go "over the top" in how they responded. Still, things are as they are. The case *was* his. It *was* Friday evening. For better or worse, *he* had to decide what in all the circumstances to do. And for better or worse, after much deliberation, he *did* decide what to do.

As we indicated earlier, it might seem easy with hindsight to criticize Dr. Chew's decision. Was he overconcerned about exposure to possible criticism on the grounds of over-reacting? Was he realistic about the risks of exposing himself to criticism for his decision not to raise the alarm? Additionally, you might criticize Dr. Chew on grounds of accessibility, responsibility and professionalism in giving his own phone number – if he does this, can he really be accessible all the time? Has he missed the opportunity for taking vital swabs on this Friday evening (a point picked up later by the pediatric consultant)?

Few decisions are perfect, just as few are beyond the reach of criticism in retrospect, but – and this is where the extended multidisciplinary team comes in – he could not have made *the actual decision he ended up making* on his own. It is always reassuring to have the support of others, even when we accept full responsibility and accountability for a difficult decision. But here there was more than support. Crucial to his decision was the balance of *values as well as skills* of a teamwork approach.

Lyndsey Carlton's role in the interview

This is where Lyndsey Carlton's role was critical. We saw this earlier in the chapter when her intervention defused a developing standoff between Jade Spence and Dr. Chew. The operative aspect of her role at this stage as we also saw was her values. She exercised

similar knowledge and skills as Dr. Chew. But as a mother her "family over safeguarding" values chimed with Jade's and for the moment partially reassured her, thus getting the interview back on a constructive footing. We noted the importance of values in this "conflict-resolving" respect in Chapter 7. In the present case, though, it is important to remember that Dr. Chew's complementary "safeguarding over family" values were equally important in ensuring that the hard issues were picked up from that point in the interview rather than being ducked.

So it "takes two," as we said. Neither Lyndsey Carlton nor Dr. Chew had, in some sense external to the situation, the "right" values. *Both* sets of values were important. Similar considerations applied again later on in the interview when Lyndsey Carlton offered to take Jade to the next-door consulting room so that she could breast-feed Brit. Her offer was motivated partly by simple fellow feeling for Jade: Lyndsey had breast-fed her own babies. But she had also grasped the moment for the more directly professional reason that she wanted to see what Jade had to say about things when she was with her on her own. She knew from experience that patients often opened up to her as a nurse about things that they had felt inhibited for one reason or another to say to a doctor (and of course this also works the other way).

Lyndsey Carlton's role in the decision

This proved to be the case here, as we have seen. The more positive picture of the family that Lyndsey Carlton in her role as a nurse and mother was able to build up resulted in a more balanced understanding of the problem. Non-verbally, she communicated a higher level of confidence to Dr. Chew and from this there came a more balanced decision about what to do.

Again, it was Lyndsey Carlton's role as mediated by her values that was crucial. We can see this if we remind ourselves briefly of the steps in Dr. Chew's thinking. Initially, before Brit intervenes with her demands to be fed, Dr. Chew is moving towards starting the safeguarding process. There is no problem with that in principle, of course. But his initial reflections on what to do when he is left on his own (as represented in our cloud diagram) suggest that, had he started a safeguarding process at this stage, his decision would have been driven not by a balanced view of Brit's best interests but rather by his fear of finding himself at the center of a media frenzy over the next safeguarding scandal.

Reading the PCT guidelines actually made a decision to start the safeguarding process more likely (by focusing more or less exclusively on the clinician's responsibilities), and even when Dr. Chew was helped to focus on relationships and trust by the *Keep Me Safe* guidance, he was very far from actually feeling brave enough to, as he puts it, "risk it": take Brit away and whatever long-term harms follow will not so far as the world is concerned be laid at his door, but leave Brit with Jade at home and things go wrong and he will be in the firing line. Dr. Chew would not have been happy with himself had he decided to take Brit away (he knew in his heart by this stage that on clinical grounds it was not the right thing to do), but would he (or any of us similarly placed) have done other than this had he been on his own?

A balanced decision

What makes the difference, what finally brings Dr. Chew to his decision to leave Brit with Jade over the weekend, is the smiling relaxed family that Lyndsey Carlton brings back into the room. When the door opens, remember, Dr. Chew is still agonizing over what to do. It is not clear to him exactly when he decides to "risk it." There is indeed no "crunch" big decision consciously taken. Rather, his mind is made up for him at this moment when he sees Jade and her children coming back into his room, no longer as a "problem" to be solved but as a family.

Dr. Chew still has to test his decision, of course. Here, the confident way in which Lyndsey Carlton felt able to endorse Jade's ability to keep Brit safe over the weekend was an important reality check for Dr. Chew. He had come to his decision to trust Jade still with a feeling of putting his professional reputation on the line. But now Lyndsey Carlton's supportive endorsement gave him confidence that he had not "lost it" (and Dr. Chew's confidence in turn was not lost on Jade). And the plan that they agreed between them (Jade now very much included) for managing the situation over the weekend reflected a balanced combination of the values that Dr. Chew and Lyndsey Carlton had respectively brought to the consultation. In other words, Dr. Chew's "safeguarding over family" values working together with Lyndsey Carlton's "family over safeguarding" values had produced a well-balanced "family *plus* safeguarding" risk-management plan to which Jade was fully committed.

Clearly, they still needed to find out what was really going on at home. But that could now be picked up properly on Monday with a foundation of trust on which to build and hence with much improved prospects for taking things forward with the family in a way that would be genuinely helpful to them in the long term. They would be keeping their fingers crossed meantime. But with the additional positive background information about the family that Dr. Chew got from Lyndsey Carlton in their subsequent de-briefing session, he felt he would sleep more easily over the intervening weekend.

It takes two

It takes two then, as we said. Again, this really does mean, in contexts of this kind, two different sets of *values*. Dr. Chew, however empathic and experienced he might have been, simply could not (literally could not) be in Lyndsey Carlton's shoes as well as his own. A balanced understanding of the presenting problem depended on bringing together his values as the clinician responsible for safeguarding with Lyndsey Carlton's values as a nurse and with her background as a mother. Their knowledge and skills were, of course, also important. But in this instance they were on a par in terms of knowledge and skills. It was their different values that provided the crucial balance in how they deployed their shared knowledge and skills.

The "two" that it takes, furthermore, really does mean, in contexts of this kind, two *different* sets of values. A mere second opinion from the same perspective won't do. This is one reason why the extended multidisciplinary team of values-based practice really does have to be *multi*disciplinary. We saw in Chapter 6 (on knowledge of values) the remarkable extent to which people with different professional roles and backgrounds bring different values as well as different knowledge and skills to their work (Colombo *et al.*, 2003). In the present case, the critical balance of values that Dr. Chew and Lyndsey Carlton brought to the situation directly reflected their distinct professional backgrounds and roles in the consultation. But had Lyndsey Carlton gone home and had Dr. Chew consequently been thrown back on a second opinion from his GP colleague, Steve Fawcett, things would have gone very differently.

We can see this from the way Steve Fawcett reacted to the decision later when he and Lee Chew talked briefly as they were closing the practice down for the evening.

"You're right out on a limb there, Lee." Steve Fawcett said looking worried. "Why on earth didn't you ring the duty social worker and talk it over straight away?"

Dr. Chew was not actually asking for a second opinion here. But had he been, Dr. Fawcett's view, far from providing a balancing perspective, would have unbalanced it further. As we have emphasized several times, this is not a matter of a right or wrong perspective. The point is that Dr. Fawcett's view of the problem reflected the same "clinician responsible for safeguarding" perspective as Dr. Chew's and without the benefit of a balancing perspective from Lyndsey Carlton.

It takes a team

Finally then, and briefly, in reply to our third question at the start of this section, although we have focused on Dr. Chew and Lyndsey Carlton as a team of two, they were, of course, not working in isolation. The extended multidisciplinary team of values-based practice is, if we may put it this way, extended in form (extending to non-clinical as well as clinical team members) as well as function (extending to team values as well as team knowledge and skills).

We have had examples of this in earlier chapters (recall, for example, the key role played by Jenny Khan, the non-professionally aligned Support Time and Recovery (STR) mental health worker in raising awareness of Sally Coombs' true aspirations in Chapter 4) and it is clear too in this story. In the first place, Jade herself had to have the courage to ask for help. Then again, her confidence in coming to the practice for help was born partly of her earlier experience of how she had been treated. Dr. Chew's support for her when she first came back to the area was important here. So, too, was that of the health visitor, Beth Stokes, in sorting out the practical aspects of managing nappies. And when Jade arrived for her appointment, the motherly way she was treated by Liz Robson, the receptionist, was foundational in setting the tone for everything else that followed: you will recall that Liz Robson was about to find Jade somewhere to breast-feed Brit when Dr. Chew's buzzer went.

Finally, Dr. Fawcett's collegial willingness to pick up a few extra patients was vital in that this gave Dr. Chew and Lyndsey Carlton the space to get to understand the situation properly and thus to come to a decision about what to do based on what the family was really like rather than the opening narratives they brought with them. What Dr. Chew knew (as we put it at the start of this chapter) by way of background was all true. But it was what he did *not* know at this stage (in particular about the family's potential strengths) that was to prove crucial to the

way the consultation came out and indeed to how the story went on from there.

A progress report

So how did things go? In this final section, we will be giving our promised progress report. In a word, things went well. Dr. Chew marshaled his forces early the following Monday: he alerted Beth Stokes, the health visitor; he rang his pediatric colleague at the local hospital, Dr. Dev Chowdhury; and he liaised with the consortium lead for safeguarding, Dr. Fauzia Hussein. Jade Spence turned up on time and on this occasion with her partner, Wayne Ball, by her side (they had taken Griff to his nursery en route). Brit's soreness was improved but Jade welcomed a check-up from Dr. Chowdhury at the hospital, which he had offered later that morning. A practice case conference was convened for the next day after morning surgery that Dr. Chowdhury also came in on by telephone.

There were a number of outcomes from the case conference, but we will focus here on just two in particular that highlight two key "take away" messages about the extended multidisciplinary team. These two take away messages are in effect two counterpart messages that run through this book as a whole. They are: (i) the importance of evidence-based practice as a partner to values-based practice, and, conversely, (ii) the importance of values-based practice as a partner to evidence-based practice.

Evidence-based practice as a partner to values-based practice

Although focusing in this chapter on the importance of diverse team values, we have repeatedly emphasized the parallel importance of diverse knowledge and skills. As in all other areas of practice then, values (and thus values-based practice) and evidence (and thus evidence-based practice) are complementary.

The importance of the evidence side of multidisciplinary teamwork was apparent in the case conference from the contributions in particular of the pediatrician, Dr. Dev Chowdhury. He had seen Jade Spence and Brit by the time of the case conference, but his written report had not yet come through. Dr. Chew and his colleagues were thus relieved that, apart from a reminder that swabs and perhaps (with the mother's consent) a photograph might have been taken on the Friday evening, he was very supportive of the way the presentation had been managed and agreed that, on balance, it was unlikely that there had been any sexual abuse. He then went on to fill out his view. Here is part of what he said:

"I am pleased to say that, as I expected, I found no evidence of sexual abuse of this infant. We can't be absolutely sure, of course, but the usual forms of penetrative abuse (penile, digital or using an object) result in small tears around the fragile mucosa. I found no evidence of this and I gather, Lee, that you saw nothing like this on Friday evening." (Lee nods confirmation.) "By far and away the most common vulvovaginitis that we see is a form of nappy rash, either infective or ammoniacal. We've taken routine swabs and will also check for sexually transmitted organisms. But in fact things have settled down quite a lot already on your Cetraben treatment, Lee, and we are not expecting any surprises from the swabs. Rachel Wadd, our lead nurse who gets involved with most of our sexual abuse cases, also saw Brit and she too was quite happy that there was really no evidence of abuse."

A new aspect of the case

Thus far then, Dr. Chowdhury's input confirmed on the basis of his and Rachel Wadd's expertise in this area the conclusions that Dr. Chew and Lyndsey Carlton had come to originally (that abuse was very unlikely) and this had given them a more secure basis from which to plan their further intervention with the family. Drawing on this same expertise, however, Dr. Chew went on to make a further suggestion that was also to prove crucial in relation to future management but for a quite different reason. Again, we will give you his suggestion in his own words.

"My only slight concern from the safeguarding angle is the circumstances of the presentation. Was this a cry for help? The home is far from a haven of safety and we should work out how we can support but also monitor this family. My feeling is that, even if the swabs are negative, as I suspect they will be, we should still involve Social Services. I think it is going to work well that you didn't pull the alarm cord straight away, Lee, but when we are sure of what we are and are not dealing with, it will be a good idea to plan future care for this family together with them."

After Dr. Chowdhury had rung off, the conference discussed his suggestion of involving Social Services at some length. Several in the group were against this fearing that the response would be "over the top" and arguing that this could prejudice the good relationship

with Jade, which was their main asset in being able to help them in the future (including the clearly important monitoring). But it was Dr. Fauzia Hussein, the consortium lead for safeguarding, who insisted, pointing out that, even without Dr. Chowdhury's comments, they would be flying in the face of all the evidence for the importance of joined-up working if they left Social Services out of the loop altogether.

Values-based practice as a partner to evidence-based practice

The result was that they agreed to have a "significant event review" meeting and to involve Social Services in this, so that they were put in the picture. The case worker assigned by Social Services, Obioma Abiola, prioritized coming to the practice for the meeting, despite a very heavy caseload, and he listened intently to all the discussion. Far from going in feet first, he adopted a softly-softly approach, talking more in terms of help than safeguarding, and in the event he brought a completely new dimension to the help that between them they were able to offer.

Obioma Abiola had cut his teeth originally as a social worker with a third-sector social enterprise organization called Turning Point, which (among other work) offers practical help and support to ex-offenders, including those with problems of drug misuse. He was thus tailor-made in knowledge and skills to help Wayne Ball, who had been at best on the margins of events and at worst cast as the villain. But there was more. For Obioma Abiola's experience of working with this group of (mostly) young men had given him a particular passion for what he called the "forgotten fathers." Since coming to the area, he had set up a parenting group specifically aimed at fathers (although not excluding their partners) that had proved a great success with a surprisingly high take-up from among the most deprived local communities.

The outcome was that Beth Stokes, the health visitor, who already knew Jade Spence well, and Obioma Abiola agreed that they would see Jade and Wayne together and work out with them what help they themselves felt they needed as a family. There were again no guarantees of a successful outcome. But the "forgotten fathers" values that Obioma Abiola brought with him together with the knowledge and skills he had acquired from his training with Turning Point added a vital additional dimension to the resources that the team as a whole brought to their ongoing work with the family.

A turning point indeed

> **A final reflection**
>
> Obioma Abiola is a latecomer to the team. Social Services would not have been involved at all but for Dr. Chowdhury's expertise and Dr. Fauzia Hussein's evidence-based insistence on joined-up working.
>
> How significant do you think Obioma Abiola's "forgotten fathers" values might be as a resource for the team in giving Jade Spence and her family the help they really needed?
>
> And what is the connection between Obioma Abiola's "forgotten fathers" values and the person-values-practice that we looked at in the last chapter?

Jade Spence came for help and she got it. But Dr. Chowdhury had been right. It was not for her baby, Brit, that Jade had been seeking help but for her partner, Wayne. It had taken all her (considerable) courage to keep her appointment at the practice that Friday evening. She knew, none better, that she risked pulling the roof down on their heads. Wayne had repeatedly warned her about what would happen if they got involved with anyone "official." This was why he had always refused to ask for help for himself. But Jade was desperate. She could see Wayne sliding inevitably down a spiral of demoralization towards another spell in prison. And Dr. Chew had helped her before.

So she came. And Dr. Chew's decision to trust her to keep Brit safe over the weekend had been the turning point. The decision in the difficult circumstances of that Friday night consultation had required the shared knowledge and skills of Dr. Chew and Lyndsey Carlton, together with their crucially different values. It was not without risks. Brit might have come to harm. As it was, Dr. Chew's decision opened up a route that led ultimately to the social worker Obioma Abiola and his "forgotten fathers" values. And these values were crucial to the provision of what we called in the last chapter person-values-centered care. For Obioma Abiola's "forgotten fathers" values were the key to giving Jade the help (for Wayne) for which, under the umbrella of Brit's nappy rash, she had been seeking that Friday evening. Again, there was no guarantee of success. Wayne and Obioma Abiola might not get on. But we can only imagine what harms would have followed – for Jade, Wayne and Griff, not to mention Brit herself – had Jade come looking for help for Wayne and instead had her baby taken needlessly away.

Chapter summary

The story in this chapter of a young mother, Jade Spence, and her family, and the help they received from Dr. Chew, his nursing colleague Lyndsey Carlton and others, has illustrated the importance of diverse team values in an area like safeguarding where difficult judgment calls have to be made about risk and safety.

Jade Spence came to see Dr. Chew because she was worried that her four-month-old baby, Brit, had become sore "down below." Dr. Chew was an experienced and conscientious GP. But had he been working on his own and unsupported other than by practice guidelines and protocols, he would have made a wrong judgment call. "Wrong" not in any sense for which he could later have been called to account. Indeed, his dilemma was precisely that a defensive decision to initiate safeguarding although not, he had come to believe, justified on clinical grounds was for him as the clinician responsible the only safe option. As it was, he and Lyndsey Carlton came together in a decision-making process that balanced the different risks involved and gave Dr. Chew, as the clinician responsible for safeguarding, the support of shared ownership.

What was critical here was not that one or the other of Dr. Chew or Lyndsey Carlton had the "right" values but rather the balance between them of their *different* values. Dr. Chew and Lyndsey Carlton both brought a considerable resource of shared knowledge and skills to how they managed the situation. But the eventual outcome was a reflection rather of the way in which Lyndsey Carlton's "family over safeguarding" values and Dr. Chew's "safeguarding over family" values balanced each other in different ways at different stages in the consultation. Both were needed. Neither on its own would have resulted in a well-balanced robust risk management plan.

Risk management is, of course, only one area in which different team values offer a resource for balanced decision-making and shared ownership. We noted at the start of this chapter that, with the increasing complexity of values as well as evidence in all areas of medicine, the different team values represented by multidisciplinary teams are essential in an increasingly wide variety of clinical contexts. Nor are balanced decision-making and shared ownership the only aspects of practice to which different team values are important. In this story, for example, communication skills (as evidenced in Lyndsey Carlton's time out with Jade Spence) and person-centered practice (through Obioma Abiola's potential support for Jade's partner, Wayne) were both facilitated by the respective values of different team members.

Running through the story as a whole, moreover, has been the essential interplay between the resources offered by different team values and the corresponding resources of their different knowledge and skills. In team work, then, as in all other aspects of practice, values-based and evidence-based approaches are complementary. It is to three particular aspects of the complementary relationship between values-based practice and evidence-based practice that we turn in the next part of this book.

References

Colombo, A., Bendelow, G., Fulford, K. W. M. and Williams, S. (2003). Evaluating the influence of implicit models of mental disorder on processes of shared decision-making within community-based multi-disciplinary teams. *Social Science & Medicine* **56**, 1557–70.

Websites

- This chapter draws heavily on the BMA's Child Protection Tool accessed by Dr. Chew during his Friday evening consultation with Jade Spence at http://www.bma.org.uk/images/childprotectiontoolkitmay2009_tcm41–184943.pdf and also on that of the RCGP toolkit at http://www.rcgp.org.uk/clinical_and_research/safeguarding_children_tookit.aspx and the work of the RCGP and NSPCC in the *Keep Me Safe* document.
- *Good Medical Practice* by the General Medical Council (2006) is available at http://www.gmc-uk.org/static/documents/content/GMP_0910.pdf.
- See also the many BMA guidance websites, available through http://www.bma.org.uk/.

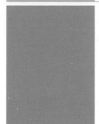

Introduction to Part 4

Values-based practice, as we have emphasized, is very much a partner to evidence-based practice as a support tool for clinical decision-making. The stories in earlier chapters all illustrate the close connections between values and evidence in clinical care and related areas of training and research.

So close indeed is the relationship between them that values and evidence may each in different ways sometimes come to mask or eclipse the other, with adverse consequences for practice. The three chapters in this part of the book illustrate three distinct ways in which this may happen and the importance of maintaining a balanced approach that keeps both values and evidence always equally in view:

- In Chapter 10, the Two-feet Principle underlines the point made in Chapter 1 that in medicine *all* decisions are both values and evidence driven. All decisions, then, in the terms of this principle stand on the two feet, respectively, of values and of evidence. In practice, however, where a decision is strongly evidence-based, important values may get overlooked – we may become, as this chapter will show, "values blinded by the evidence."

  This is what happened to Dr. Jane Hilary, the GP in this chapter, in her management of a middle-aged man, Jim Burns, with essential hypertension. So focused was Dr. Hilary on the evidence guiding her management that she failed to recognize the crucial impact of her own and Jim Burns' values. The consequence, as we will see, was that her evidence-based treatment actually increased rather than reducing Jim Burns' cardiovascular risk. Hence, the bottom line of the Two-feet Principle for practice is the reminder to "Think evidence, think values too!"

- Where the Two-feet Principle reminds us to "Think evidence, think values too!" the Squeaky-wheel Principle, discussed in Chapter 11, reminds us that it is equally important clinically to "Think values, think evidence too!" The Squeaky-wheel Principle is about values getting noticed when they cause trouble (when they squeak). But the risk is that, in paying attention to the (squeaking) values, we may lose sight of the evidence.

  Such, indeed, was the experience of the skilled and caring Charge Nurse, Matthew Cruickshank, at the heart of the story in this chapter. In a moment of understandable (although for him wholly atypical) moral outrage, he comes within a whisker of missing an otherwise self-evident acute abdomen.

- Chapter 12, the final chapter in this part, brings evidence and values together in the context of high-tech clinical interventions. The Science-driven Principle, as you will recall from Chapter 3, is about advances in medical science and technology increasing the choices available to us and thereby driving the need not only for evidence-based but also for values-based practice.

  A current high-profile example of the Science-driven Principle is assisted fertility, the subject of this chapter. Bob and Hilary Swann, referred by their GP to the local infertility clinic, find themselves caught between the science-focused approach of the research-oriented consultant, Barry Winterbottom, and his ethics-oriented senior registrar, Kathy Millar. Barry Winterbottom "thinks evidence"; Kathy Millar "thinks values." Bob and Hilary Swann need someone who "thinks values *and* evidence." As we will see, it is a perhaps rather unlikely member of what we called in Chapter 8 the extended multidisciplinary team, Bob and Hilary's local vicar, Benedict Brown, who rides to the rescue.

There is clearly a good deal more to the relationship between values and evidence than just the three principles outlined here. The principles themselves, as we indicated in Chapter 2, indeed have wider implications than the mainly practical points on which we have focused in these chapters. But the practical points are important nonetheless. Taken separately, each is a "red-light warning" of when we are at risk of losing sight either of the values or of the evidence bearing on a case. Taken together, they remind us once again that good practice is neither evidence based nor values based but evidence and values based.

Further reading on the relationship between evidence and values is given on the website supporting the series.

Map of values-based practice – the Two-feet Principle.

Chapter

10

The reluctant hypertensive: think evidence, think values too!
Values-based practice element 7: the Two-feet Principle

Take-away message for practice

*When you are focusing on the evidence, remind yourself to pay attention also to values. So, **think evidence, think values too!***

This chapter follows the story of Jim Burns, aged 56, a car sales manager recently diagnosed with essential hypertension. Failing to follow the evidence-based advice of his GP, Dr. Jane Hilary, for the management of his hypertension, Jim becomes increasingly anxious and depressed, starts to drink more and puts himself at risk of losing his job, all with a corresponding sharp deterioration in his cardiovascular risk profile.

Jim Burns finds a way out, however, when he is referred through an occupational health scheme to a cardiologist, Dr. Martin Winner, who specializes in cardiovascular risk. Dr. Winner draws on the same evidence base as Dr. Hilary but now with an awareness and understanding of Jim Burns' unique values. Combining values with evidence in this way allows Jim Burns to engage actively with the lifestyle and other preventive strategies proposed.

The clinical context

Jim Burns, a 56-year-old car sales manager, positively bounced out of his latest appointment with "his" cardiologist, Dr. Martin Winner, feeling, as he put it to himself, "turbocharged." Dr. Winner was pleased too. This was a different Jim Burns from the rundown character who had walked into his consulting room six months ago. That Jim Burns had been close to giving up on life. This Jim Burns was ready to take on the world. Not a bad result for a change of antihypertensive and a few statins. "I should have been a psychiatrist!" he thought to himself.

Dr. Winner was being too modest here – there was a bit more to his success with Jim Burns than just a change of medication. But to see how we got to the upbeat character leaving Dr. Winner's consulting room in such high spirits, we need to go back a few months to an earlier stage in Jim Burns' story.

Nine months earlier – where it all began

Jim Burns, a 56-year-old sales manager for a national car dealership firm, was sitting in the waiting room of his local GP surgery. This was a new and not entirely welcome experience for Jim. Generally in good health, and a keen rugby player as a young man, he felt he had little in common with what he saw as the "poor specimens" around him. He had been aware of drinking more than he should recently and that his waistline was creeping outwards. But he had been having a difficult year: the economic downturn had affected car sales and his largely commission related income had fallen substantially. He had taken his continued well-being despite these pressures as a sign that he remained fitter than most men his age and could get away with a few bad habits. So it was something of a shock to find himself here waiting to see his GP.

The trouble had started about a month earlier. Jim was a successful amateur racing car driver and had first been found to have high blood pressure at a routine medical examination to renew his British Automobile Racing Drivers Club (BARDC) competition license. He had been allowed to continue racing for another year but was told to see his GP, with the clear implication that unless he got his blood pressure down, his racing days were over. An "action this day" man, he had telephoned the practice as soon as he got into work the following Monday and was surprised to find that before he could get an appointment with his GP he had to see the nurse practitioner for two further checks of his blood pressure and for blood tests and an ECG. He had found "all the fuss" a bit irritating as he had had to take time off from work to attend the appointments, which had increased his work pressures, and he was anyway proud of the fact that throughout his working life he had hardly ever taken time off for illness.

Dr. Jane Hilary

As Jim Burns sat worrying about what was going on at work, Dr. Hilary, his GP, was also feeling under pressure. Hypertension was seen as "her thing" in the practice. Drawing on recent National Institute for Health and Clinical Excellence (NICE) guidelines (NICE, 2006), she had taken the lead in revising how they managed hypertension in an effort to minimize duplication of work and to make sure they achieved better Quality Outcomes Framework (QOF) points (see Chapter 7). One of the partners had a "more relaxed" attitude to hypertension, and she felt it was important for the team that she was seen to be doing the right thing herself.

Looking through Jim Burns' results and the notes from the practice nurse, there was no doubt in her mind that his hypertension needed treatment. True, it seemed he had given up smoking a few years ago and his ECG looked fine, but he had a significant family history, his weight was up and his lipid levels were raised. Yet her experience of men of Jim Burns' age and background was not good – she usually found them resistant to treatment, and as for lifestyle advice, it was "a waste of time." Only earlier that day, she had seen the daughter of a 54-year-old man who had no previous history but had died of a massive myocardial infarction the previous week. When she had reviewed his notes, she noticed that he had had significantly raised blood pressure readings on three occasions in the past year. He had repeatedly declined to take up her offers of treatment, but all the same, "Was there nothing you could have done, Doctor?" had been very difficult to answer.

Still, with the computer-based risk-modeling program she had got all the partners using, at least decision-making was now clear cut; and the new nurse practitioner was evangelical about healthy living advice and was doing really good work in the hypertension clinic – so she could tackle all that side of things later.

His and hers – one consultation, two agendas

Jim Burns and Dr. Hilary were clearly approaching the coming consultation with very different perceptions of what it was all about. Before we look at how the consultation went, it will be worth reflecting for a moment in a little more detail on their pre-consultation agendas.

> **Reflection point**
>
> The consultation that is about to begin is critical to Jim Burns' future cardiovascular risk. But how the consultation actually goes will be determined to an important extent by what Dr. Hilary and Jim Burns respectively bring to it.
>
> You may find it helpful to think about their different perspectives for a moment before reading on.
>
> One way to structure your thinking here is to list a few key points about how each of them understands the problem presented by Jim Burns, the associated risks and the need for treatment.

As with any interpretive exercise of this kind, there are no absolutely right or wrong answers here. But something along the lines of the key points given in Fig. 10.1 seems likely to have been not far from the truth. As this indicates, Jim Burns and Dr. Hilary were entering the consultation essentially at odds on all points:

- For Jim Burns, the *problem* was the *risk* to his racing car driving. At the back of his mind, he was aware of cardiovascular risk in people of his age (among family and friends), but he did not associate this with his own self-perception of robust health; and while he recognized that he might (reluctantly) have to accept treatment to keep the BARDC race officials happy, he regarded this as just a *temporary measure* until his work pressures lessened.
- Dr. Hilary, by contrast, saw Jim Burns as being there because his health was at risk: the *problem* in her mind was straightforwardly that Jim Burns had a disease – hypertension – which, if left untreated, put

	Jim Burns' perceptions	Jane Hilary's perceptions
The problem	Raised blood pressure is a threat to his racing car driving But he feels well and is proud of his robust health Probably due to stress at work	Three high readings mean clinically significant hypertension Evidence suggests drinking and weight gain are contributing Need to set an example of good practice with colleagues
Risk perception	Aware of colleagues/ family with heart attacks and strokes but does not identify this with his own robust health	Evidence-based computer-based model shows raised ten-year risk of cardiovascular disease
Need for treatment	May have to accept treatment for a while just to get his blood pressure down and keep the race officials happy But blood pressure is likely to come down anyway when his work pressures lessen	Long term medication is clearly indicated Follow evidence-based guidelines for choosing the most effective and well-tolerated treatment Lifestyle advice is needed, again based on evidence

Fig. 10.1. Jim Burns' and his GP, Dr. Jane Hilary's, pre-consultation perceptions.

him at significantly increased *clinical risk* of a stroke or myocardial infarct; he thus fell clearly within established evidence-based guidelines for *long-term treatment* with an antihypertensive combined with lifestyle advice. Dr. Hilary also had the additional problem of setting a good example within the practice with a patient who from her previous experience she expected would be likely to be non-compliant.

One consultation with two agendas, then: Jim Burns' agenda is to protect his racing car driving, while Dr. Hilary's agenda is an exercise in evidence-based medicine. So how did things go?

The consultation with Dr. Hilary

Dr. Hilary decided on a "no nonsense" approach. She had little time and felt that "giving it straight" was the best way to get Jim Burns to accept the need for treatment. So after the usual pleasantries, she opened with, "I gather your blood pressure is up – let's see what it is this morning. Hmm . . . (*looking serious as she checks it*), yes, well up . . . (*after checking his pulse and listening to his chest*) . . . OK, pop your jacket back on."

As Jim Burns sat down again, Dr. Hilary started running through the usual lifestyle factors while at the same time filling in the computer template for assessing cardiovascular risk. He had stopped smoking five years ago after his elder brother had had a heart attack. ("Good," she thinks, "one less hurdle.") However, he admits some weight gain. She fills in his weight from the practice nurse's notes, and then, adding his blood test results and noting raised gamma-glutamyl transpeptidase (GGT) and slight macrocytosis, asks, "And what about alcohol?"

"Gone up a bit lately, I suppose," Jim admits. "A lot of stress from work." She suspects that "a bit" is an understatement but moves swiftly on to ask him about exercise – "You must be joking. I don't have time nowadays" – and diet – "We get sandwiches delivered at work."

Pressing the Return button, the computer template confirms Dr. Hilary's expectations – Jim Burns has a significantly increased risk of a stroke or heart attack within the next ten years. He thus falls firmly within the guidelines for treatment for hypertension. Checking the practice protocol, she starts to prepare a prescription for lisinopril as she turns from the computer towards Jim Burns. "Well," she starts, "your blood pressure is certainly up and . . ." gesturing back to the computer screen ". . . what all our tests show is that it is really important to get it down if you want to avoid a heart attack in the next few years. But . . ." seeing the look on Jim Burns' face ". . . don't worry, we can deal with blood pressure really very effectively nowadays."

In reply to Jim Burns' question, she goes on to explain that what treatment means is "nothing drastic . . . it's just taking a couple of pills morning and evening." She adds some brisk advice about ". . . lots of things you can do for yourself that will really help. Cut back on your salt and alcohol . . . and try to eat more healthily. Obviously the extra weight doesn't help either, so try to be more active."

Jim Burns took the proffered prescription without much enthusiasm as Dr. Hilary explained the need to monitor renal function. She usually avoided mentioning too many side effects as in her experience this tended to result in anxiety and a flood of consultations for tiredness or other minor non-specific symptoms, which she doubted were ever related to the medication. But she asked if Jim had any questions – he hadn't – and recommended he came back if there were any problems with the medication. She got up to open the door with "So I'll see you in a month, to see how you're getting on."

Values blinded by the evidence

Dr. Hilary appears heavy-handed in this consultation. She has given Jim Burns little chance to discuss let alone absorb the implications of what the tests show about his cardiovascular risk. Worse, she uses repeated inappropriate diminutives, thus reinforcing Jim Burns' anxiety, such as "Don't worry," "Nothing drastic," "It's just . . ." and so on. It is thus small wonder that Jim Burns left the consultation feeling dazed.

Many of us may feel that we would never run a first consultation for hypertension like this. The variety of patient-related factors influencing compliance with hypertension medication has after all been well known for some time (Benson and Britten, 2002; Gascón et al., 2004). But the evidence is against us. A study of patients' evaluation of the management of their hypertension (Morecroft et al., 2006) found that, like Jim Burns, most were considerably taken aback to find that they were hypertensive. In this study, diagnosis was found to lead to anxieties for younger people who previously regarded themselves as healthy or "normal," while older patients were more likely to see their hypertension as a consequence of aging.

At 56, Jim Burns was no longer "young," but his self-perception was that he still had the strength of a much younger man. So the news was a double whammy: it was a blow to his self-image, and, unlike a younger man, it seemed the threat of a stroke or heart attack was imminent ("Hadn't the doctor said something about five years?"). Jim Burns also shared other anxieties with those identified in Morecroft's study: he had concerns about the effects of hypertension and its consequences on his life, and feelings related to memories of family members who had previously been diagnosed. Indeed, his first thought was of his mother after her stroke – frustrated, disabled and incontinent.

There are many factors that may contribute to this apparent widespread failure of the hypertension consultation (Gascón et al., 2004; Morecroft et al., 2006). In the present case, the consultation fails essentially because Dr. Hilary fails to connect with what is important to her patient. Again, there are many possible reasons for this "values blindness." True, Dr. Hilary like most GPs was busy. True, and again like most GPs she was under pressure to deliver evidence-based treatment (as well as QOF points, she felt her own credibility was on the line). We noted in earlier case studies that such pressures make the need for values-based practice the more urgent, and they were clearly a factor in this case.

An additional factor in this case was Dr. Hilary's own values: like Dr. Charles Mangate, the GP in Chapter 5 dealing with teenage acne, Dr. Hilary was largely unaware of her own values and of the extent to which they were coloring her interactions with Jim Burns. We will see later that her (unacknowledged) values were even more important at the follow-up consultation. But the main reason for Dr. Hilary's failure to connect with what was important to Jim Burns in this first consultation was her perception that all aspects of his presentation (the problem, risks and treatment) were sufficiently understood in terms of well-established evidence. If she was values blinded then, in this case, she was values blinded by the evidence.

We need to be clear here. The problem was not Dr. Hilary's attention to the evidence. Far from it, the consultation was exemplary in this respect. The problem was that, in attending to the evidence, Dr. Hilary neglected the operative values, her own and Jim Burns' values.

> **Reflection point**
>
> We are all blind to our own values some of the time, yet much of what we have discussed in this book has reinforced the message that values awareness is Element 1 for a good reason. Without awareness of the values at play (our own values and those of the others involved), it is difficult to make headway.
>
> If Dr. Hilary, having been values blinded by the evidence, were to wake up one day and think, "The problem may well be my values awareness," how would you advise her, as her mentor, to identify the relevant values?
>
> We will come back to this later.

The blind leading the blind

The result, as we have seen, was that Jim Burns left the consultation apparently acquiescing to Dr. Hilary's treatment but in fact deeply shocked and having taken in very little of what she had said. He spent the day immersed in his work and was reticent when his wife asked him that evening how he had got on (more on Mrs. Burns below). He finally got off to sleep after tossing and turning for what seemed like most of the night.

Waking with a start to the alarm the next morning, he felt at first angry and then dismissive. With part of his mind, he knew that the doctor was just doing her job. But he felt he had been "nannied" and was now deeply unconvinced about the whole thing. He was very aware of the stress he was under at work and believed this must be the reason for his blood pressure, which was fine before. Also, he knew he got worked up at the doctor's and was sure this must have pushed his blood pressure up when they checked it. The same happened with his medicals for his BARDC competition license. He did not feel ill and he hated the thought of being on tablets for the rest of his life. Strokes and heart attacks scared him, though. And he just *had* to get through his next car racing medical. So he decided "to give the pills a go." But as for trying to be more active, someone at work who had been "fit as a fiddle" dropped down dead with a heart attack on the golf course aged 49. "So much for exercise," he thought. And all that business about his diet and so on, "That's all very well, but how am I supposed to do that, especially when I'm working twelve hours a day?"

In his own way, Jim Burns thus came to terms with having to take medication, at least until things settled down. Matching the action to the thought, he got his prescription on the way to work. But then there came a second shock. Being the kind of man who reads the small print – one of the qualities that had made him a successful manager – he read the prescribing leaflet before taking his first pill and was immediately alarmed both by the long list of side effects and the fact that he would need regular blood tests to check that the medication was not causing kidney problems.

He had not really taken this in when Dr. Hilary had mentioned it the day before. But now seeing it in black and white, it seemed to confirm his doubts. He had always mistrusted long-term medication, believing that any powerful medicine must have a degree of toxicity ("Taking things just isn't natural.") He was also worried about getting "hooked" on them: he was aware that with some treatments (sleeping pills, for example), you start by taking them to cure a problem and end up not being able to manage without them. "But what option do I have?" he thought. So he started taking lisinopril.

One month into treatment

Jim Burns came back to see Dr. Hilary a week sooner than planned. He was still taking the tablets but wanted to stop them as he blamed them for making him impotent. He had already been worried about this because he had begun to have occasional difficulties before the problems with his blood pressure blew up. He had consequently been alarmed to find sexual difficulties on the list of side effects in the prescribing leaflet and he had later spotted a piece in the Sunday papers, which said that blood pressure tablets can cause impotence.

Dr. Hilary did not see this as a major issue. Particularly given Jim Burns' earlier sexual difficulties, she thought that it was more likely that his hypertension with its possible associated vascular disease, and more importantly his drinking, were the causes of his difficulties. In addition, she knew that lisinopril is less likely than many other antihypertensives to cause sexual problems and dreaded embarking on a fruitless search for the "perfect medication."

So she checked his blood pressure – "Much improved," she said encouragingly – and then sat him down. She explained that she did not think the tablets were the cause of his problems and that she was reluctant to abandon what had proved to be an effective treatment for a potentially fatal condition. She asked whether he had managed to reduce his alcohol intake.

"Well, not much. Still a lot of pressures at work . . ." he answered. Explaining that this was more likely to be the problem, together with lack of exercise and working too hard, she suggested he made an appointment with the nurse practitioner in their hypertension clinic and came back to see her again in a month.

His and hers in the second consultation

As noted earlier, Dr. Hilary's own values were clearly important in how she responded to Jim Burns: in her scale of priorities, impotence was a minor problem compared with a 20% increase in ten-year cardiovascular risk. But for Jim Burns it had been devastating. He was deeply distressed and felt emasculated. His confidence generally had taken a knocking and he was less effective at work. Worse still, he felt his marriage, which was important to him, was at risk. He had been through a bad divorce ten years earlier and had remarried three years ago after a whirl wind romance with a woman, Jean, ten years his junior. Their difference in age had seemed unimportant at the time – indeed, his continued sexual vigor was very much part of his self-image of being fitter than most men his age – and now *this* had happened. He felt that Dr. Hilary should have warned him about this originally, and what he now saw as her dismissive attitude left him feeling angry and dissatisfied. Car racing or not, he would stop the tablets.

As with the first consultation, many of us may feel that few doctors would be as insensitive as Dr. Hilary in the way they dealt with a patient's concerns about impotence. But again, the evidence is against us (see for example, Tomlinson and Wright, 2004). Doctors tend to underestimate just how profoundly impotence may affect men's confidence and self-esteem and their ability to function at work and in other contexts well beyond their sexual relationships as such. There could be many reasons for this. In Dr. Hilary's case, she found consultations with male patients about sexual problems awkward and embarrassing and usually tried to pass them on to one of her male partners. In this instance, she felt unable to do this because of her lead role in managing hypertension, and anyway she felt that a 20% risk of a stroke or heart attack was the priority.

Both shall fall into the pit

When the blind lead the blind, as St. Matthew's gospel puts it, both shall fall into the pit. Dr. Hilary was well aware that things were not going well with Jim Burns. True, his blood pressure was down. But he had not lost any weight and she suspected that he would give up on the medication. "Another Hilary failure," she thought gloomily, reflecting that she had not done much to reduce his cardiovascular risk. He seemed to her to be in denial. Yet despite her brisk attitude with Jim Burns, she blamed herself for this. She remembered again her other patient, the 54-year-old who had failed to take up her offers of treatment and ended up with a fatal heart attack. For the sake of the staff and her colleagues in the practice, as well as her patients, she felt she had to keep up a confident appearance. But when she thought of the look on Jim Burns' face as he walked out of her door, she surprised herself by coming just for a moment unaccountably close to tears. Pulling herself together, she called in her next patient.

If Dr. Hilary felt guilty and incompetent, Jim Burns, as we have seen, felt angry and resentful. But more dangerously still, from the point of view of his cardiovascular risk, his stress levels were rising as he was also increasingly at his wit's end. First time around, he had been able to find his own way to come to terms with his diagnosis and the need for treatment. Now he felt that

he was caught in a trap with no way out. If he took the tablets, he would be able to carry on racing but his marriage was at risk: drop the tablets and his marriage was OK but his racing was at risk. And anyway, feeling as he did, he doubted if he would still be able to compete effectively – racing was a high-testosterone sport, and he couldn't even concentrate properly at work.

Reflecting angrily on where his life was going, Jim Burns found that he had somehow wandered into a pub and was ordering a whisky. He missed a key sales meeting that afternoon.

Back from the brink

Two months later, Jim Burns had an appointment with a cardiologist specializing in cardiovascular risk, Dr. Martin Winner. Jim Burns' life had gone rapidly downhill in the interim. He did stop taking the tablets. But after a couple of weeks in his by now deeply demoralized state, and with the fear of a heart attack or stroke fuelled by memories of what had happened to his mother strong upon him, he restarted them. With continuing sexual problems, he drank more and became increasingly unreliable at work. He and his wife, Jean, fell to rowing: not over his sexual problems but over his reluctance to talk about what was wrong (Jean secretly feared he was getting involved with someone else).

The referral to Dr. Winner

The crunch and as it proved watershed in Jim Burns' fortunes came with his annual appraisal at work with his line manager, Alan Banks, the Managing Director of the firm. Alan Banks believed in straight talking. He liked Jim Burns and had known him for many years as a reliable and conscientious manager. Also, they had a shared enthusiasm for racing car driving. So it was not difficult for him to open the conversation with a direct question about what was wrong. Jim Burns reacted at first with his usual denial but faced with the inevitable "We'll have to do something about this, Jim, if things don't improve," he admitted that he had problems with his blood pressure and that it was "worrying him sick."

Alan Banks did not press Jim Burns further on what exactly was wrong. Instead he told him that he had been having blood pressure treatment himself for some years. He had done really well on it and had a lot of confidence in the doctor, Dr. Winner, he had seen through the firm's private health scheme – would Jim like to see Dr. Winner? Jim Burns jumped at the lifeline. The referral was made through the firm's occupational health doctor who, with Jim Burns' agreement, liaised with Dr. Hilary and included a report from her on his treatment to date.

The consultation with Dr. Winner

Dr. Winner was confident in his medical skin. In his middle 40s and with a string of awards already under his belt, he was widely recognized among his peers as a high flyer. Reading carefully through Dr. Hilary's report, he noted that Jim Burns had "done well on lisinopril"; however, although he had given up smoking some years earlier, he had been resistant to lifestyle advice and appeared to have a growing alcohol problem. There was a mention (no more) of Jim Burns' sexual problems, with a comment that these had preceded the start of his medication.

The tenor of Dr. Hilary's report struck Dr. Winner as odd. It was well written, concise and detailed (it was particularly helpful that she had included a series of blood pressure readings over a period of time and the results of all the tests they had done). But as to Jim Burns himself, he had got a very different picture from the occupational health doctor – the highly valued employee with an excellent health record to date was a very different character from Dr. Hilary's non-compliant patient. It was clear that Dr. Hilary had done exactly the right thing in starting Jim Burns on treatment. But from his excellent work record, he would have expected Jim Burns to do rather well. Clearly, there was something else going on. "Perhaps," he thought, thinking of other middle-aged men he had seen in similar circumstances, "those sexual problems have something to do with it."

Last-chance saloon

Jim Burns arrived in good time for his appointment. As he walked in, Dr. Winner noted his formal suit and tie and clean-shaven smartness – no ketones on his breath, either. Before the appointment, Jim Burns had made up his mind to "make a clean breast of it." He had thought this would be difficult. But Dr. Winner had a happy knack of focused attention that quickly put Jim Burns at his ease. Far from being difficult, Jim Burns actually found it a welcome relief to talk openly about his sexual problems and how these threatened to ruin everything he had worked so hard to build up in his life.

"I want to come back to the sexual problems . . ." Dr. Winner responded, "but let's have a look at your blood pressure first." He examined him carefully and then went through the lifestyle factors, much as Dr. Hilary had done.

"What do you know about blood pressure?" he now asked. Jim Burns explained that he thought his blood pressure was up because of pressures at work. Instead of contradicting him, Dr. Winner encouraged him by endorsing his belief while at the same time leading him back to the need for treatment. "You may well be right; blood pressure certainly does go up with stress. You're a racing car driver, I see," glancing at the referral letter, "so you know all about the adrenaline rush!" Jim Burns smiled in agreement. "But you know, Dr. Hilary was absolutely right to be worried about you because the evidence now is that if your blood pressure goes up a lot with stress, it can be as bad as having it up all the time."

Jim Burns' face fell again. "But what can I do, Doctor? I'd rather risk a heart attack than lose my marriage – I've got to the point I'd happily give up racing." Again, instead of picking this up directly, Dr. Winner asked Jim Burns when his next racing fitness medical was due. "Not for nine months? Good, you've obviously got on with things – so we've plenty of time to see what we can do. Let's start with the sexual difficulties . . ."

A turning point in understanding

Dr. Winner again started by asking Jim Burns how much he knew, in this case about how an erection is maintained. As with his understanding of hypertension, Jim Burns' response was close to but not on the mark. He believed that blood pressure drives an erection directly "A bit like blowing up a tyre?" Martin Winner asked. "That's on the right lines," he continued as Jim Burns nodded agreement, "but it's a bit more complicated. It's more like this . . ." Dr. Winner drew a simple diagram as he explained the key point that the blood vessels to the penis actually have to *relax* to allow the penis to fill up properly.

"So it's more like opening a valve . . .?" Jim Burns said with growing interest. This was a new idea to him, but it made complete sense from his knowledge and understanding of cars. From this point on, the messages flowed easily: high blood pressure is one of the things that can harden the blood vessels, stopping the "valve" relaxing fully ("So that's why I was having some problems before I knew about the blood pressure . . ."); exercise and a good diet help to keep the blood vessels healthy and flexible ("Like looking after a vintage E-type Jaguar carefully . . . and taking it out for a regular spin!"); and people react differently to different treatments so there are other treatments we can try that may suit you better ("I see, like choosing the right oil for the right car . . .").

139

Back to the future

From this shared understanding of the problem, there was a straight-line route back to the high-spirited Jim Burns that we met leaving Dr. Winners' consulting rooms at the start of this chapter.

Rather than tackling the hypertension head on, Dr. Winner decided on a softly-softly approach. This allowed him to build up Jim Burns' confidence essentially by giving him the support he needed to extend his skills as a manager to *self*-management. Stage 1 of this approach was to come off lisinopril and see how he got on with lifestyle changes alone. Jim Burns now tackled this with his old energy: he had already agreed with his Managing Director, Alan Banks, on no alcohol in working hours, and he and Jean (with whom he had now come clean about his loss of sexual confidence) cut their intake further to no more than two glasses of wine in an evening (although they shared a bottle on a Friday night); he started walking to and from work (half an hour each way); and Jean organized a daily fruit and salad lunch box for him.

A month later, he was back on form at work and much encouraged at his follow-up with Dr. Winner to find that his weight was down over half a stone and that there had already been a small improvement in his lipids. His blood pressure was unchanged. Martin Winner showed him how his cardiovascular risk had already improved significantly. The only "fly in the ointment," Jim Burns explained on this occasion was that he and Jean were still having some problems. At the suggestion that he try Viagra, Jim Burns was initially reluctant, having "never had to rely on anything like that . . ." But he agreed to give it a try after Dr. Winner had explained its effect on the "valve" (Jim Burns had brought Dr. Winners' diagram with him) and that Viagra was "no use at all if you didn't still have petrol in the engine." It proved fully effective.

Stage 2 of Dr. Winner's management plan was to start Jim Burns on statins. He prefaced this with a discussion of how statins worked by restoring the flexibility of the blood vessels and hence of the "valve" that was essential to an erection. Jim Burns tolerated statins well and, maintaining his lifestyle changes, was delighted by the further considerable improvement in his cardiovascular risk from a much improved lipid profile by the time of his next appointment. His blood pressure, however, although encouragingly down a few points, was still too high. But Jim Burns was by now so thoroughly hooked on the project of improving his cardiovascular risk that he actually took the initiative of asking whether they might try medication again.

Stage 3 was thus a trial of losartan with an explanation from Dr. Winner that this was the usual second line of treatment after starting, as Dr. Hilary had correctly done, with lisinopril. Anticipating Jim Burns' concerns about sexual function, Dr. Winner explained (again using his original diagram) that losartan, unlike lisinopril, brought blood pressure down by relaxing the blood vessels, "So if anything it should help rather than hinder sexually . . . but" again building on their first consultation, "everyone is different and we can always switch to something else if this doesn't suit you."

Losartan did suit Jim Burns. Thus it was that three months later, with his blood pressure now within the normal range and his lifestyle changes well maintained, a "turbocharged" Jim Burns left his final consultation with Dr. Winner, a man ready to take on the world.

His and her risk

The outcome for Jim Burns, then, was good. But it was a close run thing. To see just how close, we have only to track his cardiovascular risk.

Reflection point: tools and how we use them

Before reading on you, may want to draw a rough graph of how Jim Burns' cardiovascular risk varied over the nine months of his life outlined in this story.

The clinical usefulness of cardiovascular risk tools usually relates more to making an initial decision on whether to treat, and can be used to show (theoretically) how a reduction in blood pressure/giving up smoking/reducing cholesterol could improve the individual's risk. The relative risk as compared to the rest of the population is more useful than the absolute risk (identifying those at high risk; see http://www.assign-score.com/about/beginners/).

However, it is worth remembering that some risks are not included in common risk tools, including the risks associated with depression.

Communicating risk is one of the difficult arts in medicine, with much written on the topic. Combining science with values is clearly essential.

Jim Burns' cardiovascular risk profile

Although Jim did not reach the maximum risk levels for cardiovascular events, he came close to it when his lifestyle factors deteriorated in a vicious spiral. Add to these lifestyle factors his depressed mental state (he was threatened with no less than three major losses, his marriage, his job and his racing car driving), and the risk of a heart attack or stroke over this period was real indeed.

Dr. Hilary's risk profile

The outcome was a close run thing for Dr. Hilary too. Imagine if Jim Burns had had a heart attack or stroke. How would she have felt? As a caring and conscientious GP, she had had many successes with patients who, like her, were naturally health conscious and risk averse. But she was all too aware that she had also had many failures too: remember how she had been affected by her other patient who had died of a heart attack recently and her self-deprecating "Another Hilary failure" as Jim Burns walked out of his second consultation with her. Thus far, she had maintained her strong front. But her morale was on a knife edge.

Dr. Hilary, then, no less than Jim Burns had reason to be grateful to Dr. Winner. There was no malpractice here, of course, in any conventional sense of the term. Far from it: she had done a good evidence-based job. But all the same, if Jim Burns had had a heart attack over this period, this would have been in no small part a result of Dr. Hilary's failure to use the evidence-based guidelines for the management of hypertension in a person-centered and specifically in what we called in Chapter 7 a person-*values*-centered way. As it was, Dr. Winners' professionalism – his endorsement of her evidence-based management in his consultations with Jim Burns and his regular reports to her on progress – meant that Dr. Hilary ended up feeling that the outcome had been a good result for her too. Indeed, without realizing it, she had absorbed something of Dr. Winner's approach and found herself subsequently more confident and capable in managing hypertension in middle-aged men.

This wake-up call meant that Dr. Hilary was now sensitized generally to trying to pick up on her patients' individual points of view. As soon as she had an inkling that a consultation was not going well, she got into the habit of (without calling it as such) "thinking values." She became expert at finding a little reflective pause (perhaps by sticking her stethoscope in her ears with the other end on the patient's chest) and asking herself "What is going on here?" This in turn led to her starting to become more aware of her own relevant values and how they were playing out in consultation.

Chapter summary

In this chapter, we have taken the values-awareness message of values-based practice to a new level. Building on the experience of Jim Burns and of his GP, Dr. Jane Hilary, we have seen that it is never more important to "think values" than with a clinical decision that *appears* to be purely evidence-based:

- Dr. Hilary "thought evidence" but failed to "think values": she was, as we said, values blinded by the evidence. The result was that her evidence-based management of Jim Burns' hypertension, far from reducing his cardiovascular risk, actually increased it.
- Dr. Winner by contrast "thought values as well as evidence": by starting from what was important to Jim Burns, his person-values-centered use of the same evidence base as Dr. Hilary resulted in Jim Burns engaging positively with treatment, including an active program of self-management of his lifestyle factors, and a consequent marked reduction in his cardiovascular risk.

There are many other reasons for "thinking values as well as evidence": other chapters illustrate other reasons, ranging from improved experience of staff as well as of patients, through to compliance and the cost-effective use of resources. But what Jim Burns' story shows most directly is that good *clinical* outcomes too, including so-called "hard outcomes" such as relapse rates and risk of death, may also depend critically on remembering to "Think evidence, think values too!"

References

Benson, J. and Britten, N. (2002). Patients' decisions about whether or not to take antihypertensive drugs: qualitative study. *British Medical Journal* **325**, 873.

Gascón, J. J., Sánchez-Ortuño, M., Llor, B., Skidmore, D., Saturno, P. J. and the Treatment Compliance in Hypertension Study Group (2004). Why hypertensive patients do not comply with the treatment: results from a qualitative study. *Family Practice* **21**, 125–30.

Morecroft, C., Cantrill, J. and Tully, M. (2006). Patients' evaluation of the appropriateness of their hypertension management: a qualitative study. *Research in Social and Administrative Pharmacy* **2**, 186–211.

NICE (2006). *Hypertension: Management of Hypertension in Adults in Primary Care*. Guideline 34 (partial update of Guideline 18). London: National Institute for Health and Clinical Excellence

Tomlinson, J. and Wright, D. (2004). Impact of erectile dysfunction and its subsequent treatment with sildenafil: a qualitative study. *British Medical Journal* **328**, 1037.

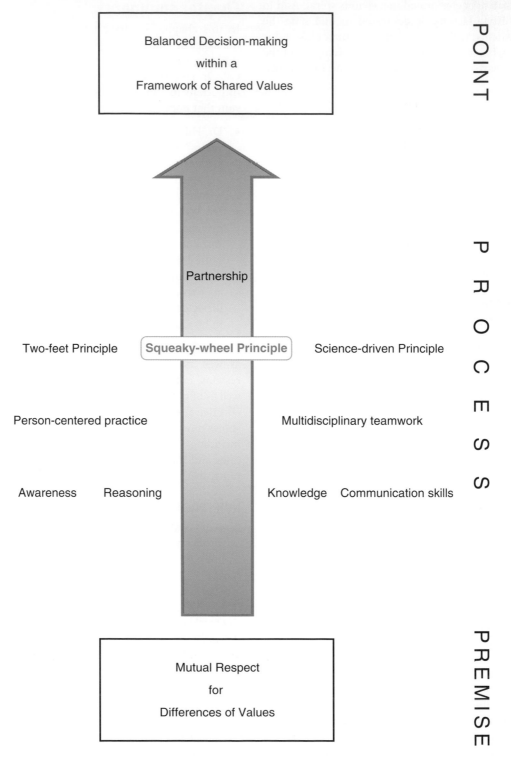

Map of values-based practice – the Squeaky-wheel Principle.

11 Unexplainable abdominal pain: think values, think evidence too!

Values-based practice element 8: the Squeaky-wheel Principle

Topics covered in this chapter

This chapter discusses the Squeaky-wheel Principle and how it reminds us not to lose sight of the evidence when we are focusing on values. Other topics include:

- Targets and care – are the goals the same?
- "Inappropriate" attendance and misuse of resources
- Use of interpreters and the role of family
- Intercultural medicine and varying patient expectations
- The role of third-sector organizations.

Take-away message for practice

*When you are focusing on values (ethical or otherwise), never lose sight of the evidence. So, **think values, think evidence too!***

The Squeaky-wheel Principle as we noted in Chapter 3 reminds us that values, although always there and important, tend to get our attention particularly when they cause trouble: it is, as they say, "the squeaky wheel that gets the grease." This is an important reminder clinically because we are always at risk of losing sight of the evidence when the values are "squeaking" and hence grabbing our attention. Just as therefore the clinical bottom line of the last chapter was to "Think evidence, think values too!" so the clinical bottom line of this chapter is that it is equally important to "Think values, think evidence too!"

We illustrate the importance of "Think values, think evidence too!" with the story of a senior emergency care nurse, Matthew Cruickshank, and his

problems with a non-English-speaking patient, Fatima Mahmood.

The clinical context

It had been a long day in the Blackstone A&E, the accident and emergency department of a large district general hospital. "Call this Accident and Emergency?" charge nurse Matthew Cruickshank was reflecting ruefully as he tidied up in his office at the end of a long shift "More like all-comers and everything." Among the mixed bag of injuries and fractures, poorly kids and a drunk or two, they had had only one genuine emergency admission since he came on at lunchtime. Still, he had the match on TV to look forward to that evening. And then Matthew Cruickshank hit a heart-sink moment. "Oh no! Not again!" he thought as he heard the all-too-familiar voice of Fatima Mahmood crying out querulously from an ambulance trolley as she was being wheeled in across the other side of the department from the street . . .

A disaster in the making

Fatima Mahmood, aged 29, had been brought in by ambulance accompanied by her 11-year-old son, Ali. She was crying on the trolley and was holding her abdomen. Ali stayed close by her side. He was composed but looked frightened. His mother kept calling out loudly in Arabic and was clearly distressed.

This is not, you may think, the stuff of which – provided the correct clinical procedures are followed – disasters are made. Indeed, as we will see, it was correct clinical procedures that saved Matthew Cruickshank on this occasion. But to understand his and Fatima Mahmood's close call with disaster we need to look more closely at the characters involved.

Charge nurse Matthew Cruickshank

Matthew Cruickshank had taken charge of the nursing at Blackstone A&E three years earlier as a run-down and demoralized department. A local boy, he had trained in London before returning to his home town, and he had since done a tremendous job rebuilding the department more or less from scratch. But he was tired. Struggling with limited resources, with often challenging and sometimes violent patients, and with many language difficulties and intercultural problems, it required all of his not inconsiderable resources of patience and dedication to maintain the high standards he had set.

Add to all that a constant pressure from the hospital managers to improve the throughput of patients and to "weed out" inappropriate referrals and it was well nigh impossible to keep everyone – clinicians, patients and managers – happy.

Reflection point

From what you have read thus far, you may find it helpful to reflect for a moment at this point on exactly why Matthew Cruickshank felt under such pressure from "management" as he heard Fatima Mahmood being wheeled in yet again to A&E.

Think in particular about any potential discrepancies there might be between his priorities as a clinician and those of the hospital managers, and about the implications of both sets of priorities (positive and negative) for their patients.

How do you think discrepancies between his and the management's priorities might affect how Matthew Cruickshank responded to Fatima Mahmood?

Matthew Cruickshank had shown himself in the past well able to handle the work load and other pressures that all busy clinicians experience. Indeed, his ability to deal effectively with difficult patients, not to mention difficult colleagues, had been an important factor in his success in rebuilding Blackstone A&E. Matthew Cruickshank was not one of those clinicians who found himself generally at odds with the priorities of "management." He recognized in particular the importance of record keeping: indeed, he was a meticulous record keeper himself when it came to patients' records and he demanded the same of others. The problem was that he felt trapped in a system that required him to compromise his own standards of clinical care in order to get the resources that were essential to deliver on those same standards.

The resources trap

Fig. 11.1 sets out the elements of the resources trap in which Matthew Cruickshank found himself in the form of a values map. As this indicates, the trap arose not from the operation of ill-directed values: there was no malpractice here on anybody's part, clinicians or managers. To the contrary, the very force of the trap came from the extent to which it arose from the tensions between their different but equally well-intentioned priorities for delivering a first-class service to patients:

- Matthew Cruickshank's priorities as a clinician were to provide person-centered care appropriate to the wide range of very diverse patients who used A&E and to make that care available to anyone within the NHS who needed it.
- The priorities of the hospital managers, on the other hand, were to reduce waiting times and to limit as far as possible the misuse of NHS resources through inappropriate use of A&E.

As Fig. 11.1 also indicates, both sets of priorities had potentially positive impacts from the perspective of patients, although importantly neither came free of cost. That is to say, both sets of priorities had negative as well as positive impacts. This is by now as we should expect of anything to do with values. As we described in Part 1, it is in the very nature of values that they tend to be in tension. This inherent tension, you will recall, is the basis of Beauchamp and Childress's Four Principles account of biomedical ethics and their emphasis on the need for "situational judgment" in applying their approach in practice. The inherent tensions between values are the basis similarly of the need for values-based practice (or something like it) to support balanced decision-making in individual cases.

Certainly "tensions of values" had been Matthew Cruickshank's experience. In his scale of priorities, it was important that A&E should be an easily accessible source of quality care to which any patient who was eligible could self-refer. But he was a victim of his own success in creating an accessible and personalized service, which meant that the department was often overwhelmed with patients, many of them bypassing their GPs.

To this extent, then, Matthew Cruickshank could just about buy into the hospital managers' priorities for reducing waiting times and cutting out misuses of the service. But the "games" that as a department they had to play to meet national and local targets and hence to compete successfully for resources went very much against the grain of his (Matthew Cruickshank's) principles: these games included longer waits in ambulances (in which he felt complicit) and resources being made available by management for extra staff to be drafted in over the auditing period (resources he felt unable to refuse).

The games people play

It is important to be clear here about the nature of the trap in which Matthew Cruickshank as a conscientious and skilled clinician found himself. It was not merely that he had to balance his aspirations for an open and person-centered service against the realities of limited resources. This, after all, is part of his job (Bevan and Hood, 2006). Nor was the trap for Matthew Cruickshank the need (merely) to meet targets. Again, he was a target setter himself and he recognized the importance of meeting management's targets if the managers were to do their job effectively of raising the resources he needed to run his department.

The trap for Matthew Cruickshank came rather from that "game playing." In the first place, this was for him a compromise too far, not only with his clinical values but also with his personal values of honesty and fair play. In the second place – and this is where the trap bit deep – he felt he had no option but to play these games if their department was to compete effectively for resources. The essence of the problem

was that resources were allocated nationally on the basis of success in meeting targets, and Matthew Cruickshank knew only too well that similar games were being played by departments up and down the country. Unless you played by the same rules therefore, it was inevitable that you would appear to be performing badly relative to other departments. Only that week, they had had a departmental meeting at which the managers were emphasizing the renewed threat to A&E departments with the economic downturn and the consequent need to maintain their recent excellent performance in achieving 97% of patients spending less than four hours waiting in the department.

"No hospital is an island," then, and it would be of little benefit to anyone (least of all to Matthew Cruickshank's often very deprived patients) to stand on his principles. But all the same, the necessity for playing the target game went against the grain.

The pressure builds

It is against this background of an exhausted Matthew Cruickshank feeling deeply frustrated and compromised by forces beyond his control that we can understand his reaction to Fatima Mahmood. For here at least, it seemed to Matthew Cruickshank at that moment, was a clear-cut case of misuse of the casualty department's services.

This was no less than the tenth occasion in the past year when Fatima Mahmood had arrived at A&E like this, complaining of abdominal pain. They had persevered on each previous occasion with the same time-

Priorities	Impact of priorities on patients	
	Positive	**Negative**
Management: • To reduce waiting times • To limit misuse of resources	• More focused clinical pathways • Reduction in waiting times for patients	• Increased pressure on staff reduces patience for slow or "inappropriate" cases • Experiences of rejection if complicated (e.g. by language barriers) • Denial of healthcare if deemed ineligible
Clinician: • To provide personalized care • To offer access to all	• Patient's experience is of individual care • Healthcare available even if "outside the system" • Clinician sense of being valued reflected in positive patient experience	• Waiting time may be longer • Diversion of resources away from other healthcare priorities

Fig. 11.1 A values map of Matthew Cruickshank's resources trap.

consuming and expensive rigmarole of translators, gynecological or surgical referral and so on, but always with nothing being found. There had also been innumerable visits with one or other of her four young children. To make things worse, there were no shortcuts with Fatima Mahmood. She was especially frustrating to "clerk" because she spoke no English and her answers through a variety of translators made little sense and anyway changed from one occasion to the next. It would not have been so bad if Fatima Mahmood had come via her GP. But she had no GP and, despite several warnings, she seemed unable to get the message that she had to register with a GP and not use A&E and the ambulance service as a convenient shortcut.

And there was more. For that business with the GP made Matthew Cruickshank suspicious that Fatima Mahmood was an illegal immigrant. He had some experience of this: of inexplicable (at the time) resistance to using appropriate resources (usually Social Services) and the person concerned then suddenly being deported. He did not doubt that Fatima Mahmood's distress was genuine, but he was coming to believe that her repeated self-referrals were directed towards building up a (misconceived) medical case for not being "sent home."

So here was a situation where he and the hospital managers were entirely at one. At that same departmental meeting earlier that week, they had gone over their new guidelines for treatment of "international patients"; and the management had highlighted the importance of identifying those ineligible for free care and making sure that they were billed for the care they received. Matthew Cruickshank was well prepared to bend the rules with genuine emergencies: no one was going to be faced with demands to produce insurance certificates in the ambulance before they were admitted to *his* department. But Fatima Mahmood was too much!

The dam bursts

These considerations were, of course, not spelled out explicitly in Matthew Cruickshank's mind in this well-organized way as he heard Fatima Mahmood crying out. But they were there all the same as the focus of the pent-up pressures he had been working under. Again, had Matthew Cruickshank not been in an exhausted state, he would not have reacted as he did. As it was, the dam burst. With "right on his side," he jumped at the opportunity to deal for once decisively with a case

that on clinical as well as managerial grounds appeared unambiguously an abuse of the service.

Walking purposefully out of his office and across the department, he rehearsed in his mind how he would set an example of "drawing the line." There would be no pandering to Fatima Mahmood this time. He would put her in a side room to cool off and leave it to the next shift when they came on in half an hour to deal with her when things had settled down a bit. It was in her best interests, after all, he thought. Her best interests were surely *not* served by reinforcing this hypochondriacal cycle of behavior. He knew the junior doctor on the night shift as someone who was not likely to take any nonsense. He could give her a quick check over in due course.

Fatima Mahmood

Fatima Mahmood had lived too long with fear. She had had recurrent episodes of lower abdominal pain for some months now, but this was the worst yet. She was sure that something must be badly wrong to cause such pain and was worried that she might die if she did not seek treatment . . . and then who would look after her children.

Fatima Mahmood's story

So far so neurotic, then, some may think. But Fatima Mahmood had in fact good reason to be afraid. She and her four young children had fled to the UK four years previously after her husband was killed in front of his family when their town was caught up in ethnic conflict. She had never spoken to a doctor about what the rebels did to her shortly after (she was repeatedly raped) but wondered if it might have something to do with the pains she had had ever since.

In some respects, things had started to go better recently: as a family they had finally been granted refugee status earlier that year (contrary to Matthew Cruickshank's not unreasonable assumptions) and the children were now doing well at school. Yet, even as her other worries lessened, Fatima Mahmood became more preoccupied with her health problems and fear of dying. She came from a rural and close-knit community where she had lived with an extended family circle and many friends always at close call. Here in the UK she had few such supports. She felt lonely and vulnerable and had become increasingly tearful and sad much of the time.

Fatima Mahmood's situation was complicated by her difficulties in understanding how the UK health system worked. She felt instinctively that, as a large modern hospital, Blackstone was the safest place to be. But her fears were now becoming further aggravated by the fact that even they (the staff) seemed unable to help her. Worse still, she had picked up their growing frustration as she struggled to explain what was wrong and she had become increasingly fearful that next time they might refuse to see her at all (Olsson and Hansagi, 2001).

Lost in translation

> **Reflection point**
>
> Before reading on, it will be worthwhile reflecting for a moment on the problems of working across language barriers in health care.
>
> Translators, either professional or family members, are often used, but this has disadvantages as well as advantages.
>
> Think about the use of translators with Fatima Mahmood. Draw on any personal experience you may have had of working with translators and look at the issues for you as a clinician as well as for the patient.

There is a growing body of evidence from a number of disciplines on the problems of translation between cultures in health care contexts showing that Matthew Cruickshank's and Fatima Mahmood's experiences were far from unusual. Matthew Cruickshank was like many others in his position in finding it deeply frustrating to have to work through language barriers (Haffner, 1992). He was well aware that best practice demanded the use of professional translators attuned to reconciling different explanatory models of illness and other cultural aspects of translation (Bhui and Bhugra, 2004). But there was virtually no statutory provision available to him and, despite his best efforts, he had been unable to identify a reliable resource among local voluntary sector organizations (Thomas *et al.*, 2009). Besides which, waiting for a translator seemed to him a waste of precious time and he had had experiences of patients (including Fatima Mahmood) refusing to use particular translators after he had gone to a lot of trouble to find one.

There was also a gender issue in this case: Matthew Cruickshank was aware that the fact that he was a man might make Fatima Mahmood feel awkward; but as a male nurse he had stood his fair share of stick for his choice of career and he felt it was important for patients not to be prejudiced against male nurses, or female doctors for that matter.

From Fatima Mahmood's perspective, she was well aware that the problems she experienced every time she came to Blackstone hospital were in part a result of her lack of ability to speak English. Yet, as a perceived failure on her behalf, this only served to deepen her sense of demoralization. In truth, she had been doing well in English classes at the local college. But when, already feeling ill and frightened, she found herself in the overwhelming environment of the hospital, such language skills as she had acquired just slipped away. Moreover, as a Muslim woman she felt deeply inhibited talking to male staff (the staff always seemed to be male) and she had consequently not been able even to try telling anyone about some of her symptoms. The result was that she had found herself at times inventing other reasons for her attendance, which she was aware had inevitably complicated things further.

They had used translators, of course. But she feared being blamed for what had happened and had found it impossible to talk about it. The last translator she had been offered was a man whose name and dialect quickly identified him as coming from the ethnic group whose violence had led to their seeking asylum. Her son Ali had proved adept at languages and could now translate for them successfully in everyday contexts. But how could she talk openly about what had happened through her son?

A disaster averted

All the elements necessary for a clinical disaster were thus present: an exhausted Matthew Cruickshank striding across his department in high dudgeon at what he had come to believe was a flagrant misuse of the service, and an increasingly hysterical Fatima Mahmood now in severe pain and terrified that her last hope of getting help was slipping away.

In the event, both Matthew and Fatima were saved by robust clinical procedures. But disaster would even so not have been averted had it not been for Fatima Mahmood's son Ali.

Ali Mahmood

Ali Mahmood was strong. A slightly built 11-year-old, he had taken increasingly seriously his role as the male head of the family as he began to grow up in his new country. He now recalled very little of what had happened to them four years earlier and was doing well at school, despite the problems at home. He was also helped by his culture: it was natural for him to take up his role as "head of the family," and it gave him a clear context in which to make sense of his new situation and move on from the past. His religion provided additional stability and purpose – his father had taught him their daily cycle of prayer and the local Imam had been impressed with his knowledge of the Koran and encouraged him in his studies.

Robust clinical procedures

It was thus an Ali Mahmood mature beyond his years who called the ambulance, despite his mother's protestations, when she collapsed as she was serving their evening meal. The ambulance crew, when they arrived, was impressed with his quiet presence ("dignified" one of them described him later). They could see at once that he had done the right thing: Fatima Mahmood was by then clearly very ill – sweating, unable to stand and with a thin racing pulse. With Ali translating, they managed to persuade Fatima Mahmood that, notwithstanding her previous experiences and fear of rejection, they really did need to get her to hospital, and quickly too. She finally agreed after a neighbor (who was from a similar background) offered to look after Fatima Mahmood's daughters. Ali Mahmood insisted on coming with them in the ambulance.

Mathew Cruickshank had been delayed leaving his office and following the stretcher into the assessment room by a call about another patient. By the time he arrived on the scene, the clinical procedures he had himself put in place for expediting emergency admissions were already in full swing, and Fatima was responding to the expert and very necessary resuscitation of a patient in shock. Matthew hesitated for a moment on the edge of the circle of well-organized activity. Then turning, he walked quietly away.

The diagnosis

Later that evening, Matthew Cruickshank telephoned the gynecology ward to ask if Fatima Mahmood was all OK. She was. However, in addition to a ruptured ovarian cyst, they had found extensive perineal scarring and fistulae, probably related to the violence she had suffered and subsequent infections before coming to UK.

Moving on

Matthew Cruickshank was in a place where as clinicians we have surely all been at one time or another – thanking our lucky stars for narrowly avoiding an egregious error and having learnt a vital lesson from one of our patients.

Fatima Mahmood's troubles were not over. But the fact that they had found something "really wrong" had restored her belief in herself: better a serious physical problem than to be written off as "neurotic." Before she left hospital, she was visited by the Imam (Ali had told him what had happened) who encouraged her to join a new women's group that had been set up in their mosque. Her confidence thus restored and her social network re-established, she was soon well on the way to finally moving on from the past and to building a new life for herself and her family.

Chapter summary

This chapter has offered a cautionary tale about the dangers in health care of losing site of the evidence when values – ethical values in this case – are strongly in play. The strong (if uncharacteristic) moral outrage of an A&E charge nurse, Matthew Cruickshank, provoked by an apparently inappropriate use of NHS resources, put him at risk of missing a genuine emergency in a case of unexplained abdominal pain.

Clinically then, the message of this chapter is complementary to the message of the last:

- Chapter 10, applying the Two-feet Principle of values-based practice, illustrated the dangers of focusing on the evidence at the expense of values – so the message was "Think evidence, think values too!"
- This chapter, applying the Squeaky-wheel Principle of values-based practice, has illustrated the equal and opposite dangers, clinically speaking, of focusing on values at the expense of the evidence – so the counterpart message is "Think values, think evidence too!"

Taken together, these two principles reflect the importance of maintaining a positive interplay between values and evidence in all areas of health care. This is self-evidently so in intercultural medicine: the story of Matthew Cruickshank and Fatima Mahmood shows the central importance here of looking at the evidence rather than falling back on assumptions and stereotypes in which, as the British psychiatrist and expert on cultural medicine Kamaldeep Bhui has put it, "default values trigger actions and oversights" (personal communication).

In recognizing the importance of the interplay between values and evidence, intercultural medicine is thus well ahead of many other areas of health care in combining values-based with evidence-based approaches. Bhui and his colleagues have indeed developed practical tools to support intercultural consultations, which we believe have much wider application (see websites, below). In the next chapter, we will find that the interplay between values and evidence is no less important in relation to the very different challenges presented by high-tech medical interventions.

References

Bevan, G. and Hood, C. (2006). Have targets improved performance in the English NHS? *British Medical Journal* **332**, 419–21.

Bhui, K. S. and Bhugra, D. (2004). Communication with patients from other cultures: the place of explanatory models. *Advances in Psychiatric Treatment* **10**, 474–8.

Haffner, L. (1992). Translation is not enough: interpreting in a medical setting. *Western Journal of Medicine* **157**, 255–9.

National Institute for Mental Health in England (NIMHE) and the Care Services Improvement Partnership (2008). *3 Keys to a Shared Approach in Mental Health Assessment*. London: Department of Health.

Olsson, M. and Hansagi, H. (2001). Repeated use of the emergency department: a qualitative study of the patient's perspective. *Journal of Emergency Medicine* **18**, 430–4.

Thomas, P., Shah, A. and Thornton, T. (2009). Language, games and the role of interpreters in psychiatric diagnosis: a Wittgensteinian thought experiment. *Medical Humanities* **35**, 13–18.

Websites

- Websites giving further information relevant to intercultural medicine include: www.medact. org.uk areas on global health education and on refugee and asylum seeker health resources; and HARPWEB www.harpweb.org.uk for resources on multicultural health and refugee and asylum seeker needs in health care, in a UK context.

- The materials developed by Kamaldeep Bhui and others to support intercultural consultations (see text) are available at: www.culturalconsultation. org-if.

- Many practical examples of the important role played by Imams and other local leaders and voluntary sector organizations in helping with translation and similar challenges of intercultural medicine are given in the Department of Health consultation, *3 Keys to Assessment in Mental Health* (National Institute for Mental Health in England (NIMHE) and the Care Services Improvement Partnership, 2008, which is also available as a downloadable pdf on the website supporting this series).

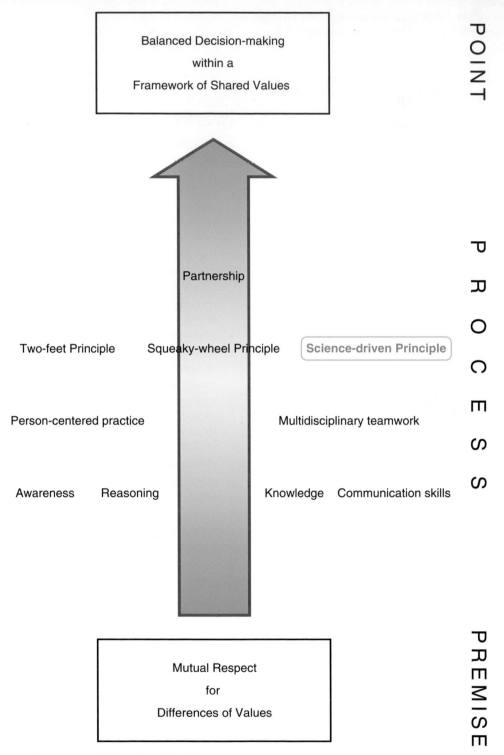

Balanced Decision-making
within a
Framework of Shared Values

Partnership

Two-feet Principle   Squeaky-wheel Principle   Science-driven Principle

Person-centered practice   Multidisciplinary teamwork

Awareness   Reasoning   Knowledge   Communication skills

Mutual Respect
for
Differences of Values

Map of values-based practice – the Science-driven Principle.

12

Elective fertility: think high-tech, think evidence *and* values!

Values-based practice element 9: the Science-driven Principle

Topics covered in this chapter

The Science-driven Principle – that advances in medical science and technology drive the need equally for values-based as for evidence-based practice – is illustrated by the experience of a couple seeking treatment for infertility.

Other topics include:

- Patients' experiences of infertility treatment
- Clinicians' experiences of infertility treatment
- NICE guidelines
- Spiritual direction
- Importance of the extended multidisciplinary team.

Take-away message for practice

*It is above all in a high-tech area of medicine (like IVF) that it is important to adopt a balanced "values **plus** evidence" approach. So, "think high-tech, think values **and** evidence!"*

Organ transplants, prosthetic limbs, laser surgery, in vitro fertilization – these are just some of the growing list of new high-tech resources now available in everyday clinical practice driven by the unprecedented advances in medical science and technology in recent decades. Nor is there any sign of the rate of advance slowing. Gene therapy, it is true, heralded over 20 years ago as the next big thing, is only just beginning to get under way, but getting underway it is.

Two high-tech challenges

Advances in high-tech medicine clearly hold out the promise of great benefits for patients. But these same advances raise many challenges for practitioners, both scientific and ethical. On the science side, there is the challenge of keeping up to date with the evidence: here the resources of evidence-based practice guidelines are helpful. Whatever the limitations of locally or nationally agreed guidelines, they at least set mutual limits on our options.

More troubling though, on the ethics side, are the challenges from high-tech medicine to strongly held moral convictions about our very nature as human beings. Adopting a term attributed to the American bioethicist, Leon Kass, the philosopher and ethicist Baroness Warnock described this as the "yuk factor" (Jasanoff, 2005). The "yuk factor" it is true tends to diminish with time. It is difficult now to recall the moral uproar that greeted Robert Edwards and Patrick Steptoe's announcement in 1978 of the birth in the UK of Louise Brown, the first test-tube baby, or, further back, the first successful human heart transplant in 1967 by Christian Barnard at Groote Schuur Hospital in Cape Town.

From ethics to values

Both advances were, of course, also greeted with acclaim for the benefits they offered patients (Robert Edwards finally received the Nobel Prize for Medicine in 2010). And there's the rub. High-tech medical advances take us straight into the contested territory between the benefits of science and the claims of morality.

One response to this is regulation. Baroness Warnock made her comments about the "yuk factor" when she was Chair of the government committee of enquiry that resulted in the establishment of the UK's Human Fertilisation and Embryology Authority (HFEA). But as we saw in Part 1, regulation alone can never cover the wide diversity of situations faced by individual patients and clinicians in practice. And the danger if the competing claims of the sciences and morality are carried over into the clinic is that patients end up getting caught in the cross fire. This at any rate was the experience of Hilary and Bob Swann.

The clinical context

Hilary and Bob Swann looked anxious as they sat holding hands awkwardly in the infertility clinic of their local hospital. The consultant, Mr. Barry Winterbottom, who had seen them on a previous occasion, was away and they were booked to see his senior registrar, Dr. Kathy Millar. They had mixed feelings about this. It was hard enough coping with "this infertility thing" without having to see someone new. They had talked last night about going private or even just giving up. But they were here now and would at least hear what Dr. Millar had to say.

Different individuals, different narratives

In this chapter, we are going to depart from our usual practice and move straight to a reflection point before providing more in the way of background about the characters involved, Hilary and Bob Swann, their friends and families, and their attendant clinicians.

The point of this reflection is to underline the starting point for values-based practice in individually unique values. Recall here from Chapter 2 David Sackett and his colleagues' definition of evidence-based medicine as integrating best research evidence with each individual patient's unique values (their "... unique preferences, concerns and expectations ..." as Sackett *et al.*, 2000, put it). The message of this chapter is that it is above all in high-tech medicine that evidence and values have to be integrated if our decisions are (as Sackett also put it) to "serve the patient."

So, in the reflection that follows, the idea is to try building your own background narrative, your own particular and individual "Hilary and Bob Swann," and your own particular and individual cast of professionals and others involved. You might try writing down brief profiles of each of these characters. You can then refer back to these profiles later on when we ask you to imagine how your cast of characters might have reacted in the story that follows in the rest of the chapter.

Reflection point

Before reading on then, try imagining what lay behind Hilary and Bob Swann's feelings as they waited to see Dr. Millar: think about the characters involved and the experiences they might have been through. Be specific (e.g. give your characters specific ages).

Let your imagination range freely but "keep it real" by drawing on your own background and experience (whether personal or professional) and any knowledge you may have of patients' and clinicians' experiences of infertility treatment.

In the sections that follow, we introduce our own versions of Hilary and Bob Swann and follow their experiences with a supporting cast of friends and professionals as they navigate their way through the early stages of infertility treatment. As we will see, they come at one point close to being torn apart by the apparently conflicting imperatives of science and ethics as represented, respectively, by the consultant in charge of the local NHS infertility clinic, Mr. Barry Winterbottom, and his registrar, Dr. Kathy Millar.

In this case, Hilary and Bob Swann's story has a happy (interim) ending. We leave them before they actually start IVF treatment. As many others have found (witness the patients' stories on the HFEA website, see below), they eventually reached a decision about what to do with their relationship actually strengthened (Wilkes *et al.*, 2009). But the key to this, as we will see, was an approach in which, consistent with the Science-driven Principle, evidence and values were equally in play in a well-balanced and fully integrated way. In the final section of the chapter, we reflect on exactly why high-tech areas of medicine above all demand a well-balanced "evidence plus values" approach of the kind that proved so pivotal in Hilary and Bob Swann's story.

Poor-quality sperm

Hilary and Bob Swann

Hilary and Bob Swann were both in their mid-30s. They had been together for five years and got married three years previously. Hilary was a primary school teacher and Bob an IT technician working for the local council. They stopped using contraception about two and a half years ago and had presumed that a baby would soon follow. They were active members of their local church and believed having a family of their own to be integral to what life and marriage are about. Their congregation was full of young families. Hilary had run the Sunday school for many years and for some time had been looking forward to bringing her own children into it.

Initially, they put their failure to conceive down to stress, as they both worked hard, and had decided to just "wait and see." But with Hilary's ongoing failure to fall pregnant, they decided to see their GP, Dr. Chandra.

Dr. Chandra

Dr. Chandra seemed understanding, although the photo of his four smiling children on his desk showed that he had not experienced infertility first hand. He told them that this was a common problem and that many couples did not even come forward to ask for help. He suggested that he arrange some initial tests and would then see them again.

The tests were organized through the clinic nurse and were carried out quite promptly. Bob Swann knew from what he and Hilary had already read about infertility treatment that he would have to produce a semen sample, but he nonetheless found the process surprisingly stressful. It left him feeling, as many men in his situation have felt (Carmeli and Birenbaum-Carmeli, 1994), that his masculinity was on trial; and when at their second appointment with Dr. Chandra they were told the sample showed "poor-quality" sperm, it hit him hard as a personal failure.

> **Reflection point**
>
> This is clearly an important point in Hilary and Bob Swann's experience of the early stages of treatment for infertility.
>
> How do you think they reacted? And how did the reactions of other people – their GP for example, Dr. Chandra, and their family and friends – influence them.
>
> Try thinking about this for our Bob and Hilary Swann and then imagine how things might have gone (the same or differently) for the characters you developed yourself in the reflection point earlier in the chapter.

Again, Dr. Chandra was understanding and took time to talk through their options and next steps. He emphasized the good news that they had found nothing to prevent them having a baby. This could still happen in the natural course of events but with long waiting lists (one to two years locally), he suggested he got the process going with a referral to the local infertility clinic. Was there anything they could do in the meantime? Just try to relax about it all, Dr. Chandra had advised, continue having regular intercourse, and avoid all those ovulation kits – they will just make you worry more! He also gave them the leaflet the local clinic had produced about infertility and its treatments.

Friends and family

Twelve months later, Hilary and Bob Swann received an appointment to see Mr. Winterbottom at the infertility clinic in two weeks' time. Their reaction was mixed. The appointment was earlier than they had expected and they were glad that the waiting was over. But over the previous year, they had begun to have doubts about the whole thing: they feared that if they tried to put off the appointment, they would go to the bottom of the waiting list, but all the same, two weeks felt like a short call to crunch time.

Their doubts had started when they began to find out more about infertility treatment following up the websites in the infertility leaflet Dr. Chandra had given them, and other resources (as a teacher and IT specialist, respectively, they were both competent with web-based resources). Official sources such as the NICE guidance (with its appendix for patients) and the HFEA website (with its many stories from patients) were full of information. But all this information also made the process sound incredibly challenging: relationships under strain, roller-coaster emotions, the many side effects of the drugs used, and rather terrifying-sounding procedures (whatever was "ovarian drilling"?). They also picked up that to go private would cost tens of thousands of pounds.

The dawning realities of infertility treatment in turn increased the pressure on them to conceive naturally. Despite Dr. Chandra's warnings, they did buy an ovulation kit from the chemist. But this had made sex feel like a scientific process that neither of them was particularly enjoying any more. Their awareness that this loss of sexual satisfaction was likely to reduce still further the chances of Hilary getting pregnant gave a further twist to their growing anxieties.

Friends and family in this instance were no help at all. A rather self-contained couple, they had decided not to tell anyone about their difficulties in conceiving and their plans for getting infertility treatment. But Hilary's three sisters were all busy looking after their own small children, and Hilary has found it increasingly hard to get excited as her sisters and their friends seemed to be announcing one pregnancy after another. Both sets of parents were keen to have lots of grandchildren and had started dropping ill-disguised hints about when they were going to start a family. Hilary's mum had told her many times how "I only needed to look at your dad to get pregnant." Bob had had a few digs from football friends about "firing blanks." Ever conscious of his poor-quality sperm, these had upset him a good deal more than he had let on at the time.

Doubts and dilemmas

Their doubts had come to a head when, a few days earlier, a work colleague of Hilary's had talked in a frank and unapologetic way in the school staffroom about her recent termination for a pregnancy that came at the "wrong time" for her career. Hilary and Bob Swann were not fundamentalist Christians. But even before their difficulties conceiving, they had been broadly anti-abortion, and this casual attitude to, as they saw it, ending a baby's life now struck them with renewed force. It was all the more difficult to accept in someone that Hilary had come to admire as a hard-working and caring teacher. And then, when they talked about it that evening, they made the unwelcome link to the spare embryos that were an inevitable part of IVF.

They had already been well aware of this aspect of IVF, of course. But somehow Hilary's colleague's talk of her abortion had brought it home to them. True, their situations were different. Hilary's colleague had sacrificed a baby for her career: spare embryos (the irony of that term "spare" was not lost on them) were sacrificed to give a baby life. But some of their friends from church believed that "killing" embryos that are not implanted was morally no different from abortion. This, they now realized, was one reason why they had held back from sharing their problems with their vicar or with other members of their congregation.

They had not discussed this previously, but they now recognized that their reluctance to talk about their plans with others in their congregation was something about which they had both felt uneasy all along. After all, this was a congregation that made a point of supporting each other and indeed the wider community in an open and always non-judgmental way (look at how hard they had worked to help that underage "single mum"). There were differences of views among them, but no one (least of all their vicar, the Reverend Benedict Brown) tried to claim the moral high ground. This was one reason why, as a couple, they had felt drawn to this particular church. So the

"problem" they now recognized was their own ambivalence. Was this a test? Was it right? They desperately wanted a baby. But was that really so much better than desperately wanting a career? Who were they to judge? And there was that word again, "judge."

Mr. Barry Winterbottom

Mr. Winterbottom, when they saw him two weeks later, had had a professional and business-like manner that they found initially reassuring. He had been a medical student at a London teaching hospital when Edwards and Steptoe announced the birth of Louise Brown and he had gone on to do research in the early IVF movement. Now a consultant gynecologist, he had remained active as a clinical researcher and was well on top of the latest scientific developments in this still rapidly evolving field. His evident grasp of the technical issues and clear explanations of some of the more complex aspects of IVF gave Hilary and Bob Swann immediate confidence that they were in safe hands.

They were also impressed by Barry Winterbottom's enthusiasm and commitment to his work. They already knew (from the HFEA website) that his clinic achieved consistently above-national-average results for both waiting times and success rates. This was a man, they felt, of integrity.

Yet in the end, they left the appointment still undecided what to do. Confident as Barry Winterbottom had been on the technical issues, he had given them little encouragement to talk about their doubts and concerns. He had seemed perplexed, even perhaps a little impatient, when with their growing concerns about "spare embryos" they had tried to press him on exactly why several embryos had to be produced, when (as they had read on the HFEA website) only three (at most) would be transferred for implantation.

"Actually," Barry Winterbottom had replied, taking their concerns here as a request for further technical information, "in this clinic we are looking at going for single-embryo implantation." And he had launched into a detailed explanation of the latest evidence on the costs (emotional and financial) of multiple pregnancies, the medical risks (he had been involved in collaborative research on ovarian hyperstimulation syndrome) and the growing conviction among those in the field that multiple transfers did little to increase the chances of a successful pregnancy. "After all," he concluded, finishing with an odd narrative sideslip, "over half of spontaneous pregnancies abort naturally."

A relationship under pressure

Bob and Hilary Swann had to get back to work after their appointment with Barry Winterbottom, but they had time that evening to go over what he had said. They found that they had both been unimpressed with his enthusiastic lecture on single embryo transfer. Obviously, he was the expert, and they had seen similar if less forcefully expressed ideas about the potential benefits of this approach on the websites they had looked at. But the claim that transferring only a single embryo made little difference to the chances of a successful pregnancy simply did not square, so far as they could see, with their concerns about spare embryos.

This inconsistency somewhat undermined their otherwise very positive first impressions. But here their feelings about what to do had started to diverge. Thus far, they had had shared concerns about whether they were doing the right thing to go for IVF. What Barry Winterbottom had said about single-embryo transfer was indeed relevant to those concerns but in ways that Hilary and Bob had respectively taken in very different directions over the course of the day:

- Hilary had decided she wanted to "go for it." Her initial reaction to what Barry Winterbottom had said (and the rather zealous way he had said it) was a sense that she was going to be "maneuvered" into a procedure (single-embryo transfer) that would reduce her chances of a successful pregnancy – not by much perhaps (if Barry Winterbottom's reassurances were to be believed), but now in her mid-30s (they had already lost another year waiting

for the appointment) and with only three cycles on offer from the NHS, she could not afford to waste any opportunity. And like others in this situation, the possibility of more than one baby (whatever the risks) suddenly began to look like a bonus. And then, finding herself thinking along these lines, she realized suddenly and with a sense of relief, that moral dilemmas or not, and medical risks or not, *she wanted that baby*; and if necessary they would blow their savings and go private.

- Bob, by contrast, had decided that they should pull out. Still influenced by that poor-quality sperm result, he too had picked up that, like it or not, they were going to end up with a procedure (Barry Winterbottom's single-embryo transfer) that would give them even less chance of success.
- Was it all worth it? The risks to Hilary's health of multiple pregnancies sounded to him very real. But single-embryo transfer meant that, in the process of trying for a baby, probably (as he now increasingly felt) unsuccessfully, they would only end up being responsible for even more "spare embryos."

Bob and Hilary Swann were not at this stage actually falling out. But it was a shock to them both to find that they, who had been until now so close, were for the first time at serious odds. It was in this new and unfamiliar state of mind, anxious as much for their relationship as for their chances of starting a family, that they went into the consultation with Dr. Kathy Millar.

Dr. Kathy Millar

Dr. Millar inadvertently made things worse. Barry Winterbottom had asked her to see if Bob and Hilary Swann would be willing to be included in a multicenter randomized trial of single-embryo transfer that he had been asked to take part in. He was keen that the clinic should be included as a collaborating center in this project to maintain its status as a research-oriented center of excellence. It would also bring in extra resources that would help to bring down waiting times still further.

Dr. Millar dealt with Bob and Hilary Swann's questions about the technical aspects of the proposed research in a competent and professional way. But when Bob Swann had asked her straight out whether she (Kathy Millar) was happy with single-embryo transfer, she had found herself revealing more of her personal feelings than she had intended. It was true, she said, that there was a case for this approach. But she could not help feeling that the recent push for it was being driven as much by concerns about the burden on the benefits budget of multiple births (child allowance was at that time paid on a per capita basis without any cap) as by purely clinical considerations. After all, there had been no change in the basic science, no new techniques had been introduced and the clinical data about the risks of multiple pregnancies had been there almost from the start.

Of course, she went on, she knew first hand from her experience of working in the termination clinic that there was much less public concern nowadays about the rights and wrongs of abortion ... though, she added hastily seeing the look on Bob's face, that was certainly not *her* view ...

Reflection point

Why do you think Dr. Millar responded like this? What lay behind her moment of self-revelation?

If you wrote a character for Dr. Millar earlier, how would your Dr. Millar have dealt with Bob's question?

Dr. Millar was a young obstetrics and gynecology registrar who worked in the fertility clinic as part of her many duties. She enjoyed this aspect of her work and shared the team's pride in the high standard of the service they provided. Although still single, she hoped to have children of her own one day and she was glad to have the opportunity to help other couples achieve this. She was aware that many had long and desperate histories of trying for a baby for many years, and felt that, as a woman, she understood, perhaps rather better than her consultant, why their patients were so often anxious and tearful.

She was less happy with having to cover the so-called "social gynecology" clinic. The very need for a euphemism, she felt, said it all; and she had found the direct contrast between the two clinics increasingly hard to manage, particularly as they were run back-to-back in the same rooms. In the morning, she was helping couples desperate to have a baby. In the afternoon, she was helping couples desperate to get rid of a baby. In theory, she could opt out of dealing with terminations. But she could not claim a religious objection (as a Roman Catholic colleague had done) and she knew that (in practice) it would put a big question mark in her otherwise exemplary CV. And now her concerns had been given a further twist by this new plan to get involved in a trial of single-embryo transfer.

Having no close friends in her field, she had not been able to share her growing unhappiness about this with anyone. She had thus far seen next to nothing of her educational supervisor and certainly had not built up enough of a relationship to feel able to share her feelings. Mr. Winterbottom was not an option. They got along tolerably well but without much in the way of mutual understanding. When she was appointed, Dr. Millar had been delighted to get the chance to work with a recognized expert in the infertility field, but she had found him in the event rather overwhelmingly male – "Too outdoors," she once described him to a friend.

Mr. Winterbottom too had been delighted to recruit a first-class doctor who he had believed would be as keen as he was on research, but he in his turn had found Dr. Millar's rather serious manner a little daunting – "Not one for a joke," was how he had summed her up in his mind – and he had been disappointed by her apparent disinterest (as he saw it) in their latest research (the single-embryo trial).

Seeing ourselves in our patients

Thus, it was a relief for Dr. Millar to off-load with a couple she assumed from Bob Swann's question shared her concerns. But like Mr. Winterbottom, she had been misled in this by her own preoccupations. Mr. Winterbottom had responded to Bob and Hilary's attempt to raise their concerns about single-embryo transfer as a request for more *technical information* (his passion being the science of infertility treatment). Dr. Millar had taken Bob Swann's direct question as a sign that he and Hilary both shared her *moral concerns*, and, these having been bottled up for so long, it was perhaps not surprising that this young doctor ended up saying too much.

A relationship at breaking point

Dr. Millar, like Mr. Winterbottom, was in no sense an ideologue. Neither of them had subjected Bob and Hilary Swann to anything in the way of a diatribe (*for* science or *for* morality). But just as Mr. Winterbottom's enthusiasm for the science of infertility had led him (inadvertently) to open up a rift between Bob and Hilary Swann, so Dr. Millar's ill-judged sharing of her moral doubts had (also, of course, inadvertently) widened the rift.

The contrast between the two clinics (infertility and "social gynecology") and the discovery that they were in the very same rooms was bad enough for Bob Swann. But the fact that this clearly dedicated doctor, Dr. Millar, could be dealing with terminations one minute and then, after, as Bob Swann put it to himself, a cup of coffee, go straight on and deal with infertility treatment rubbed a considerable quantity of salt into the already sore wounds of his moral doubts. It was the coldly deliberate nature of the arrangements that got to him. Was this, he felt, what as a society we had come to? Bright and obviously caring young doctors obliged to go so transparently against their consciences . . . and not in a moment of weakness or under extreme duress but in a planned and wholly deliberate way?

And wasn't that just the point – no one tried to justify the deliberate induction of abortion on the grounds that most natural pregnancies ended in spontaneous abortion. To the contrary, it was precisely that it was *deliberate* that made abortion morally suspect. So how could the equally deliberate creation of "spare embryos" be justified merely on the same grounds, of the high rate of spontaneous abortions? It was, he now realized uncomfortably, the deliberate nature of IVF that made it in both senses of the word – moral and biological – *un*-natural.

But even as Bob Swann's moral doubts became more acute, so, in response, did Hilary Swann's determination to have a baby become the more desperate. They found it increasingly difficult even to talk about what to do. And then one evening a few days later, it all came to a head. In a fit of exasperation, Bob had ended up making the potentially fatal (for their relationship) mistake of saying, alright then, he would do it for her. "But it's *our* baby," she had shouted at him, now in tears . . . and neither had known what to say next.

An (interim) happy ending

At the start of this chapter, we promised you what we described as an (interim) happy ending. So how did Bob and Hilary Swann get from this unhappy standoff, with their relationship at risk, to a shared decision about whether to go ahead with the next stages of IVF treatment?

As the patients' stories on the HFEA website testify, many couples find themselves under strain in different ways from the trials and tribulations of IVF. But as these stories also show, they often end up with their relationships deepened by the experience of working through the problems together. The details vary from case to case. But a common theme is the need for someone outside their immediate relationship to share their feelings with. In some instances, friends and family can provide this role. More often, it is someone beyond the couple's personal circle: a counselor experienced in this area perhaps, or a patient support group.

There was neither patient group nor counseling service connected with the infertility clinic to which Bob and Hilary Swann had been referred. This was a perhaps surprising omission given that the NICE guidelines recommend counseling should be available.

The omission perhaps reflected Mr. Winterbottom's particular focus on the basic science. From time to time, the clinic nursing team had suggested setting up a support group, but he had not encouraged this, fearing that such initiatives tended to get taken over by pressure groups: he also felt that "self-help" meant inaccurate science (how could a patients' group, however well read, match his 30 years of research and clinical experience?). A counseling service was a more reliable option from Mr. Winterbottom's point of view but would divert much needed and increasingly limited resources from front-line clinical services (keeping their waiting list down to one year did not come cheap). At all events, Bob and Hilary Swann had to find their own way forward.

> ### Reflection point
>
> Try thinking for a moment here about how you imagine they might have done this. How did Hilary and Bob Swann get from standoff to a shared decision about IVF?
>
> Clearly, your own versions of Hilary and Bob Swann are likely to have reached a very different point in their particular stories by this stage. We will be leaving Hilary and Bob (in all their instantiations) shortly. So try completing your own version of their story and then, as you read on, consider how and why this differed from the version of their story in this chapter.
>
> The diversity of different stories will be important when we consider in the final section of the chapter exactly why it is so important to bring values and evidence together in high-tech areas of medical practice.

The Reverend Benedict Brown

As already noted, every couple is different. In the case of our Hilary and Bob Swann, it was their religion that gave them a way forward, and in the person of their vicar, Benedict Brown. They both recognized that they could not go on without help. Friends and family were out of the question. Dr. Chandra might have recommended a counselor but they knew from what other people had told them of their experiences that unless you had a serious mental illness it was likely to be months before they would get an appointment; and with no counseling service or self-help group available through the clinic, they were anyway reluctant to take what they saw as the gamble of seeing someone who might not really understand their feelings about IVF.

So the obvious choice was their vicar. Although unmarried and a little younger than them, they knew Benedict Brown to be a caring and thoughtful person and they felt that he would at least understand Bob's continuing moral dilemmas over IVF. In the event, he turned out to be, as they had anticipated, entirely non-judgmental. He was also and more surprisingly from their point of view entirely non-directive. He listened carefully to their concerns and encouraged them to talk openly about their fear that this would "drive them apart," but he quietly but firmly refused to get drawn on the moral issues.

He did, however, reassure them about the theology (he was a Reverend Doctor). In their tradition, he reminded them, care of the body went hand in hand with care of the soul (look at the way Jesus always had an eye to the health and welfare of his followers). He encouraged them to talk further about things and made an appointment for them to see him again in a week.

Spiritual direction

When they got together a week later, Benedict Brown continued his strategy of refusing to take sides in their moral argument, thus opening up a space for Hilary and Bob Swann to air and explore their different takes on where they had got to about whether to go ahead with IVF. Benedict Brown did not think of this as counseling. He was drawing rather on a deep tradition of spiritual direction that, in tracing its origins to the desert fathers of Christianity, preceded the "invention" of counseling by some 2000 years. Like counseling, however, and contrary to the all-too-common stereotypes of religious ideologies, the primary aim of spiritual direction (and of other similar traditions within all the major religions; see Atwell and Fulford, 2006) is not to "direct" but to provide a safe and non-judgmental environment in which those concerned can find a way forward that is right for them.

At the end of their second session, Benedict Brown offered to lend Hilary and Bob Swann a copy of Phillip Sheldrake's (1998) *Befriending our Desires*. He had picked up that their growing rift over the rights and wrongs of IVF was surprisingly out of touch with the realities of the science: despite clearly being well informed, they did not seem to be aware (and certainly had not mentioned) the growing opportunities for spare embryos to be frozen for future use by themselves or as a gift to others. This raised its own dilemmas, no doubt, but it at least showed the parallels between IVF and abortion in a very different light. He suspected, therefore, that there was some unspoken factor, a hidden variable of which, likely as not, they were as yet unaware, driving their inability to come together in a decision about what to do.

He could have raised this possibility directly. But as a skilled counselor (in all but name), he recognized that if he was right, he risked reinforcing whatever denials and defenses were in play. His suggestion that they had a look at Phillip Sheldrake's book was thus aimed at distracting them from what risked becoming a (dangerously irresolvable) sideshow and allowing them to get to their real agenda for themselves and by their own route. He knew them both well and felt confident that their relationship remained basically very strong – it had, after all, been the driving force behind this very private couple's decision to break cover and seek help. They needed, he felt, to stop beating themselves up morally and come back to understanding their self-worth as individuals and as a couple. This book, by a widely respected authority, an ecumenical theologian within their shared spiritual tradition, could help them do just that: the message of *Befriending our Desires* was a message of inclusion and of respect for the diversity of individual beliefs and values.

Discernment

Bob and Hilary Swann started to read *Befriending our Desires* initially as required homework, but by the time they saw Benedict Brown again, they had both devoured it from cover to cover. The key word of the title, "befriending," had given them the lifeline they needed: suddenly their desire for a baby ceased to be "selfish" (how could it have got to this?) and became something they could own together. But a second word, "discernment," had allowed them (extending the metaphor) to climb the lifeline.

Reflection point

Before reading on, you may want to think what "discernment" might mean in this context and why it proved so helpful to Bob and Hilary Swann.

Would Benedict Brown have been able to help your versions of Bob and Hilary Swann? And what would they have understood by "discernment"?

Discernment in the tradition of spiritual direction can be thought of as a response to the challenge of "anything goes." As we discussed in Part 1, this is a challenge that must be met by any liberal and inclusive approach, not least values-based practice. As a term of art in the tradition of spiritual direction, discernment is a process of reflection on where our desires are taking us and hence whether they are desires we should follow or resist.

For Hilary and Bob Swann, such reflection, combined with a coincidental report in a national newspaper of a new "record" being set for the time a frozen embryo had been kept before successful transfer to a non-donor recipient, took them back to the realities of the basic science: yes, some embryos might still be lost (as happens naturally, Mr. Winterbottom as they now recalled had pointed out), but "befriending" their desire to have a baby by way of IVF could help others as well as themselves. This obvious yet thus far blocked insight gave them both the confidence to think about IVF as a positive option rather than as an unfortunate (or, as Bob Swann had come to believe, morally dubious) necessity. Their whole approach thus shifted from anxious preoccupation to positive engagement, with a corresponding increase in their chances of success.

For Bob Swann, the process of reflection, and the now more relaxed and realistic atmosphere in which as a couple they found themselves, had a further and equally important outcome. He now saw clearly for the first time that at the back of his reluctance to go ahead with IVF was not really moral doubt but plain fear, fear of failure. That poor-quality sperm result and the feelings that it evoked had hurt him more than even he had realized. It had meant that deep inside and without acknowledging it, he had come to fear every future failure to conceive (and he knew there were likely to be many failures to conceive) as *his* failure to conceive.

As is the way with such fears, however, to name them is to tame them. By the time of their third (and as it proved final) appointment with Benedict Brown, they had found their way forward. The moral arguments were unchanged. In his orderly mathematical way, Bob Swann could still lay them out clearly before his mind's eye. But seeing them now for what they were, a shield against his fear of failure, they had lost their hold on him. Hilary Swann, too, although in a different way, had "befriended" her desires. Reassured by the authority of Benedict Brown's theology, she no longer felt morally compromised by her wish for a baby and was thus no longer driven to fight her corner merely defensively. Bob and Hilary Swann both knew perfectly well that there was no guarantee of a successful pregnancy. But, thus befriended, they were indeed friends once more.

Individuals and individual narratives

Benedict Brown, being a single man who was a little younger than Bob and Hilary Swann and an ordained priest at that, was, you may feel, an unlikely hero in a story about IVF. After all, the "churches," of all religions, were among the fiercest opponents of Robert Edwards and Patrick Steptoe in the early days of their work although there was opposition too from the scientific and medical communities of the day – they had to fund much of their early research privately. But Benedict Brown had spent some years in one of the great medieval contemplative orders before finding his vocation as a parish priest, and he had learned at first hand the skills of spiritual direction. He had his own demons to slay. But they were not the demons of either scientism or moralism.

Your version of Hilary and Bob Swann's story with a cast of perhaps very different characters may well have developed in a very different way. This is important. It is the *uniqueness* of individual narratives that is at the heart of values-based practice:

- In one version of the story, it might have been the clinic nursing staff who gave Bob and Hilary Swann the support they needed: as the patients' stories on the HFEA website testify, IVF clinic nurses, who generally do much of the routine history taking and follow-up once IVF starts, often provide the understanding and support that couples going through this stressful process so desperately need.
- In another version of the story, Dr. Millar might have come to understand what it had meant for Mr. Winterbottom as a young man to fight alongside Edwards and Steptoe for the science of

infertility. The ethical and legal battles they had to win in those early days represented no small risk to his career.

- In yet another version, Mr. Winterbottom might have found ways of channeling Dr. Millar's moral energies into more productive channels – perhaps getting her to set up a patient support group or counseling service (NICE guidelines would have given them a shared basis for promoting this). In this way, with her feelings less dangerously bottled up, Dr. Millar would have been less likely to have mismanaged her consultation with Bob and Hilary Swann.

The possible narratives are as diverse as the diversity of individual human values.

Science . . . and values?

Before moving on to the next chapter, it will be worth reflecting for a few moments on the Science-driven Principle in light of Bob and Hilary Swann's story. The Science-driven Principle, you will recall from Chapter 3, states that advances in medical science and technology drive the need equally for values-based practice as for evidence-based practice. But we left unanswered the question of why this should be so.

Reflection point

You may find it helpful to think for a moment about this question for yourself before reading on.

That advances in medical science and technology drive the need for ethical debate seems now (with hindsight at least) self-evident. Baroness Warnock's "yuk factor" (as above, this chapter) is sufficient to explain why science drives ethics.

But values-based practice is about *values* more broadly construed. So the question is, what have advances in medical science and technology got to do with driving values in the broad sense implied by values-based practice?

Science, *choices* and values

The short answer to this question is *choices*: advances in medical science and technology open up an ever wider range of choices for patients and clinicians alike, and with choices go values.

Reproductive medicine provides a clear example of how science and technology open up new choices and thus bring an ever wider range of values into clinical

decision-making. Before Robert Edwards and Patrick Steptoe's success with Louise Brown, there was little that medicine could offer infertile couples beyond excluding obvious causes. How different the situation is now, *post*-Louise Brown:

- Pre-Louise Brown, values were certainly in play and strong values at that. Infertility is widely (although, of course, not universally) strongly negatively evaluated – this is why there was and continues to be such an active research program in this area. But this was a value that, in the absence of anything much in the way of effective treatment for infertility, meant that its impact on clinical decision-making was relatively uncomplicated.

- Post-Louise Brown, and with the ever widening range of choices opened up by subsequent rapid developments in the science of assisted fertility, the choices opened up in reproductive medicine have increasingly become (as in Hilary and Bob Swann's story) wide indeed.

With this widened range of choices then, as those involved in this story illustrate, the diversity of human values is brought directly into play in clinical decision-making, and with this diversity goes the need for values-based practice.

Chapter summary

Hilary and Bob Swann's story in this chapter has illustrated the extent to which, in high-tech areas of medical practice, patients are ill served by polarized "ethics versus science" attitudes. Dr. Millar and her consultant boss, Mr. Winterbottom, as we have seen, were very far from the ideological extremes. Both were furthermore caring and skilled doctors. Yet between their respective preoccupations, with ethics and with science, they came close to tearing Bob and Hilary Swann apart.

In our version of Bob and Hilary Swann's story, it was their vicar, the Reverend Doctor Benedict Brown, who rode to the rescue. But this, as we have indicated, is only one "possible world." Different individuals (different clinicians as well as different patients) would have made different choices based on different values and resulting in different narratives. The stories on the HFEA and other websites richly illustrate the variety of these individual narratives. And as the Science-driven Principle reminds us, it is the *science* that is driving this diversity, the science in this instance being Robert Edwards and Patrick Steptoe's remarkable technical achievement with the birth of Louise Brown in the 1970s.

So the red-light warning from this chapter is "Think high-tech, think evidence *and* values." In the next chapter, we will find that "Think evidence *and* values" is no less important in low-tech death than in this chapter it has proved to be in high-tech birth.

References

Atwell, R. and Fulford, K. W. M. (2006). The Christian tradition of spiritual direction as a sketch for a strong theology of diversity. In J. Cox, A. V. Campbell, and K. W. M. Fulford, eds, *Medicine of the Person: Faith, Science and Values in Health Care Provision*. London: Jessica Kingsley Publishers. pp. 83–95.

Carmeli, Y. S. and Birenbaum-Carmeli, D. (1994). The predicament of masculinity: towards understanding the male's experience of infertility treatments. *Sex Roles* **30**, 663–7.

Jasanoff, S. (2005). *Designs on Nature: Science and Democracy in Europe and the United States*. New Jersey: Princeton University Press.

National Collaborating Centre for Women's and Children's Health (commissioned by the National Institute for Clinical Excellence) (2004). *Fertility: Assessment and Treatment for People with Fertility Problems*. London: RCOG Press at the Royal College of Obstetricians and Gynaecologists.

Sheldrake, P. (1994). *Befriending our Desires*. London: Darton, Longman & Todd.

Sackett, D. L. Straus, S. E., Scott Richardson, W., Rosenberg, W. and Haynes, R. B. (2000). *Evidence-based Medicine: How to Practice and Teach EBM*, 2nd edn. Edinburgh and London: Churchill Livingstone.

Wilkes, S., Hall, N., Crosland, A., Murdoch, A. and Rubin, G. (2009). Patient experience of infertility management in primary care: an in-depth study. *Family Practice* **26**, 309–16.

Websites

- The HFEA website (http:\\www.hfea.gov.uk) as well as providing detailed information about all aspects of IVF includes many stories from a wide range of different couples about their experiences in working through the stages of infertility treatment.
- The NICE Clinical Guideline on fertility treatment was produced by the National Collaborating Centre for Women's and Children's Health (2004). Information on elective single embryo transfer can be found at www.oneatatime.org.uk.

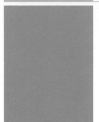

Introduction to Part 5

The elements of values-based practice taken separately, as the stories in Parts 2–4 of this book illustrate, may each be helpful in their own right in supporting good practice. Bring these elements together, however, and use them in a well-joined-up way, and you get a turbo-charging effect. It is this turbo-charging effect that is shown in different ways by the two chapters in this final part of the book.

- Chapter 13: one way in which the elements of values-based practice come together in practice is through the tenth element of the process itself, dissensus. We introduced the idea of dissensus and how it differs from the more familiar consensus in our overview of values-base practice in Chapter 2. Briefly:
  - In consensual decision-making, differences of values are merged (this is what it means to "come to a consensus").
  - In dissensual decision-making, by contrast, differences of values remain in play as a resource for balanced decision-making according to the particular circumstances presented by each individual case.

  The story in this chapter shows how the elements of values-based practice came together to support a positive process of dissensus in the story of a dying man, Joe Monaghan, and the decisions that he and his family made in partnership with an in-reach palliative care consultant, Dr. Emma Barnes, and other members of the multidisciplinary team.
- Chapter 14: a second way in which the elements of values-based practice come together in practice is through the development of shared frameworks of values. We gave two examples of such frameworks from mental health in Chapter 2:
  - The NIMHE Values Framework developed to support balanced decision-making in the implementation of policy under the first National Service Framework for Mental Health.
  - The "round table" framework of Guiding Principles developed to support balanced decision-making on the use of involuntary treatment under the Mental Health Act 2007.

  In this chapter, we return to the story of Dr. Gulati from Part 1 to see how, working with her colleagues and the local Patients' Forum, she used an explicitly values-based approach to develop a shared framework of values. The original trigger for this, you will recall, was her unresolved dilemma about how to manage the inappropriate demand of her patient, Roy Walker, for an off-work certificate. Having developed their shared framework of values, however, this becomes a resource for a number of other values-complex challenges for the practice (including the recently announced GP commissioning).

In focusing on the elements of values-based practice in these two chapters in the contexts, respectively, of palliative care and of general practice, we may appear to have neglected the important role of other decision support tools. This was not our intention. Values-based practice used in whole or in part is, as we emphasized in Part 1, only one tool in medicine's values toolbox – and we need all the tools we can get if we are to respond adequately to the increasingly complex challenges raised by current clinical practice

POINT

PROCESS

PREMISE

Balanced Decision-making
within a
Framework of Shared Values

Partnership

Two-feet Principle　　Squeaky-wheel Principle　　Science-driven Principle

Person-centered practice　　　　　Multidisciplinary teamwork

Awareness　　Reasoning　　　　Knowledge　　Communication skills

Mutual Respect
for
Differences of Values

Map of values-based practice – partnership.

13

A good (enough) death: dissensus in end-of-life care

Values-based practice element 10: partnership in decision-making

Take-away message for practice

Dissensual decision-making can help usx to build genuine partnerships in working with other team members and with patients and their families.

Partnership between stakeholders in decision-making, although coming tenth in the list of process elements of values-based practice, is last but definitely not least in importance. We will see in this chapter that, as the tenth element, partnership draws together and underpins the process of values-based practice as a whole.

The importance of partnership in values-based decision-making is illustrated in this chapter through the story of a 69-year-old man, Joe Monaghan, after he is found to have disseminated bowel cancer following an emergency admission with acute abdominal symptoms. There has been much talk in such situations of a "good death." But the surgical team and Joe Monaghan's various family members, as we will see, had very different perspectives on what a "good death" would mean, with Joe Monaghan himself, as is so often the case, at risk of becoming caught between their conflicting best intentions.

Consensus, dissensus and partnership in decision-making

One way to resolve a potentially conflicting situation of the kind presented by Joe Monaghan would be to agree (to come to a consensus) on whose values should be pre-eminent in deciding what to do. As we saw in Chapter 8 on person-centered care, recent policy and practice has shifted from the traditional "doctor knows best" (where the doctor's values are pre-eminent) to the currently pervasive "patient knows best" (where the patient's values are pre-eminent).

Neither a "doctor knows best" nor a "patient knows best" consensus, however, is a basis for partnership between those concerned. Genuine partnership, as we outlined briefly in Chapter 3, requires a dissensual model in which the values of those concerned, instead of being subordinated one to another, remain in play to be balanced according to the circumstances presented by a given decision. (Consensus, as we will describe later, is also important to partnership in decision-making but through its role rather in *evidence*-based practice.)

Dissensus, values-based practice and palliative care

The care plan that emerges towards the end of this chapter from Joe Monaghan's story is a dissensual care plan. As such it builds on and draws together many of the process elements of values-based practice described separately in earlier chapters. At various points in the story, we will thus be pointing out a number of these elements as they are reflected in the way those concerned work together with Joe Monaghan and his family (we will call these values-based practice (VBP) flashbacks).

As with previous chapters in this book, the elements of values-based practice in Joe Monaghan's story reflect and build on best practice, in this case in palliative care. As we emphasized in Part 1, values-based practice as a whole (like evidence-based practice) reflects and builds on best practice. Palliative care in particular is an area in which, without calling it as such, a strong tradition of combining values-based with evidence-based approaches is already well established (see, for example, Chochinov, 2002 and Schattner, 2009), although even in palliative care, as we will find, there is further values-based work to do in building genuine partnership between patients and clinicians in decision-making.

Three clinical stages

The chapter is in three sections, corresponding to three key stages in the early management of Joe Monaghan's cancer: a first cancer multidisciplinary team (MDT) meeting, a palliative care referral and a second cancer MDT meeting:

- Section 1, the first cancer MDT meeting, looks at the different perspectives of the surgeon and others involved and how these perspectives influenced their respective interpretations of the clinical and pathological findings for Joe Monaghan's subsequent care.
- Section 2, the palliative care referral, follows a palliative care consultant, Dr. Emma Barnes, as she comes to understand what Joe Monaghan himself wants but also to appreciate the points of view of Joe Monaghan's family and of the various staff involved.
- Section 3, the second (ward-based) cancer MDT meeting, follows Dr. Barnes as she works with others to produce a care plan that, in focusing on what Joe Monaghan wants but also reflecting the needs and

concerns of his family and the staff involved, provides a dissensual basis for genuine partnership between them in the difficult times that lie ahead.

In a brief concluding section, we show how this "dissensual care plan" (as we will call it) drew critically on the elements of values-based practice shown by Dr. Barnes and others in the way they had worked with Joe Monaghan and his family.

The clinical context

It is 4.00 p.m. at the James Chadwick District General Hospital. Mr. Charlie Bennett, the surgeon, is pleased with the way the lower gastrointestinal cancer MDT meeting is going. His patient, 69-year-old Joe Monaghan, had been admitted as an emergency from his GP during the night two weeks ago, when his team was on call, with acute abdominal pain and a recent history of constipation. Emergency surgery for a large-bowel obstruction with early perforation had revealed a primary cancer in his colon, which had already spread to his local lymph nodes and liver (with early lung secondaries shown by a subsequent CT scan). It was a challenging operation technically, but he had managed to remove the primary and to form an effective colostomy.

The problem now was that he was stuck with Joe Monaghan in a general surgical bed that was urgently needed for other patients on his ever growing list. Joe Monaghan was doing reasonably well post-operatively, all things considered, but his wife was clearly worried about having him home and the occupational therapy assessment had supported her anxieties about their lack of facilities (notably a downstairs toilet). Still, the good news was that the clinical oncologist, Dr. Watts, had agreed to see Joe Monaghan and his wife with a view to taking him over for chemotherapy. The only potential fly in the ointment was that Dr. Watts seemed keen on pulling in the palliative care in-reach team. Normally he would have welcomed this, but in this case he had his doubts.

Section 1: the first cancer MDT meeting

Site-specific cancer MDT meetings are now widely accepted as being essential to the process of care planning for patients with cancer. These meetings concentrate on clarifying the diagnosis and deciding on recommendations for treatment, with the patient then being referred on as appropriate, although, as in Joe Monaghan's case (see below), patients may be reviewed at a second MDT meeting if there are matters that require further discussion.

A particular focus of cancer MDT meetings is whether, based on the balance of risks and benefits, chemotherapy should be offered. It is up to the patient concerned (or parent in the case of a child) to decide whether or not to accept it.

Values in the MDT

The MDT meeting (a "lower gastrointestinal tract MDT meeting") considering Joe Monaghan's case in the clinical scenario outlined above was thus very much following a standard pattern. As noted above, the meeting included Mr. Charlie Bennett, the surgeon with clinical responsibility for Joe Monaghan at this stage, and the oncologist, Dr. Watts, as well as a radiologist and histopathologist; also present was a gastrointestinal clinical nurse specialist (CNS), Gina Morris, who had spoken with Sister Clancy from the nursing staff on the surgical ward. Not present in person, but of course very much in everyone's minds, were Joe Monaghan and his family.

> **VBP flashback**
>
> In Chapter 1, we made three background points about values in medicine. Before reading on, you may find it helpful to think for a moment about these background points about values and how they relate to Joe Monaghan's cancer MDT meeting.

The three key points about values in medicine that we looked at in Chapter 1 are all clearly relevant here. Values, we said, are wider than ethics, they are everywhere and (alongside evidence) they are action-guiding:

1. *Values are wider than ethics.* The issues here are not, as such, ethical issues but they certainly extend to include the *needs, wishes, preferences and other values* of those concerned.
2. *Values are everywhere.* Those concerned here include the clinicians (Mr. Bennett, the nursing team, the oncologist and others), the patient (Joe Monaghan) and his family; their values are both *foreground* and, as we will see, importantly *background*; and their values are set within a wider *network of values* represented by, for example, local and national policy guidelines and issues of resourcing.
3. *Values are action-guiding.* The overt focus of the MDT meeting as we have seen is the evidence (clinical and pathological) and how it bears on the

treatment options for Joe Monaghan, in particular whether he should be offered chemotherapy; but it is the *values* in play (the "balance of risks and benefits," as we put it above) that are guiding the MDT in applying the evidence in Joe Monaghan's case.

In Chapter 2, we described the process by which evidence and values come together to guide clinical judgment in a particular case as "squaring down." In the sections that follow, we look first at the evidence and then at the values guiding those present in the MDT meeting as they "squared down" on what to do in Joe Monaghan's case.

Evidence in the MDT meeting

The evidence available to those present in the MDT meeting presented them with a dilemma. On the one hand, although carcinoma of the bowel is generally chemosensitive, the pathology reports, together with the fact that the cancer had already spread widely with secondaries in Joe Monaghan's lymph nodes, liver and lungs, suggested that chemotherapy was likely to be at best of temporary benefit. On the other hand, Joe Monaghan had relatively strong pre-operative functioning, suggesting that he might nonetheless benefit from chemotherapy, as reported by the National Confidential Enquiry into Patient Outcomes and Death (NCEPOD, 2008).

So from an evidence-based point of view, there was no obvious conclusion about whether or not Joe Monaghan should be offered chemotherapy. The evidence as such was equivocal: the nature and stage of the cancer argued on balance against the appropriateness of offering chemotherapy, while Joe Monaghan's good pre-operative functioning argued on balance in favor of chemotherapy.

Also in play in the MDT meeting, however, and influencing the way the team were "squaring down" in Joe Monaghan's case, was, as we have seen, a complex values base reflecting the different perspectives of those present. We will look at these different value perspectives in turn.

The surgeon, Mr. Bennett's, value perspective

Joe Monaghan was Mr. Bennett's patient and it is thus no surprise that his (Charlie Bennett's) values should have been prominently in the foreground in the MDT meeting. As his reflections in the opening scenario above indicate, he and the surgical team were keen to move their patient on. They felt there was little more they could do for Joe Monaghan now that his colostomy had settled down, and there was considerable pressure on beds.

A little further back in Mr. Bennett's mind, but nonetheless deeply influencing how he saw things, was the fact that Joe Monaghan clearly had a very poor prognosis, and managing terminal patients was an area where he knew himself to be very much out of his depth. Technically, he was confident of his skills as a surgeon and felt he had served Joe Monaghan well: the operation had been challenging due to the infiltration of the tumor into adjacent structures and he was proud of the colostomy he had constructed and the fact that it was functioning well.

But his particular specialty was in laparoscopic hernia repairs and rectal incontinence surgery; he enjoyed mastering difficult technical procedures, and he liked surgery for its ability to cure and heal. Crucial to all this, in his view, was the importance of maintaining hope for the individual and a cheerful ward: he greatly admired his nursing team for their ability to remain calm and good-humored even when dealing with the most challenging clinical emergencies. As an "action this day" man himself, furthermore, he knew exactly what Joe Monaghan's wife, Brenda Monaghan, meant when she had told him that "Joe had always been a fighter" and that "they were not going to let this one beat them." He admired their courage when, despite (he believed) knowing that Joe probably had only a few weeks to live, they were pressing on with their plans for a first trip to Australia to see their grandchildren.

So all in all, Mr. Bennett was glad that the oncologist, Dr. Watts, seemed ready to take Joe Monaghan over for further treatment. As for Dr. Watts' suggestion of involving the palliative care team, although he would normally have welcomed this, it was not his preferred option at this stage in this case – it seemed to be sending the wrong message to Joe Monaghan and his family, and it might delay a transfer to Dr. Watts'care.

On the other hand, he was reassured by what Gina Morris (the gastrointestinal CNS) had said about palliative care referrals now being dealt with expeditiously following the recent appointment of a new in-reach consultant. And he was mindful of what Sister Clancy (the senior surgical ward sister) had told him earlier about concerns from the night staff over pain control. No one deserved to be in pain unnecessarily, least of all someone in Joe Monaghan's position. So from this point of view, he could see that a palliative care referral could be a good idea.

Charlie Bennett and values-based practice

> **VBP flashback**
>
> Mr. Bennett's perspective in the cancer MDT meeting illustrates a number of key points about values-based practice.
>
> Before reading on, you may find it helpful to think about his perspective, drawing briefly on what we have covered in earlier chapters.
>
> In terms of a values-based approach, what is helpful about Mr. Bennett's perspective and what might cause problems?

A key feature of Mr. Bennett's perspective from the point of view of values-based practice is that he is firmly person-centered (values-based practice element 5, Chapter 8). Mr. Bennett's concern to get back his acute surgical bed and his personal ambivalence about dealing with patients who are terminally ill could easily have led him to resist the palliative care referral as something to be picked up later. As it was, he took the nursing team's concerns seriously and made Joe Monaghan's immediate need for pain control his person-centered (or as we called it in Chapter 8 his person-*values*-centered) priority. We will see later that this was to prove crucial to Joe Monaghan's care, although not in the way that Mr. Bennett and the surgical team expected.

A more problematic aspect of Mr. Bennett's perspective, on the other hand, from the point of view of values-based practice, was (in the terminology of Chapter 4) his "delusion of sameness." As a man of action, Mr. Bennett's values were about dealing with problems in a pro-active and assertive way. In much of his professional life, these values served him, his team and his patients well. Small wonder, then, that he picked up readily on Brenda Monaghan's fighting spirit and – which is where, as we will see, the delusion of sameness became a problem – assumed that this was Joe Monaghan's perspective as well.

The nursing team's perspective

Sister Clancy (as is usual) was not present in person at Joe Monaghan's MDT meeting but she and Mr. Bennett had discussed the issues beforehand. About ten years older than Mr. Bennett, she had behind her a distinguished career as a surgical nurse in the armed forces including battle-front experience. The disciplines of a surgical team suited her temperament well, and she and her colleagues shared Mr. Bennett's positive "action this day" approach: their shared values and mutual respect were essential to their effectiveness as a first-class surgical team with excellent results and a reputation for decisive action in emergencies. Also like Mr. Bennett, Sister Clancy and the nursing team were concerned about Joe Monaghan blocking a bed.

There were also differences between her and Mr. Bennett's perspectives, however, arising from the fact that most of the day-to-day care on the ward was provided by the nursing team. These differences between the nursing team and Mr. Bennett's perspectives had allowed a natural division of labor to develop: the nursing team dealt with difficult communication and relationship issues allowing Mr. Bennett to concentrate on solving the more technical aspects of management.

> **VBP flashback**
>
> Which element of values-based practice does this division of labor between Charlie Bennett and the nursing team remind you of?
>
> How might the division of labor play out in Joe Monaghan's case?

Divisions of labor of the kind that had developed between Mr. Bennett and the nursing team reflect the importance of differences of perspective as well as differences of skills in what we called in Chapter 9 the "extended multidisciplinary team." In the present case, the nursing team's greater contact with Joe Monaghan and his family meant that they were more aware than Mr. Bennett of tensions within the family. Yes, the occupational therapist had said that their terraced house with its steep steps and an upstairs bath was unsuitable until various adjustments had been made, but they were concerned that Brenda Monaghan anyway did not seem confident about having her husband home and might not cope well.

In the last day or two, there had been further issues. The nursing team could see that, despite Joe Monaghan's initially good post-operative recovery, he was becoming steadily frailer and his pain had been harder to control through the night. The ward rounds were not much help here: Mr. Bennett concentrated on checking the surgical dressings and the colostomy, and seemed reluctant to pick up their

concerns. They felt that Joe Monaghan was more seriously ill than was being acknowledged. Mr. Bennett talked with Joe and Brenda Monaghan soon after the operation. But the nursing staff felt increasingly strongly that as a family they needed time and more open discussion of the issues if they were to be able to cope during the coming weeks.

We will see later when we come to the perspective of the oncologist, Dr. Watts, that the nursing team's observations of the family would make a crucial contribution to a balanced view on the key issue for the MDT about chemotherapy.

Sister Clancy and values-based practice

With the nursing team's concerns about the family in mind, Sister Clancy had taken the opportunity to try to open up the issues with Joe and Brenda Monaghan when a chance remark suggested that, like her, they were Roman Catholics. She had come to check Joe Monaghan's dressings (which one of the nursing auxiliaries had reported was weeping). Brenda Monaghan was visiting at the time, and as they chatted they discovered that they had a shared background in the armed services. Joe had done his National Service as a young man in the Royal Engineers (it was there that he had learned his trade as an electrician) and it turned out that the couple had been married by a Roman Catholic Army Chaplain whom Sister Clancy had known.

When this came up, it seemed to Sister Clancy to be a golden opportunity for them to start facing some of the issues that she and her colleagues felt everyone had been avoiding. Consistent with the literature showing the value of spiritual and religious beliefs for many people at the end of life (Gilbert, 2011), she had found her shared background with other Roman Catholic families a powerful basis from which to talk about death and dying. As a way of moving the conversation in this direction, she thus made a comment to Joe and Brenda Monaghan about how she had found their faith a great support in times like this. But far from opening up the conversation, Brenda politely but firmly went on to talk about their planned trip to Australia.

Sister Clancy tried to open up the issues again with Brenda Monaghan as she was leaving the ward by offering to contact the hospital chaplain or perhaps their parish priest. But Brenda Monaghan had brusquely rejected this offer; and she had walked off angrily when Sister Clancy persisted by saying she would remember them anyway in her prayers.

Faith and values-based practice

The red-light warning that Sister Clancy missed was what we described in Chapter 11 as "Think values, think evidence too!" In Chapter 11, a skilled and normally caring charge nurse, Matthew Cruickshank, was "thinking values" (in a moment of uncharacteristic moral outrage) to the extent that he stopped "thinking evidence" and thus came perilously close to missing an acute abdomen. Sister Clancy, at this point in Joe Monaghan's story, was also "thinking values" (religious values in this case). There is no problem with "thinking values," of course. It is in a sense what values-based practice is all about. And used with care, religious and spiritual values have an important role in palliative care (Walter *et al.*, 2002). The problem was that, like Matthew Cruickshank in Chapter 11, Sister Clancy, in "thinking values," stopped paying attention to the evidence.

Sister Clancy's faith, as we noted earlier, had served her and many of her like-minded patients well in previous similar situations. It was thus appropriate that when the opportunity came up she should have gently introduced the idea of their apparently shared religious background. The warning she missed was that Brenda (and tacitly Joe) Monaghan not only failed to take up her overture but firmly ignored it (Brenda went on to talk about their planned trip to Australia). This was clear evidence, then, that in this area at least Joe and Brenda Monaghan's values were very different from those of Sister Clancy (they were in fact lapsed Catholics).

Had Sister Clancy remained attentive to the evidence, she would have backed off at the first rebuff and left it open for them to pick up the issues in some other way. As it was, with her final comment to Brenda Monaghan about remembering them in her prayers, she effectively alienated the couple from further engagement with her on these or on any other sensitive issues.

The oncologist, Dr. Watts', perspective

At the time of the first MDT meeting, the oncologist, Dr. Watts, had not seen Joe Monaghan, although he had reviewed the histology, CT scan and other reports. A quiet, scholarly man, he had worked with his more colorful (as he saw him) colleague, Mr. Bennett, before and shared the general view of his skills as a surgeon.

Dr. Watts was less persuaded, however, than Mr. Bennett about the merits of chemotherapy for Joe Monaghan. Certainly, Joe Monaghan appeared to have a surprisingly good pre-operative status. But the extent to which the cancer had already spread and its histological appearance suggested that he was not likely to maintain his good post-operative course for long. Indeed, Sister Clancy clearly also had a less optimistic picture than Mr. Bennett, and Dr. Watts had learned the value of the nursing team's more intimate understanding of how a patient was feeling. Dr. Watts, however, understood better than most the uncertainties in cancer care (Christiakis, 1999): embarking on chemotherapy could well be disastrous but it could just work. If Joe Monaghan and his family really were as insistent on chemotherapy as was being suggested, this was going to be a difficult call to make.

That said, it was clear on present showing that there was a good chance that one way or another he, as the oncologist, would be taking over further management from the surgical team. But he would insist on involving the palliative care team now at this early stage. There was the issue of pain control, but there was also good evidence that early involvement of palliative care made it more likely that end-of-life issues would be more appropriately dealt with (NCEPOD, 2008). Reading between the lines, Dr. Watts felt, this was just the kind of case where an unrealistic view of the options could lead to decisions being made that turned out badly from the patient's point of view.

Dr. Watts and *evidence*-based practice

What lay behind Dr. Watts' use of these overtly *value*-laden terms ("more appropriately" and "turned out badly") were all three elements of David Sackett's definition of evidence-based practice: best research evidence, clinical experience and patients' values:

- *Best research evidence*. Dr. Watts was familiar with several excellent studies showing that all too often the values of those most deeply concerned, the patient and their family, were not well served by the decisions that were made by clinicians. For example, a far higher proportion of patients wanting to die at home than actually doing so. Worse still, 19% of patients (admittedly with worse pre-operative performance status than Joe Monaghan) actually died prematurely from the effects of chemotherapy (NCEPOD, 2008).
- *Clinical experience*. As an oncologist, Dr. Watts had wide clinical experience of dealing with end-of-life decisions and the difficulties of establishing a realistic understanding of the risks and benefits of different treatments: the issues at stake made it inevitable that everyone, clinicians as well as patients and their families, tended to hear what they wanted to hear.
- *Patients' values*. Dr. Watts had yet to talk to Joe Monaghan and his family, but, as noted earlier, current guidance supported his experience that early involvement of the palliative care team made it much more likely that a care plan would eventually be agreed that was based on a realistic understanding not only of the treatment options available but also of the actual (rather than supposed) priorities of Joe Monaghan and his family (National End of Life Care Programme, 2010).

These three elements of Sackett's definition of evidence-based medicine are important for partnership in decision-making because, as the definition continues, "When these three elements are integrated, clinicians and patients form a diagnostic and therapeutic alliance which optimizes clinical outcomes and quality of life."

The next step, then, Dr. Watts insisted, was to involve the palliative care team in the person of the recently appointed in-reach consultant, Dr. Emma Barnes.

Section 2: the palliative care referral

Dr. Barnes arrived on the surgical ward a couple of days later. As this was her first referral from Mr. Bennett and the surgical team, she had arranged to come at a time when she could meet with them before seeing Joe Monaghan. The team made her welcome. They spoke warmly of Joe Monaghan's stoical approach and his family's support for his fighting spirit. They discussed the problems of appropriate discharge and the night staff's concerns about pain control.

Dr. Barnes asked what Joe Monaghan and his family had been told about her visit and who else she might talk to. Mr. Bennett replied that he had not seen Brenda Monaghan but had told Joe Monaghan that she, Dr. Barnes, was one of the people who could help with his post-operative care. Sister Clancy said that, although she had met Brenda Monaghan, she had not seemed keen to talk with them. They had seen one of Joe Monaghan's daughters (Molly, Joe had called her) when she visited, but she had not asked to see them and no one had talked with her. Dr. Barnes offered to come back for a further talk with the team after seeing Joe Monaghan, and they welcomed this.

From cure to care

Dr. Barnes opted for a career in palliative care because as a junior doctor she had found that her particular strengths were in dealing with people rather than in the more practical aspect of medicine. This was partly a matter of competencies: Dr. Barnes' skills were empathic and personal rather than technical (she had joked with Mr. Bennett about how she had been "rubbish at surgery"). But it was also a matter of values: Mr. Bennett and the nursing team's "cure values" of optimism and action orientation were essential to their success as an acute surgical team; Dr. Barnes' "care values" of openness and giving time were equally essential to her success as a palliative care clinician.

So, to come to the second question in the reflection above, how might these differences of values affect how Dr. Barnes and the surgical team, respectively, worked with Joe Monaghan and his family? Here, as we saw in Chapter 9 on team working, we need to be careful. This is clear from Fig. 13.1. The words in this figure are taken from a seminar in values-based practice for palliative care clinicians with different professional backgrounds. The groups of words were their respective responses when they were asked to write down "three or four words or short phrases" that they thought most accurately reflected the values of palliative care.

> **Reflection point: a VBP flashback**
>
> What points about values from Chapter 9 on team working do you think are relevant to understanding how the differences between the surgical team's values of cure and Dr. Barnes' values of care might influence the way they worked with Joe Monaghan and his family?

Two points in particular stand out from Chapter 9 that are important for understanding how values come into and support effective team work:

- Complex, diverse, individual, meaningful
- Individual, whole-person care, empathy, openness
- Care, caring, do no harm, honesty
- Partnership, holistic, individualized

Fig. 13.1. The values of palliative care: bullet points from a seminar flip chart (see text).

1. *Family resemblances.* Like the team values explored in Chapter 9, the four sets of values expressed here are linked together by what we call "family resemblances." There are similarities – connections and overlaps – between the lists; and the lists are consistent with Dr. Barnes' values. But notwithstanding these family resemblances, the actual lists *are all different.*

   So there is no prescribed list of values for palliative care. There are shared values certainly (we return to the importance of shared values in the next chapter), but there are individual differences as well. And again, like families, this leaves room for overlap: Sister Clancy, you will recall, as well as being a first-class surgical nurse, reflected many of the values of palliative care in her alertness to the unspoken issues between Joe Monaghan and his family.

2. *Implicit and explicit values.* Notwithstanding their values of "cure," the nursing team and Mr. Bennett if presented with these values of "care" would no doubt have been more than ready to sign up to them. Again, this reflects the difference we explored in Chapter 8 between the values we are ready to acknowledge explicitly and the often very different implicit values that drive what we actually do.

   Both explicit and implicit values, as we have earlier emphasized, are important. Shared explicit values support mutual understanding (recall here the premise of values-based practice in "mutual respect"). Differences of implicit values, in guiding what we actually do, support an approach that is appropriately balanced to the different circumstances presented by different situations. Thus, as between Dr. Barnes and the surgical team, without mutual respect (explicitly expressed in this case), there would have been no basis for a partnership between them. And it was the differences between them in their implicit care versus cure values that would support a balanced approach to deciding on next steps, including the vexed question of chemotherapy.

Dr. Barnes' implicit values of care were already evident in what she learned from her meeting with the surgical team before seeing Joe Monaghan. From her experience in the field, as well as her knowledge of the research literature, she was well aware that when people are terminally ill the real issues they face are often not openly acknowledged and hence not properly managed.

She had picked up a sense that this might be the case here from the fact that the surgical team, although clearly warm and welcoming, had had relatively little contact with Joe Monaghan's wife and daughter. She could understand this in part: their priority was curing people, and as a surgical team, their optimism and action orientation made them good at this. Joe Monaghan, however, was beyond cure. His need now was for care and this demanded realism and time for reflection. But the gap between the team's generally positive approach and their engagement with Joe Monaghan's wife and daughter suggested that this could be one of those situations in which the move from cure to care was proving problematic for all those concerned, the ward staff included.

Dr. Barnes thus approached her first talk with Joe Monaghan conscious of what she had been told about his family's fighting spirit and the problems of discharge and pain control, but also very much with an open mind about what other issues there might be.

Dr. Barnes talks with Joe Monaghan

Dr. Barnes introduced herself to Joe Monaghan as "Dr. Barnes" saying only that Mr. Bennett had asked her to see him. As she sat down beside his bed, Joe greeted her with a smile and asked her straight out if she was from the hospice. Far from being upset when she confirmed this, he seemed relieved and responded readily when she asked him how he was getting on. This is what she learned from what he told her.

He had come round from the operation to find himself with a colostomy and a huge scar down the middle of his abdomen. When he was first brought back from theatre, the nurses had seemed reluctant to talk about his operation, and his worst fears were confirmed when the consultant came to talk to him and his wife later that day. The surgeon had told them that they had found an advanced bowel cancer that had already spread widely and that, although the operation had removed the tumor and the blocked segment of bowel, they suspected the cancer was very aggressive. He had subsequently had a scan that had shown secondaries in his liver and lungs.

Joe Monaghan talked a lot about his wife, Brenda. They had been married for 49 and a half years. They grew up together in Liverpool and had four children

and 11 grandchildren, with two more on the way. Joe had retired three years earlier – he had been a self-employed electrician – and he and Brenda had looked forward to starting a new life together. Brenda had retired from her job as a much loved dinner lady in a primary school some five years earlier. They had saved hard over the years and had been enjoying the rewards of their labor now. They could not afford to travel when they were younger but had now got the travel bug; after a trip to Florida, one to the Grand Canyon and another to South Africa last year, they had been planning a golden wedding trip to Australia in six months' time to see their youngest child, Brendan, and his wife and growing family. Brendan had recently emigrated and they had yet to meet their third grandchild as the latest addition to the family.

Joe Monaghan believed that Brenda knew he was dying but felt unable to talk with her about it because he knew how desperately upset she would be. They had dealt with many problems together in the past and Brenda now seemed determined they should fight this one in the same way. He felt that she and their daughter, Molly, were both hanging on to the idea of getting to Australia as a way of keeping up their hopes. The surgeon, too, talked about this. But Joe was far from sure he would ever make it. He had felt so tired before he was taken ill. He had tried to disguise this from his family. But the reality was that he had been dreading the long-haul flight; and now, since the operation, although the nurses all seemed pleased with how he was doing, he knew that his old strength was gone.

All in all, he felt very alone. The surgical team were all really kind and thoughtful, but he knew they were keen to get him off the ward as fast as possible; and his family, although very good at visiting him, felt increasingly distant as they chatted about the telly from last night and kept on about their Australia trip. He was frightened of dying here in hospital. He would love to be at home, and back surrounded by the reminders of his old life, but he had been afraid to say this because "Brenda will think I am giving up."

Dr. Barnes concluded the session by asking if Joe would like her to talk to his wife and maybe also his daughter and that they might then get together to talk about what to do. He said simply, "Yes, that would be good."

Dr. Barnes and the skills for values-based practice

> **VBP flashback**
>
> You can see that, although Joe Monaghan was meeting Dr. Barnes for the first time, he was very ready to open up to her.
>
> Why do you think she got so much more from him than anyone else had done?
>
> Which skills of values-based practice (described in Part 2) does Dr. Barnes show here?

Joe Monaghan's willingness to open up to Dr. Barnes was partly a matter of context. He knew perfectly well that she was from the hospice: the surgeon's evasive answer as to why she was coming to see him was enough to tell him that. Yes, he and Brenda had always solved problems together in the past. But he was no fool. He knew what was happening to him. For the sake of his family, though, he had had to keep his true feelings bottled up since coming round from the operation. It was thus a relief to be able to talk openly with someone at last.

So the context was right. But Dr. Barnes showed all four skills for values-based practice in allowing Joe Monaghan to make best use of the opportunity her visit offered to tell someone what really mattered to him. We will look briefly at each of these skills.

Awareness of values (element 1 of values-based practice)

We looked at the foundational importance of raised awareness of values in Chapter 4 with a story from mental health. In the present case, Dr. Barnes' whole approach was about allowing not only others but also Joe Monaghan himself to understand and acknowledge where his true priorities really lay.

Dr. Barnes' approach, furthermore, reflected two key aspects of values awareness that we emphasized in Chapter 4:

1. *The importance of values in diagnosis as well as in treatment.* The problem in Joe Monaghan's terms (what really mattered to him, i.e. being allowed to die at home) proved to be quite different from the referral problem of pain control. Indeed, despite a couple of strong prompts from Dr. Barnes (with questions about whether he was comfortable after the operation and how he was sleeping), Joe Monaghan did not mention pain control as a problem at all.

2. *The importance of strengths (StAR values).* Again, Dr. Barnes' approach reflected the importance of aspirations (the "A" in StAR values) as a key aspect of strengths assessment (Joe Monaghan's aspiration to die at home), although of course he and others all brought many other strengths to how they handled the situation.

Reasoning skills (element 2 of values-based practice)

Dr. Barnes' approach reflected in part her experience of previous cases. In this, she (like Dr. Watts in the first cancer MDT meeting) was in effect using what we called in Chapter 4 case-based reasoning or casuistry.

The story in Chapter 5 (about the consultation of a GP, Dr. Mangate, with a teenage patient with acne) employed an explicit use of this approach: recall that we ran the consultation twice, first without and then with Dr. Mangate having a chance to reflect on a previous case. Dr. Barnes' use of case-based reasoning, like that of Dr. Watts, was more implicit but no less powerful for that. Indeed, as we said in Chapter 5, implicit case-based reasoning is a crucial if neglected aspect of the clinical experience that as clinicians we bring to the clinical encounter; and as Sackett's definition of evidence-based medicine again reminds us, clinical experience is essential for linking science (best research evidence) with people (and their individual values).

Knowledge of values (element 3 of values-based practice)

As noted earlier, in addition to Dr. Barnes' clinical experience, her knowledge of the research literature (which was again similar to that of Dr. Watts) alerted her to the possibility that there were likely to be important issues for Joe Monaghan and his family other than those that had thus far been identified by the team.

Nothing that Joe Monaghan told Dr. Barnes thus came as a complete surprise: it is well recognized that clinicians underestimate patients' need for information (Fallowfield *et al.*, 2002); poor communication is a common factor in difficulties in end-of-life care (Lo *et al.*, 1999), and Joe Monaghan's priority to get back home as soon as possible was consistent with one of the big challenges for end-of-life care that as we noted earlier has been recently highlighted.

Communication skills (element 4 of values-based practice)

Dr. Barnes showed in good measure the two key communication skills for values-based practice noted in

Chapter 7: skills for eliciting values and skills of conflict resolution. For eliciting values, Dr. Barnes' body language alone made it easy for Joe Monaghan to talk openly with her: recall that she sat down beside his bed rather than standing, and she paid careful attention to what he was saying, making notes as they went along. Her approach of open listening and giving time rather than focusing prematurely on assumed problems (like pain control in Joe Monaghan's case) is well recognized to be important in palliative care (Lo *et al.*, 1999).

Conflict resolution as such was less evident in Dr. Barnes' first meeting with Joe Monaghan, but she laid the groundwork for this in her relationship with the surgical team when she arrived on the ward by listening carefully to what Mr. Bennett and the nursing staff had to say rather than breezing in as the "expert" (remember her good-humored exchange with Mr. Bennett about her failures as a surgeon).

Talking with the surgical team took a little time (about 20 minutes perhaps) but giving time to building relationships at this crucial stage of first contact is an investment that pays off handsomely in a number of ways later on (including overall time saved). Dr. Barnes' "time investment" was vital for establishing a positive relationship that allowed her to work in partnership with the surgical team in trying to help Joe Monaghan and his family. We return to Dr. Barnes' skills for conflict resolution shortly.

Clinical skills and relationships

None of this happened in isolation, of course. As we noted earlier, the opportunity for Dr. Barnes to talk with Joe Monaghan would not have arisen at all but for the person-centered approach of the surgeon Mr. Bennett and the nursing team (element 5 of values-based practice) combined with their established multidisciplinary ways of working (element 6 of values-based practice).

Dr. Barnes talks with Molly Monaghan

As Dr. Barnes was leaving the ward, she stopped at the nursing station to let them know that she would come back later to meet Brenda Monaghan. A young woman who had just arrived on the ward, hearing this, introduced herself as Joe Monaghan's daughter, Molly, and asked if she could have a word with her. The nurse found them a side room.

Molly Monaghan seemed very anxious. She had tried to corner the nurses and junior doctors to find out what's going on, but no one had seemed willing to talk to her. She suspected that her dad might not have long to live but when she said this in an email to her brother, Brendan, in Australia, he had accused her of "taking their hope away." Brendan seemed fixed on his parents making it to Australia to visit them. In their email exchanges, he talked of little else.

Molly Monaghan had always felt that she was more like her dad than was Brendan – they were both rather quiet, while Brendan and her mother had always been the forceful ones. She suspected that her dad did not really want to "fight on" and was afraid of the effects of chemotherapy. But she had not felt able to talk openly with him about this because she was worried that she would be seen as undermining Brendan and her mum; and then there was that accusation of taking away their hope. Molly Monaghan hoped Dr. Barnes would not tell her Mum what she had said when she saw her, but she welcomed the suggestion of a family meeting with Dr. Barnes' support.

Dr. Barnes talks with Brenda Monaghan

Later that day, Dr. Barnes got a similar story from Brenda Monaghan. The past fortnight had come as a total shock to the family. Looking back, Brenda could see signs that she felt now should have made her suspect that Joe was ill, and she wondered if Joe himself had guessed that there was something wrong and ignored it. He had lost a lot of weight in recent months and had been making excuses not to finish the work on their new conservatory – she now suspected he had been in too much discomfort.

Since the operation, the family had rallied round them. Their daughter, Molly, who still lived locally, had been in every day visiting, as had Brenda herself; and their son, Brendan, in Australia had been in touch by email nearly every day. Brenda said she knew that it didn't look good but had been encouraged by Mr. Bennett's optimism and the fact that he had told them what a success the operation had been. The stoma was "working like a dream," Mr. Bennett had said.

Brenda Monaghan did not really know what to do for the best. She felt she had to stay strong and positive for Joe. Brendan was desperate for her and Joe to keep to their plan of visiting him and their grandchildren in Australia. To be honest, she and Joe felt very cheated that after all their hopes it looked like this might never happen. Molly never said much and Brenda was worried she was taking it badly. This made conversation during their visits very difficult and uncomfortable. But "never say die" had been a life-long motto that had served them well.

Conflicts and conflict resolution

Dr. Barnes had thus heard "equal and opposite" stories on the one hand from Joe Monaghan and his daughter, Molly (who had both accepted that Joe was dying and wanted to work with the situation), and on the other from Joe's wife, Brenda and (through her) their son, Brendan, in Australia (who wanted to fight on). Yet all of them were in different ways keeping up a brave front in order to protect the others from distress.

Such situations are relatively common in palliative care and indeed, if not handled carefully, may result in difficult conflicts arising between those concerned. A report from the National End of Life Care Programme (2010, p. 6) in the UK identifies such conflicts as being among the most difficult problems faced by those working in this area: "One of the key challenges that we have is when there is a conflict between a resident's wishes and what a relative feels they would like to happen at the end of life. Building strong relationships with the relatives from the start can really help when we try to resolve these situations."

Dr. Barnes showed her skills of conflict resolution in the way she built strong relationships with those concerned. As she had done with Joe himself, Dr. Barnes gave his daughter, Molly, and then later his wife, Brenda, time to express their real concerns rather than rushing in: it would have been equally disastrous to the process of establishing genuine partnership between those concerned either to have sided with Molly Monaghan's values of care or to have sided against Brenda Monaghan's values of cure (her "never say die" attitude). As it was, when Dr. Barnes gave Brenda Monaghan a chance to talk, it became immediately clear that her motivation in "fighting on" was similar to Mr. Bennett's: both knew deep down that Joe Monaghan's condition was essentially incurable, short of a miracle, but both felt they owed it to Joe to keep up a hopeful and positive front.

Dr. Barnes showed similar skills in the way she built up her relationship with the surgical team. The conflicts here were potential (over Mr. Bennett's ongoing blocked bed) rather than actual, so we should perhaps see this as a case of conflict avoidance rather than conflict resolution. All the same, Dr. Barnes handled this very effectively: as we have seen, she allowed time to meet Mr. Bennett and the nursing staff when she first came on the ward, she adopted a listening approach, and she acknowledged in a good-humored way their very different (and hence complementary) skills sets. The scene was thus set for a constructive second cancer MDT meeting.

Section 3: the second (ward-based) cancer MDT meeting

Dr. Barnes discussed what Joe, Brenda and Molly Monaghan had told her with Mr. Bennett and the surgical nursing team after their next ward round a couple of days later. In the meantime, she had talked with the occupational therapist and also made preliminary enquiries about possible home-based nursing care from the local branch of a national cancer charity to provide additional nursing support at home. Sister Clancy reported that Joe Monaghan seemed to be sleeping better, although he remained very tired during the day, and Molly had started to say hello to the staff when she visited.

They agreed that they needed a second cancer MDT meeting, which this time would be held on the ward and include, in addition to Dr. Watts and Gina Morris (the gastrointestinal CNS), Sister Clancy, the occupational therapist and others who could contribute to aspects of the care package over and above the decision about whether to recommend chemotherapy. This was planned for early the following week.

In the rest of this part, we will be looking first at the outcomes from the second MDT meeting and then at how these outcomes reflected palliative care advance care planning (ACP) as reinforced and extended by the process elements of values-based practice. In the final part of the section, we will show how these process elements came together in a strong dissensual basis for ongoing partnership between the staff, Joe Monaghan and his family in managing the difficult months that lay ahead.

The outcomes from the second MDT meeting

The second MDT meeting was brief. It was agreed that, although chemotherapy remained an option, the next step was for Dr. Barnes to see Joe Monaghan again together with his wife and daughter if he wished to have them there (he had indicated that this was so) to discuss a care plan covering the following key areas:

1. *Joe Monaghan's and his family's priorities and preferences given the options available.* Dr. Barnes knew that Joe Monaghan wanted to get home as soon as possible (this would also cover the surgical team's concern about a blocked bed).

   Her enquiries had indicated that the community occupational therapists could offer alternatives to a stair lift by providing a commode and a hospital-style bed downstairs. There was also the likelihood of a Marie Curie nurse who could cover some night shifts, with the District Nurse coming in daily as needed, which she hoped would help Brenda Monaghan to manage Joe's care. It was possible the family would press for a stair lift (to maintain normal living as far as possible), but this would be expensive and would probably take too long to install.

2. *Treatment options in light of Joe Monaghan's likely prognosis.* It was clear from what Dr. Barnes had learned from Joe, Brenda and Molly Monaghan that they would all welcome an open and realistic discussion of treatment options (this is not always the case). A key issue would be whether or not to embark on chemotherapy and whether this would help or hinder their hopes for Joe Monaghan to see his Australian family and their new grandchild. If anything, the indications for chemotherapy were now less strong given Joe Monaghan's weakening condition: he needed to be fit enough not only to survive the journey to Australia but also to get back.

   These were issues that would benefit from further discussion between the family and Dr. Watts at a follow-up meeting. The most likely recommendation at this stage would be to go for a lower-dose "palliative treatment" regime aimed at symptom control rather than cure. Such a regime was likely to produce fewer side effects and carried fewer risks of premature death (NCEPOD, 2008).

3. *Follow-up and further information.* The MDT meeting was aware that, while Joe and his daughter Molly were likely to welcome the shift from "cure to care," Brenda Monaghan, and perhaps even more so their son, Brendan, might continue to find this very difficult.

It would be important therefore to include in the discussion with the family, sources of information and support that they could use as needed. Dr. Barnes had found that some patients and relatives welcomed quite technical and detailed information: she had in mind offering to email the link to the NCEPOD report (NCEPOD, 2008) to Brendan Monaghan in Australia. Clearly, Brendan's position was particularly difficult given that, for practical purposes, he only had email contact. (In the event, when Brendan Monaghan read the NCEPOD report and realized the risks of premature death from inappropriate chemotherapy, he decided to bring his family over to the UK rather than pressing for his parents to come to Australia.)

Dr. Barnes would write up a detailed care plan agreed with Joe Monaghan and his family and share this with their GP (who had already had a report from Mr. Bennet). Everyone involved with them would keep this up to date. This would help to establish clear lines of communication with their GP and the palliative care team (who were in the process of setting up a 24-hour help line) and thus ensure timely and well-coordinated care. It would also be a vital record for future decision-making, particularly if Joe Monaghan became unwell in a way that involved loss of decision-making capacity.

Advance care planning

Anyone working in palliative care in the UK will recognize in these outputs from the second MDT meeting many of the elements of what is called advance care planning (ACP). A recent publication from the UK's Department of Health (The NHS End of Life Care Programme, 2007, p. 4) describes ACP thus:

Advance care planning (ACP) is a voluntary process of discussion about future care between an individual and their care providers, irrespective of discipline. If the individual wishes, their family and friends may be included. It is recommended that with the individual's agreement this discussion is documented, regularly reviewed, and communicated to key persons involved in their care. An ACP discussion might include:
- *the individual's concerns and wishes,*
- *their important values or personal goals for care,*
- *their understanding about their illness and prognosis,*

- their preferences and wishes for types of care or treatment that may be beneficial in the future and the availability of these.

That ACP is all about values is clear from this statement: the first component of the care plan (summarized above) directly reflects Joe Monaghan's values as reflected in the bulleted points of the ACP statement. As a basis for partnership in decision-making, however, there are some important values missing from this statement.

VBP flashback

Before reading on, you may want to think for a moment about the values base of this statement of ACP.

One way to do this is by highlighting the value words and phrases in the statement using different colors for explicit and for implicit values (much as in Part 1 Dr. Gulati used blue highlighting and underlining, respectively, in thinking about the values base of the "yellow flags" for chronicity with low back pain; see Chapter 2).

Highlighting the text in this way will bring out the values that are included in the statement. But think also about any values that are *not* included.

We give our own marked-up version of the statement in Fig. 13.2. As already noted, the ACP statement makes clear the importance of values in palliative care planning – we can see blue and underlined text everywhere! But what stands out from the marked-up version is that the explicit values expressed (highlighted blue) are all *patients'* values. The values of carers and of staff, by contrast, if represented at all, are left implicit (appearing merely in underlined expressions like "... key persons involved in their care").

Equating values with patients' values is not unusual in healthcare contexts. Sackett's definition of evidence-based practice, as we noted in Chapter 2, although importantly including values, talks like the above ACP statement, only of patients' values. This emphasis on patients' values, as we have repeatedly emphasized, reflects an important shift towards care being patient-centered rather than being driven by the perspectives of staff or carers. But carers and indeed staff have values too. And to exclude their values is no basis for partnership.

Advance care planning (ACP) is a <u>voluntary</u> process of discussion about future care between an individual and their care providers, irrespective of discipline. If the individual wishes, their family and friends may be included. It is <u>recommended</u> that with the individual's <u>agreement</u> this discussion is documented, regularly reviewed, and communicated to <u>key</u> persons involved in their <u>care</u>. An ACP discussion might include:

- The individual's concerns and wishes.
- Their important values or personal goals for <u>care</u>.
- Their <u>understanding</u> about their illness and prognosis.
- Their preferences and wishes for types of <u>care</u> or treatment that may be beneficial in the future and the <u>availability</u> of these.

We will see in the section that follows that the values excluded are as important as those that are included to effective values-based partnership in decision-making.

Fig. 13.2. Values expressed in a summary statement of advanced care planning (blue highlight = explicit values; underlining = implicit values).

A dissensual care plan

What is needed, then, for genuine partnership in decision-making is not to exclude this or that perspective but rather a *balance* of perspectives – in a word then, dissensus. It is just such a dissensual balance of perspectives that the care plan outlined above achieved. It was focused consistently with the values base of ACP on Joe Monaghan's wish to be at home. But it provided a balanced approach to this in acknowledging:

- Brenda Monaghan's concerns as the principal carer (in the support offered through the Marie Curie nurse and other elements of the care package) and also
- the surgical team's concerns (in expediting a return home with the provision of a downstairs toilet).

On the key issue of chemotherapy, the plan provided a basis for a balanced approach through the improved lines of communication that Dr. Barnes had opened up between Joe Monaghan, his family and the professionals advising them. Here in particular, the resources of evidence-based practice would be important alongside and complementing those of values-based practice.

Dissensus and consensus

Reflection point

Throughout this book, we have noted the many similarities between evidence-based practice and values-based practice and both were clearly important in Dr. Barnes' work with Joe Monaghan, his family and the clinical team.

But at this point, you may find it helpful to think for a moment before reading on about any *differences* there might be between evidence-based practice and values-based practice when it comes to supporting partnership in decision-making.

In a word, where evidence-based practice is consensual, values-based practice is dissensual. Thus, in evidence-based practice, consensus is reached by *ironing out differences* of perspective on the evidence bearing on a given decision. Partnership in decision-making on this consensual model thus depends on those concerned coming to an agreement about which of their different perspectives on the evidence in question is best ("best evidence" in evidence-based practice is a consensual concept). In values-based practice, by contrast, differences of perspective on the values bearing on a given decision instead of being ironed out *remain fully in play* and are balanced according to the particular circumstances of the decision in question.

The difference between consensus and dissensus is not as starkly drawn as this summary might suggest. In practice, the two processes often work in concert. We had an example of this in Chapter 3 when we looked at the way in which values-based practice supports balanced decision-making within the framework of the Guiding Principles for the UK's Mental Health Act 2007. The Guiding Principles provide what we called a "round table" of values (see Fig. 3.3) within which balanced decisions can be made on individual cases. So the decision-making process is *dissensual* (the values represented by the Guiding Principles remain in play), but the framework itself is a *consensual* framework (recall that the Guiding Principles incorporate values that are shared among all stakeholders).

We discuss dissensus and the interdependence of dissensual and consensual processes in shared decision-making further in the web-based resource supporting the series. We will be exploring the role of shared frameworks of values further in the next chapter when we return to Dr. Gulati and how she resolved the

problems within her practice with off-work certification. We conclude this section by drawing together the elements of values-based practice in this story as each contributed to the dissensual care plan that came out of the second cancer MDT meeting.

The second cancer MDT meeting and the elements of values-based practice

When Dr. Barnes first arrived on the surgical ward, the stage was set for the different but unacknowledged value perspectives in play to come into conflict, with Joe Monaghan the loser:

- The action-oriented surgical team were doing their best, but the pressure to get back an urgently needed "acute" bed was growing.
- A second pressure that was building up was the surgical team's growing frustration at their inability to provide the kind of care that Joe Monaghan and his family needed (expressed in but not limited to the nursing staff's concerns about pain control).
- A third area of potential conflict was within the family itself between Joe Monaghan and his wife and son over the extent to which they should "fight on."

Yet by the time of the second cancer MDT meeting, a care plan was emerging that, as we have just seen, in balancing the different perspectives in play provided a basis for partnership instead of conflict.

VBP flashback

In this final VBP flashback, the idea is to think for a moment about which of the different elements of values-based practice in Joe Monaghan's story were important in achieving a basis for partnership rather than conflict between those involved in this story.

We have noted a number of such elements in earlier VBP flashbacks at various points in the chapter. Try running through these to see which of them were important in this respect. Also, note any elements that have *not* thus far been mentioned.

One way to organize your ideas here is to write a checklist of the elements of values-based practice and then to note against each of them where and if so with which character they come into Joe Monaghan's story.

We give our own checklist in Fig. 13.3. As this indicates there are no favorites here. The bottom line from

VBP process element	How it is reflected in this story (and by whom)
1. Awareness of values and diversity of values	Dr. Barnes (palliative care consultant): awareness of (i) strengths (StAR values, especially Joe Monaghan's aspirations), and (ii) possible conflicting values (between the surgical team and Joe Monaghan's family, and within the family) both in how the problem was understood (diagnosis) and hence how it should be dealt with (treatment).
2. Values reasoning skills	Dr. Watts (oncologist): casuistry – drawing on different case experiences from the surgical team, he suggested early palliative care referral. Similar case-based reasoning shown by Dr. Barnes.
3. Knowledge of values	Dr. Watts: knew from clinical experience and the research literature that Joe Monaghan could well be putting on a brave face for the sake of his family. Again, similarly with Dr. Barnes.
4. Specific communication skills (eliciting values and conflict resolution)	Dr. Barnes: (i) eliciting values (listening and being open with Joe Monaghan, thus giving him a chance to recognize and come to terms with what he wanted in his final months); and (ii) conflict resolution (with the surgical team and between Joe Monaghan's family members).
5. Person-values-centered practice	Mr. Bennett (surgeon): agreed to palliative care referral for pain control (reflecting Joe Monaghan's values) despite the likely delay in getting back his surgical bed (reflecting his own values). Sister Clancy and the surgical team: care for Joe Monaghan and his family (concerns about pain control; also, welcoming approach and listening).
6. Extended MDT	Surgical team, Dr. Watts and Dr. Barnes: all brought different value perspectives as well as different skills to the balanced dissensual care plan that came out of the second MDT meeting.
7. Two-feet Principle ("Think evidence, think values too!")	From the first to the second cancer MDT meeting: in the first cancer MDT meeting, the outcomes reflected focusing mainly on the evidence (research evidence on outcomes in general; clinical and laboratory reports about Joe Monaghan's condition and what "they" wanted (reports of the family's "fighting spirit"); the outcomes from the second MDT meeting, by contrast, reflected "thinking values" as well as "thinking evidence" (including what Joe really wanted).
8. Squeaky-wheel Principle ("Think values, think evidence too!")	Sister Clancy: forgot to "think evidence" when "thinking (religious) values" in her interactions with Joe and Brenda Monaghan over their religious faith.
9. Science-driven Principle ("Think high-tech, think evidence *and* values!")	Dr. Barnes: her implicit skills for values-based practice reflected the established tradition in palliative care of working with values alongside evidence: the need for this has been driven by the new and extended choices opened up at the end of life by scientific and technological advances in medicine.
10. Partnership (through dissensus) in decision-making	Dr. Barnes: uses her implicit skills for values-based practice to draw together a dissensual care plan that balances the values of all those involved (Joe Monaghan and his family, the surgical team and Dr. Watts) as a basis for partnership rather than conflict in Joe Monaghan's ongoing care.

Fig. 13.3. Summary of the ten process elements of values-based practice involved in Joe Monaghan's story.

this final VBP flashback is that *every* element of values-based practice contributes to this story in one way or another through one or more of the characters involved. This is true even of the elements that we had not thus far mentioned, elements 7 (the Two-feet Principle) and 9 (the Science-driven Principle). As Fig. 13.3 indicates, these two elements, although to this point implicit, were nonetheless present and important in the background to the story.

The premise and purpose of values-based practice

In addition to the process elements of values-based practice, its premise and purpose as outlined in Chapter 2, although not shown in Fig. 13.3, were also important in Joe Monaghan's story. Without the premise of values-based practice in mutual respect for differences of values, the very possibility of dissensual decision-making could not have arisen, while, as to the purpose of values-based practice, this just is balanced decision-making.

Consensus, dissensus and a "good enough" death

The idea of a "good enough" death guiding this chapter may have seemed at first glance a poor sort of compromise: surely, some will say, nothing less than "simply the best" should be our aim for someone who is dying. Winnicott's concept of the "good enough" mother emphasized the benefits of striving for "good enough" over perfection, and thereby leaving room for a sense of control to the baby (Winnicott, 1953). Likewise, dying patients can benefit from a sense of control. All the same, with dying patients "simply the best" is a sentiment with which few would take exception.

The problem though, as we hope this chapter has shown, is that in complex situations of the kind in which Joe Monaghan was placed there is (nor can be) no consensus on whose values are best. The result, we have suggested, is that if "simply the best" means focusing exclusively only on one value perspective (even on that of the patient), "simply the best" becomes a recipe for conflict rather than partnership between those concerned.

What is needed then, as we have suggested, is a balanced approach in which, although the values of the patient concerned remain central, the values of others involved, as family members and as staff, are also fully in play. It was this balanced approach that was achieved by those concerned in this story through the dissensual care plan that came out of the second MDT meeting. In balancing different perspectives, this dissensual care plan could not be, from the perspective of any one of those involved, "simply the best." But it was precisely in balancing the different value perspectives of all those involved that the care plan provided a basis for genuine partnership between them and thus to achieving a death that for all of them might be, if not a good death, at least a death that was "good enough."

Back with Mr. Bennett

Mr. Bennett was thinking about the second MDT meeting as he drove home. He had been worried about the early referral to the palliative care team, but it had proved to be surprisingly helpful: the ward staff were happier, there was a plan for Joe Monaghan and his family that looked feasible (and would get him his bed back), and he wasn't preached at! He would have no worries about calling in the in-reach team straight away the next time.

Chapter summary (see also Fig. 13.3)

Joe Monaghan's story in this chapter has illustrated how the process elements of values-based practice come together to provide a balanced dissensual basis for partnership in decision-making. Each of the elements of values-based practice considered separately in earlier chapters of the book has been important here:

- *Clinical skills* (elements 1–4 of values-based practice). The palliative care consultant, Dr. Emma Barnes, and the oncologist, Dr. Watts, between them showed each of these in good measure: Dr. Barnes helped *raise awareness* of the different values in play (element 1); she and Dr. Watts both used case-based *reasoning* based on their clinical experience and both were prepared with *knowledge* of what was likely to be important to Joe Monaghan (elements 2 and 3); and Dr. Barnes showed advanced *communication skills* particularly for eliciting values and of conflict resolution (element 4).
- *Relationships* (elements 5 and 6 of values-based practice). Dr. Barnes' clinical skills would have been ineffective if the relationships between those involved had not been enabling to values-based practice in the two essential respects of being *person-centered* (element 5) and *multidisciplinary* (element 6). For all the conflicting values at play in this story, the surgical team always put their patient, Joe Monaghan, first; and they were able to

181

build on their established practice of MDT work in shifting, with Dr. Barnes' help, from their team values of (surgical) cure to engage with Dr. Barnes' values of (palliative) care.

- *Links with evidence-based practice* (elements 7–9 of values-based practice). The three principles linking evidence-based practice and values-based practice were also important in this story: the Two-feet Principle, reminding us to "Think evidence, think values too!" was apparent in the first cancer MDT meeting in the different takes on the evidence being driven by (largely unacknowledged) values; the Squeaky-wheel Principle, with its counterpart reminder to "Think values, think evidence too!" was reflected in the way Sister Clancy inappropriately (in this particular instance) pushed her religious values; and the Science-driven Principle, reminding us to "Think high-tech, think evidence *and* values!" has been behind the whole story in that it is advances in medical science and technology and the new choices that these have opened up at the end of life that have driven the development of values-based practice so actively alongside evidence-based practice in palliative care.
- *Dissensus* (element 10 of values-based practice). Building on the above elements, the outcomes from the second MDT meeting, in focusing on Joe Monaghan's needs and priorities but reflecting also those of his family and of the staff involved, established a *dissensual basis* for partnership in decision-making between them.

The very natural way in which the different aspects of values-based practice came together in Joe Monaghan's story reflects the point noted at the start of the chapter that palliative care is above all an area of medicine in which the importance of values alongside evidence has been well recognized for some time. The restricted values focus of ACP noted in the chapter reminds us that there is further values-based work to do even in palliative care. All the same, palliative care is an area in which examples of what are in all but name values-based practice are not hard to find. Palliative care, then, in developing values-based alongside evidence-based ways of working, is, like mental health

and the other areas of primary care that we looked at in the opening chapters of this book, leading the way in linking science with people.

In the next chapter, we return to the story of Dr. Gulati from Part 1 to see how a more explicit use of values-based practice can be used to support partnership in decision-making in the (apparently) more prosaic circumstances of off-work certification.

References

Chochinov, H. M. (2002). Dignity-conserving care – a new model for palliative care. *Journal of the American Medical Association* **287**, 2253–60.

Christiakis, N. A. (1999). *Death Foretold: Prophecy and Prognosis in Medical Care*. Chicago: University of Chicago Press.

Fallowfield, L. J., Jenkins, V. A. and Beveridge H. A. (2002). Truth may hurt, but deceit hurts more: communication in palliative care. *Palliative Medicine* **16**, 297.

Gilbert. P. (ed.) (2011) *Spirituality and Mental Health*. Brighton: Pavilion.

Lo, B., Quill, T. and Tulsky, J. (1999). Discussing palliative care with patients. ACP-ASIM End-of-Life Care Consensus Panel. American College of Physicians-American Society of Internal Medicine. *Annals of Internal Medicine* **130**, 744–9.

National End of Life Care Programme (2010). *The Route to Success in End of Life Care – Achieving Quality in Care Homes*. London: National Health Service.

NCEPOD (2008). *For Better, for Worse? A Review of the Care of Patients Who Died Within 30 Days of Receiving Systemic Anti-cancer Therapy*. London: National Confidential Enquiry into Patient Outcomes and Death.

Schattner, A. (2009). The silent dimension: expressing humanism in each medical encounter. *Archives of Internal Medicine* **169**, 1095–9.

The NHS End of Life Care Program (2007). *Advance Care Planning: a Guide for Health and Social Care Staff* (revised 2008). London: Department of Health.

Walter, T. (2002). Spirituality in palliative care: opportunity or burden? *Palliative Medicine* **16**, 133–9.

Winnicott, D. (1953). Transitional objects and transitional phenomena, *International Journal of Psychoanalysis* **34**, 89–97.

CHAPTER 14 begins on following page

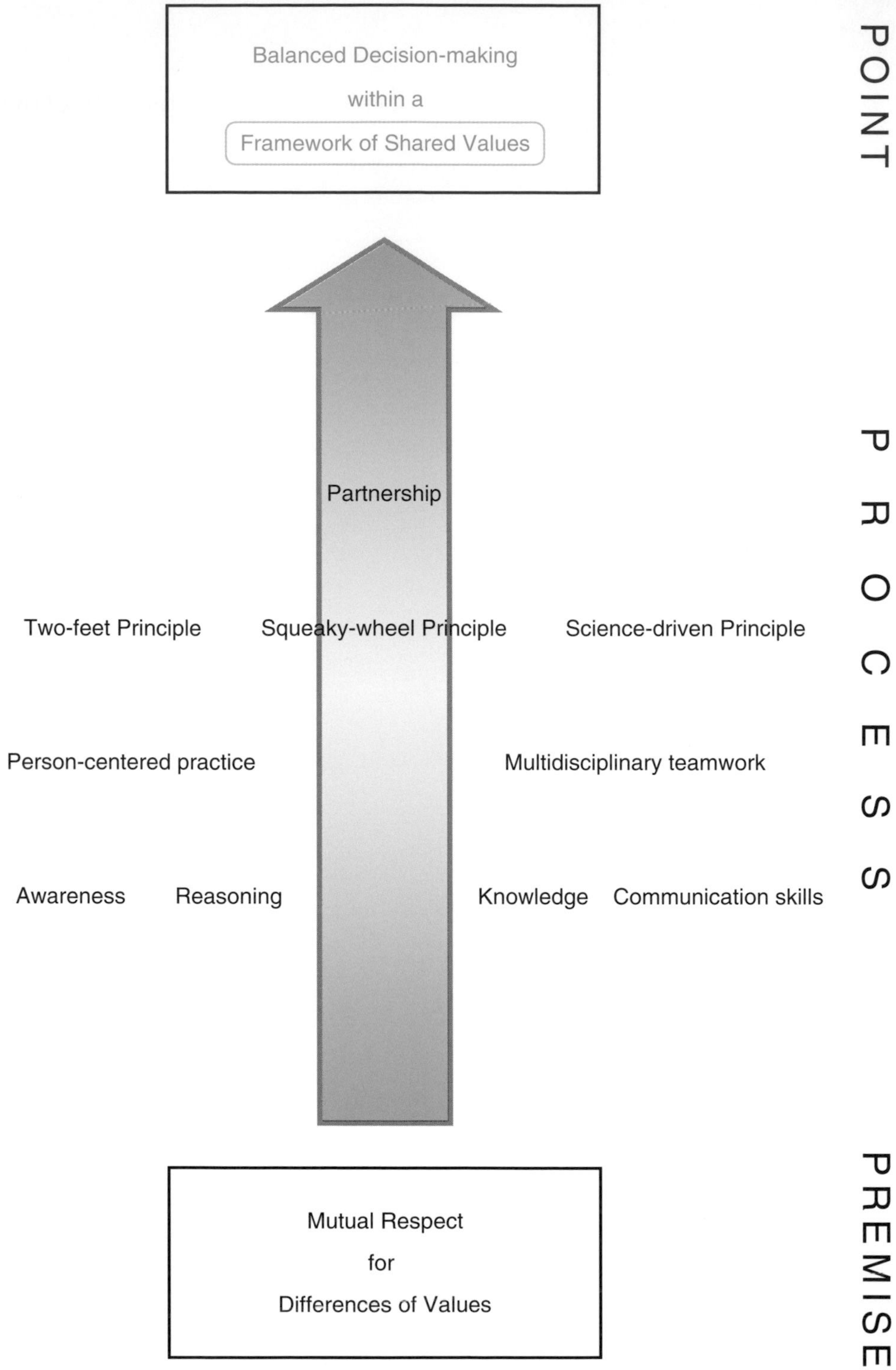

Map of values-based practice – a framework of shared values.

"It's my back, Doctor" (episode 3): building a shared framework for values-based practice

Topics covered in this chapter

This chapter describes how to bring together the elements of values-based practice within a framework of shared values to support balanced decision-making in clinical practice.

Other topics include:

- Management of chronic low back pain
- Chronicity and compliance
- Protected learning time
- Efficiency and effectiveness
- Practice policies
- Values-based commissioning

Take-away message for practice

*A **framework of shared values**, built up between clinicians, patients, carers and managers, provides a basis for balanced decision-making on contested issues.*

In this chapter, we return to the story of Dr. Gulati from Part 1 to see how the elements of values-based practice, as set out separately in the preceding chapters, came together to support her in resolving her dilemma about how to manage the demand of her patient, Roy Walker, for an off-work certificate.

The buck stops here

Dr. Gulati's reflection had helped to clarify her dilemma. There were important ancillary issues: her personal and professional obligations to Dr. Austin, and her concerns for Roy Walker's family. But the essence of her dilemma was that she was caught between two important conflicting aspects of good practice. On the one hand, she wanted to support autonomy of patient choice as an aspect of person-centered practice, while on the other hand, she had not only her societal responsibility for certification but also her responsibility to Roy Walker to act in his clinical best interests as indicated by established evidence on chronicity and low back pain.

Yet none of the resources to which Dr. Gulati turned in her period of reflection – codes of practice, ethics, decision analysis and evidence-based practice – had actually *resolved* her dilemma. Indeed, the one thing she was clear about on the Monday when he returned was that, informed as she certainly had been by these various resources, the decision about what to do was a matter ultimately for her own clinical judgment.

A route map

In bringing together the elements of values-based practice, this chapter inevitably covers a good deal of ground, but you can think of Dr. Gulati's work with Roy Walker in two broad phases, short term and longer term:

- In her short-term management of Roy Walker, Dr. Gulati built on her already well-developed clinical skills for values-based practice to steer a middle course between outright refusal of and mere acquiescence in his demands for off-work certification. The way she did this, as we will see, allowed doctor and patient to build a relationship of mutual respect as a basis for helping not only Roy Walker but also his family.
- In the longer term, Dr. Gulati worked with her colleagues and other stakeholders in the practice, including their local Patients' Forum, to develop a shared framework of values that, like the frameworks described in Chapter 3, could be used to support balanced decision-making in other difficult areas such as resource management and commissioning.

Developing a shared framework of values required a not inconsiderable investment of time and effort from those concerned. This is to be expected. As we noted at the end of Part 1, values-based practice is not an off-the-shelf one-size-fits-all "solution" to working with complex and conflicting values. Rather, it has to be developed and adapted in the particular circumstances of a given area of clinical decision-making. The upside, however, as Dr. Gulati and her colleagues found, was that, once the necessary up-front investment had been made, it paid off across a wide range of values-complex areas of decision-making within the practice.

The clinical context

Dr. Gulati had temporarily defused the situation with Roy Walker in her first appointment by asking him to come back for a double appointment a week later when they would have time to go through things properly. She gathered from the receptionist that he had turned up (this was a good sign – she had thought he might wait to see Dr. Austin) and she was about to call him in. She was still not sure exactly how she would play things, but in the course of her deliberations over the past week, she thought she had come up with at least a possible course of action.

Reflection point

Before reading on, you may want to think for a moment about what you would do in Dr. Gulati's situation.

Think about this from *your own* point of view. If Roy Walker was your patient, how would you handle the consultation with him? What would *you* do?

Waiting for Roy Walker to come in

There is, of course, no one right answer to what to do in Roy Walker's case. There is a clear evidence base about chronicity and low back pain. There is also extensive literature on compliance. But exactly how these evidence bases are applied in a given case depends, as David Sackett and his colleagues reminded us in Chapter 2, on case-specific factors including the clinician's expertise and the patient's unique values. To "patient's unique values," moreover, as Dr. Gulati's experience showed us in Part 1, we must now add the unique values of other stakeholders, not least the unique values of the *clinician*.

Clinicians' values as well as those of patients

This is why the above reflection point emphasizes thinking about what to do in Roy Walker's case, not in general terms ("In this kind of case, one should do . . ."), nor even from Dr. Gulati's point of view ("Dr. Gulati should do . . ."), but from *your own* point of view ("What I would do is . . .").

Again, each of Sackett's three elements – research evidence, clinical expertise and values – could be important here. There could be differences of view about the *evidence* (although in this case the relevant evidence on chronicity and low back pain is not at issue). There could be differences of *clinical background and experience*. To be able to draw on our experience with previous cases is an important part of what it means to have *expertise*, clinical or otherwise. Last but not least, there could be differences in the *values* that, as clinicians as well as patients, we bring to individual decision-making.

Dr. No and Dr. Yes

We can see just how much individual clinicians' values matter by considering how two hypothetical clinicians, Dr. No and Dr. Yes, both with values very different from those of Dr. Gulati, might respond to the question in the above reflection about what to do in Roy Walker's case.

- Dr. No, unlike Dr. Gulati, has a top value, i.e. a value that he considers should be paramount in all circumstances, namely "clinical best interests as guided by best evidence." Dr. No thus has no hesitation in simply refusing Roy Walker's demand straight out. In taking this course of action in Roy Walker's case, he is also guided by his clinical experience: Dr. No has had good previous experience of taking a hard line with patients like Roy Walker.
- Dr. Yes also has a top value, but in this case it is autonomy of patient choice. Dr. Yes thus has no hesitation in adopting a course of action directly contrary to Dr. No's and going along with Roy Walker's demands. Dr. Yes was no less aware than Dr. Gulati or Dr. No of the evidence on chronicity and low back pain. But Dr. Yes had found with previous patients that showing a little flexibility in areas like off-work certification gave good returns when it came to (as he saw it) more serious issues like alcohol consumption: and she felt that, particularly given the risks to Roy Walker's family, getting him to cut down on his drinking was the priority in this case.

In your own reflection on what you would do in Roy Walker's case, you may have been influenced by different values altogether from Dr. No and Dr. Yes. Dr. Austin was closer to Dr. Yes than to Dr. No. We will see later in this chapter that these and other values were expressed by Dr. Gulati's colleagues and members of the local Patients' Forum when they got together to work out how to manage these and other similarly difficult areas of decision-making.

In the present instance, however, Dr. Gulati's dilemma arose from the fact that she was poised equidistant between the two top-value extremes of Dr. No and Dr. Yes. Now, with Roy Walker about to be called back in to see her, she knew that, for good or ill, she had finally made up her mind what to do.

Short-term management

Roy Walker looked more apprehensive than aggressive as he entered Dr. Gulati's consulting room for the follow-up consultation. Dr. Gulati started by getting him settled – she made a point of asking him if his back was OK in the chair she indicated, thus making clear right from the start that she was taking his problems fully seriously. She then built on this by explaining that she had now had a chance to read all Dr. Austin's helpful notes but would like to hear from Roy Walker in his own words exactly how he had come to strain his back and what had happened since.

Reflection point

How do you think the previously truculent Roy Walker was likely to respond to this opening approach by Dr. Gulati?

Before reading on, you may find it worthwhile going back to our brief characterization of Roy Walker in Chapter 1. Look again at the section "Meet Roy Walker."

You may also want to think about why Roy Walker returned as requested rather than waiting until Dr. Austin got back from his holidays; and again, why he seemed more anxious than aggressive as he entered Dr. Gulati's consulting room.

Meet Roy Walker again

Roy Walker was surprised by Dr. Gulati's invitation to him to tell his story in his own words. Most of the people he had seen, including a back specialist at the local hospital and a physiotherapist, had started with a phrase along the lines of "I see you've got . . ." and then proceeded to tell him what they could do to help. Of course, he knew that doctors were very busy, but all the same, it had done nothing for his already limited self-confidence that no one cared about what he had to say. Even Dr. Austin after his first few visits had seemed to lose interest.

And as we noted in Chapter 1, Roy Walker had got to the point when he did indeed have something that he wanted to say. For behind the bluster, as we said, was a man who had become all too aware that he needed help and who had been plucking up courage to ask for it. In the earlier clinic, he had been wrong-footed by finding himself seeing this lady doctor instead of Dr. Austin – as we noted, this was why he reacted as aggressively as he did. But in the interim, he had found himself wondering whether this firm but clearly caring doctor might after all be someone to whom he could turn. His initial reaction to being offered a double appointment was to go along with it for the sake of getting his certificate renewed. But later that morning, he had woken up to the fact that Dr. Gulati was the first person he had seen who had actually offered him *more* time: usually, everyone seemed only too keen to get rid of him and move on to the next patient.

Roy Walker speaks up

Thus it was that this previously inarticulate and bullying man found himself pouring out his story to Dr. Gulati. There were no particular surprises. It was the usual story of an incautious lift of a load (an awkward pile of scaffold poles), the like of which he had managed effortlessly so many times before; the sudden "tearing" in his back; the embarrassment of being unable to straighten up; the good-humored ribbing from his work mates; initial sympathy from his boss, and then growing impatience and demands for a second opinion. "But what can I do?" he finished, now looking almost in tears. "My dad did his back and kept on working and he ended up in a wheelchair."

Dr. Gulati explains about backs

Rather than answering Roy Walker's question directly, Dr. Gulati said she would like to examine him again. She had examined him briefly on his first visit but now carried out a full neurological review. As with her willingness to listen to him, Roy Walker was impressed that she cared enough to take time to go through everything so thoroughly.

Finding no abnormal signs (as his notes indicated was likely), Dr. Gulati sat Roy Walker down again and now asked him what he thought happened when people "did their backs." Like many people, Roy Walker had only the vaguest of ideas about this. He had played football as a younger man and said he thought it was like spraining your ankle but in the back. "That's on the right lines," Dr. Gulati replied, "but backs are a bit different. It's like this . . ."

Getting out a piece of paper, she drew a simple diagram of the back as a column of muscles supporting the spine. As she drew, she explained about backs being, yes, like ankles made up of bones and joints, but the key difference was that with backs the bones and joints are held in place by *muscles*. So the back is really a column of strong muscles.

"Does that make sense?" Dr. Gulati asked. It did. As we saw in Chapter 1, Roy Walker knew about muscles. This was "his thing," as it were. He had prided himself on his strength as a young man and remained powerfully built. For this second appointment, he had abandoned his skinny "vest" in favor of a more modest open-necked shirt but his well-muscled physique was still evident.

Roy Walker thus felt growing confidence as Dr. Gulati went on to explain about the two stages of a back strain. First, the initial shift (as she put it) with perhaps a disc getting pushed a bit out of line, and the muscles going into spasm and "locking up" the back. Then, secondly, the recovery stage when the key thing was to *build up the muscles* to support the discs and to stop it happening again.

This was all a revelation for Roy Walker. Dr. Gulati took more time than we have indicated here to take him through it. But it all made sense to him. And Roy Walker ended up seeing for himself that if he wanted to avoid ending up like his dad in a wheelchair he had to "get himself going again."

Progress and an agreed plan

So with a shared understanding of the problem in place, they now started to work out a shared plan. With his new-found (if still fragile) confidence, Roy Walker engaged with this. He felt again for the first time that he was being listened to rather than just being ticked off and told what to do (and then being made to feel a failure when he couldn't do it). The first part of their plan came together readily enough:

1. Dr. Gulati agreed to give Roy Walker a further off-work certificate.
2. She also offered to write to his employer saying that he was engaging actively in rehabilitation.
3. In return, Roy Walker agreed to attend back classes with a physiotherapist who came to the clinic twice a week.

Thus far, now that he had got the idea of his back as a column of muscles, Roy Walker went along with the plan readily enough. He understood and indeed welcomed the prospect of being able to strengthen his back with exercises. But there was a further element of the plan that he found more challenging, namely that Dr. Gulati was encouraging him to take on some light voluntary work until he was fit again. This was partly to restore his confidence for a return to work. It was also to give him experience of other areas of work should it turn out that in the longer term his back problems made it impossible to continue with the heavy laboring that he had done all his life.

Dr. Gulati's master stroke

Initially, Roy Walker was terrified by this suggestion, but it turned out, as we will see towards the end of the chapter, to be Dr. Gulati's master stroke. In Chapter 1, we noted that, behind his bluster, Roy Walker lacked confidence and had an impoverished sense of self-worth. But he now respected Dr. Gulati sufficiently not to reject her suggestion out of hand and they spent the final few minutes of the consultation discussing what he might do.

It turned out that one of his unrecognized strengths was that he liked and had always been good with animals. They were not allowed pets where he lived, but he had had a dog as a boy and still missed the companionship of that early relationship. Aware as she was of the importance in chronicity of employment and other social factors outside the reach of the GP (Underwood, 1998), Dr. Gulati picked up on this immediately. "So why don't you go along to the local PDSA [People's Dispensary for Sick Animals] group," she suggested, adding with a smile before Roy Walker could reply, ". . . and let me know how you get on!"

We will see how Roy Walker got on later. First, we will take time out ourselves to review Dr. Gulati's management of his case from the perspective of values-based practice. We will look at what elements of values-based practice she has drawn on thus far and then at what else will be needed to carry the management plan through successfully in the longer term.

Values-based practice in Dr. Gulati's short-term management

In Part 1, we noted that values-based practice has not been conjured up "out of the blue" but builds rather, as in a similar way to how evidence-based practice builds, on best practice. Dr. Gulati was clearly a very skilled practitioner and among her other talents she had a natural ability for working with values.

To this point, however, although she was experienced in ethics and had a good working knowledge of decision analysis and of evidence-based practice, she had not even heard of values-based practice. (Dr. Gulati will come across values-based practice for the first time a little further into the story.) Nonetheless, like Dr. Emma Barnes, the in-reach palliative care consultant in the last chapter, Dr. Gulati's management of Roy Walker's case has shown a number of key features of values-based practice.

> **Reflection point**
>
> Before reading on, you may want to try reviewing for yourself what aspects of values-based practice Dr. Gulati has shown in her management of Roy Walker to this point in their story.
>
> One way to do this is in the form of a simple table like that shown in Fig. 14.1 summarizing the elements of values-based practice.
>
> We will be filling in the "blanks" as we work through the rest of the chapter. But you may find it helpful to have a go at the empty column (reflecting Dr. Gulati's management of Roy Walker's case thus far) before reading on.

Elements of values-based practice	Demonstrated in this case
Premise: mutual respect	
Skills – awareness	
Skills – knowledge	
Skills – reasoning	
Skills – communication	
Person-values-centered	
Team values	
EBP/VBP – Two-feet Principle	
EBP/VBP – Squeaky-wheel Principle	
EBP/VBP – Science-driven Principle	
Dissensus + consensus	
Point: balanced decisions	

EBP, evidence-based practice; VBP, values-based practice.

Fig. 14.1. Summary table of processes of values-based practice.

Dr. Gulati as a values-based practitioner

We give our own take on Dr. Gulati as a values-based practitioner in Fig. 14.2. As you can see, her management of Roy Walker's demand for an off-work certificate reflects the point and premise of values-based practice as well as a number of its key process elements. We will look briefly at each of these in this section before moving on to how Dr. Gulati built on all this in her longer-term management of the case.

The point of values-based practice: balanced decision-making within a framework of shared values

Dr. Gulati's dilemma was precisely the need to balance the different values in play in this case. In her time out, she came to understand that she was torn between different professional values (patient autonomy, best interests and so forth) to all of which she, like others, was committed. These values were indeed framework values in the sense that they are all values that are widely shared by clinicians, patients and other stakeholders in health care. But in this instance, these framework values were pulling Dr. Gulati in different

directions. Unlike Dr. No and Dr. Yes above, she did not know what was right.

By the end of her time out, moreover, Dr. Gulati had come to see that there would be no rule, ethical or otherwise, resolving her dilemma. The buck, as we said, stopped with her. It was a matter for her clinical judgment to decide how to balance the different framework values in play in this particular case. Thus was she brought directly to the point of values-based practice in the need for balanced decision-making within a framework of shared values.

The process of values-based practice: ten elements

In balancing the framework values in play in this case, Dr. Gulati drew (intuitively but no less effectively for that) on a number of the key process elements of values-based practice. As we have emphasized several times, these elements are important individually for values-based decision-making, but they also support and complement each other when they are used together in a well-joined-up way. It is Dr. Gulati's joined-up use of the process elements of values-based practice that we will focus on here.

189

Elements of VBP	Demonstrated in Dr. Gulati's management of Roy Walker
Premise: mutual respect	✓
Skills – awareness	✓
Skills – knowledge	
Skills – reasoning	✓
Skills – communication	✓
Person-values-centered	✓
Team values	
EBP/VBP – Two-feet Principle	✓
EBP/VBP – Squeaky-wheel Principle	✓
EBP/VBP – Science-driven Principle	
Partnership – dissensus	✓
Point: balanced decisions	✓

Fig. 14.2. Summary table of processes demonstrated by Dr. Gulati as a values-based practitioner.

Reflection point

We summarize some of the interactions between the process elements of values-based practice illustrated by Dr. Gulati's work with Roy Walker below. Before reading this, you may want to try working out some of the interactions yourself.

One way to do this is by drawing a diagram along the lines of Fig. 3.1 (and repeated at the start of this and previous chapters) and then adding extra arrows to show the interactions between elements.

How many interactions between the process elements of values-based practice can you identify in the way Dr. Gulati has worked with Roy Walker thus far?

Clearly, there are many ways in which the elements of values-based practice are interacting to support each other in Dr. Gulati's capable hands. We describe just a few of them here by way of illustration.

Start with awareness of values and communication skills . . .

Fundamental to Dr. Gulati's success in engaging Roy Walker in a positive way was her *awareness* of values, including in this instance her own values as well as those of Roy Walker – remember her self-awareness in her reaction to Roy Walker's show of flesh in her first encounter with him in his skinny vest.

We have looked at a number of tools for becoming aware of one's own values in a clinical situation. The important point is to make sure we are in touch with our values.

This self-understanding carried with it a corresponding capacity to elicit Roy Walker's values through the *communication skills* she showed by remaining open and receptive to him in their second interview. Besides her skills for *eliciting values*, Dr. Gulati showed good skills of *conflict resolution* (or avoidance in this case) in her initial containment of a potentially explosive situation by offering Roy Walker a longer appointment in her later clinic. This in turn gave her the time out she needed to think about what to do – this included using at least one form of *values reasoning*, principles reasoning, as well as dipping into the related values tools of ethics, decision analysis and evidence-based practice.

Offering Roy Walker a longer appointment also communicated to him that Dr. Gulati was ready to give time to understanding him. As we saw earlier in this chapter, she built on this effectively in their second appointment, with the result that she was able not only to understand exactly why he was so terrified of going back to work but also to elicit a number of unexpected *positive values*. These StAR values, as we called them in Chapter 4 (strengths, aspirations and resources), included an ability to work with animals that, as we will see later, turned out in the longer term to play a key role in his recovery.

. . . add person-values-centered practice . . .

The insight into Roy Walker's values (positive and negative) that Dr. Gulati's skills of awareness and communication gave her were the basis of an approach that was *person-centered* in the specifically person-*values*-centered sense described in Chapter 8, i.e. that her approach was focused on Roy Walker's values. Again, however, there was a two-way trade here. Dr. Gulati's commitment to person-centered practice was the basis of one side of the dilemma (the autonomy of patient choice side of her dilemma) that led her to deploy her skills of awareness and communication in moving towards a balanced decision about what to do.

. . . and a touch of evidence-based practice

Although not involving an area of high-tech medicine (where the Science-driven Principle applies), the importance of its "red-light warning" for practice – to "think values *and* evidence" – is clear throughout this story. The other two principles linking evidence-based and values-based practice are also clearly in play:

- *The Squeaky-wheel Principle*, reminding us to "Think values, think evidence too!", was reflected in the way Dr. Gulati recognized that one side of her dilemma ("best interests") was driven by the evidence of chronicity and low back pain. But this realization of course led her back to the Two-feet Principle.
- *The Two-feet Principle*, reminding us to "Think evidence, think values too!" was in turn evident in Dr. Gulati's further realization that the evidence on chronicity and low back pain was itself deeply values laden (recall here her highlighted copy of the "yellow flags").

So here, as in all real-life scenarios, it is not "evidence *or* values" but always "evidence *and* values" that is the basis of good clinical care.

Finally, mix with dissensus . . .

Dr. Gulati's management plan, however well founded in principle, would have been ineffective in practice unless it had been developed *in partnership* with Roy Walker. The basis of partnership in values-based decision-making, as we saw in Chapter 13, is dissensus. Dissensus differs from consensus in that differences of values instead of being ironed out (as in consensus) remain in play to be balanced according to the particular circumstances of a given decision within a framework of shared values.

Differences of values were where the story started from, but the values of patient autonomy and best interests in which Dr. Gulati formulated her dilemma turned out also to be (although of course not in the same words) Roy Walker's values: yes, he wanted Dr. Gulati to go along with what he wanted (an off-work certificate) but this, it now transpired, was because of his mistaken belief that it was in his best interests to remain off work (to avoid, as he thought, ending up in a wheelchair like his dad).

Their shared framework of values was (as we also indicated in Chapter 13) a consensual framework. Indeed, much of the action of the second interview was about establishing consensus. The story started in Chapter 1 with a potential standoff of values: Roy Walker wanted his certificate (autonomy) and Dr. Gulati wanted him to engage in rehabilitation (best interests). It was in these terms, as a standoff between autonomy and best interests, that Dr. Gulati came in Chapter 2 to understand her dilemma about what to do. But once she had understood that Roy Walker also wanted rehabilitation (or at any rate not to end up in a wheelchair like his dad), and once Roy Walker had understood that avoiding a wheelchair meant activity rather than inactivity (that his back needed strengthening), then their values were aligned, and the first three elements of Dr. Gulati's plan then followed straightforwardly from the consensus that through mutual understanding they had now reached.

But if the first three elements of the management plan were in this way consensual, the fourth, that Roy Walker had to agree to find some voluntary work, was *dis*sensual in that it balanced autonomy and best interests (as their shared values) *differently for the two of them*. If Roy Walker had had his (autonomous) way, finding some voluntary work was the last thing he would have thought of doing. Dr. Gulati, on the other hand, saw this as essential to Roy Walker's longer-term recovery (his best interests). So there was no consensus here. Rather, they were at a point of dissensus with their differences of values still in play. But it was precisely because Roy Walker felt that his values really were in play (through the way he had been listened to, the discovery of his talent for working with animals and so forth) that he left the consultation not only having agreed to look for some voluntary work but feeling genuinely motivated to "give it a go."

The premise of values-based practice: mutual respect

Here, then, as in all real-life scenarios, there was a rich interplay of the different process elements of values-based practice. None of this would have been possible, however, if Dr. Gulati and Roy Walker by the time of the second consultation had not reached a relationship of mutual respect. Again, there was a two-way interaction at work here. Had Dr. Gulati not treated Roy Walker in a respectful and professional manner from the start, despite his demanding manner and (from her point of view) unprepossessing appearance, the process could not have got off the ground, and her skills of awareness and communication (as outlined above) were crucial here.

Equally importantly, however, had Roy Walker been racist in his reaction to Dr. Gulati, had he taken against her merely as an Asian, there would have been no prospect of progress (recall from Chapter 3 that racism and other forms of discrimination and prejudice are incompatible with values-based practice). As it was, Roy Walker recognized in Dr. Gulati's firm but caring response to his initial demands something that, despite his bluster, he respected: this was why he turned up for his afternoon appointment rather than waiting until Dr. Austin got back. And by the end of that second consultation, as a man who for the first time felt he had been really listened to, he was ready to trust Dr. Gulati and to do his best to (as he put it to himself) "follow doctor's orders."

Longer-term work within the practice

The management plan that Dr. Gulati had now worked out with Roy Walker met her primary clinical objectives: it engaged Roy Walker in rehabilitation in a way that was consistent with his values and hence had a reasonable chance of being successfully carried through.

It also covered as far as possible her secondary concerns about Roy Walker's family. Clearly, she could not be sure how he would react when he got home. But she had been concerned that if she had simply refused to renew his certificate, he might have taken out his frustrations on his wife and children. She felt now that, with Roy Walker leaving her office in an encouraged rather than disappointed frame of mind, she had at least avoided, in the terms of the Four Principles (Chapter 2), "doing harm" to his family.

Carrying the plan through

Dr. Gulati remained concerned, however, about her partner, Dr. Austin. He would be pleased, she felt

sure, that she had got Roy Walker moving in the right direction. He was, as it turned out, pleased; and he suggested that Dr. Gulati should follow through with Roy Walker who had in the interim asked if he could have his next appointment with Dr. Gulati.

But this left unresolved the background issue of how as a practice they should manage off-work certification. This could be important for Roy Walker: despite his good start, they needed a joined-up approach as a practice (including the liaison physiotherapist as well as other partners) to deal with the inevitable setbacks. And then there was the wider concern about over use of fitness certificates that, as we saw in Chapter 1, had come out of their last practice audit.

> ### Reflection point
>
> What elements of values-based practice are likely to be important as Dr. Gulati works out her longer-term management of the issues raised by Roy Walker's case?
>
> Go back to your summary list (as in Fig. 14.2) and think what elements are likely to be filled in the right-hand column.

Next steps

Dr. Gulati found an opportunity to tackle the wider issues when her turn came to organize one of their monthly protected learning time (PLT; see Chapter 6) sessions. PLT sessions are organized in different ways in different practices. In Dr. Gulati's practice, they included all the clinical staff, rather than limiting them to the medical partners. They also regularly invited members of a local reference group, the Patients' Forum. So their PLT sessions provided a good opportunity to think about policies for dealing with issues like off-work certification that needed a joined-up approach, including patients and carers as well as clinicians.

Dr. Gulati had originally suggested a PLT on off-work certification when this was identified as an issue of concern in their recent practice audit. Her idea was to use the session to see if they could come up with a shared approach: this would allow them to tackle the issues without putting any particular partner on the spot. Now, fresh from her experience with Roy

Walker, Dr. Gulati saw that coming up with a shared approach meant coming up with a shared set of *values*. Being already interested in this aspect of practice, she had attended a workshop on values-based practice run by a GP colleague, Dr. Ted Real, at a recent conference, and her colleagues welcomed the suggestion that she should invite him to run a similar workshop with them, shortly after Dr. Austin's return from study leave.

The values-based practice workshop

Working together, Dr. Gulati and Dr. Real devised a two-hour PLT workshop with the specific objective of developing a shared framework of values. They would use off-work certification as an example but would not focus directly on this as an outcome from the session. This was important, Dr. Real pointed out. Focusing directly on off-work certification risked the workshop ending up as an exercise in writing yet another set of regulatory guidelines. Values-based practice, by contrast, was about skills and other factors supporting balanced decision-making where (as in the case of work certification) complex and conflicting values are in play.

Clearly, they could not do the whole "skills development thing" in one workshop, but, particularly if the Patients' Forum was also represented, they could have a go at building a shared framework of values. This would provide a basis for balanced values-based decision-making not only in relation to off-work certification but also for other contested issues within the practice.

The program that Dr. Real and Dr. Gulati devised is shown in Workshop Diagram 1. The workshop, when it took place four weeks later, was intentionally fast moving. There were 17 participants in all, with a majority of (full- and part-time) medical partners, three practice nurses, a physiotherapist,

two representatives from the Patients' Forum and the Practice Manager. It resulted in enthusiastic participation with outcomes for each part of the program as shown below.

1. Warm-up exercise: what is a "good GP"?

The workshop started with an exercise looking at participants' views on the qualities of a good GP. Although used here as a warm-up exercise, this first part of the program also served as a skills training exercise in awareness of values as the first process element of values-based practice.

Various exercises can be used for enhancing values awareness (as described in "Whose Values?" and other resources on the website). The one used by Dr. Real in this workshop asked participants to compare what we value in something as simple as an eating apple with the more complex values involved in the idea of a "good GP." The choice of this exercise thus had the additional purpose of getting the group to take their first step towards a shared framework of values but in an unselfconscious way.

The workshop was divided into two subgroups with roughly similar membership including a representative of the Patients' Forum in each. The groups were given just five minutes to make some silent personal jottings in response to the instructions in Workshop Diagram 2. The words that they came up with are given in Workshop Diagrams 3 and 4.

When describing a good apple, participants in both groups used similar terms, some of the top terms appearing on many different people's lists. (In both tables, the most frequently used terms are at the top.) There was, everyone agreed, little disagreement among participants about the qualities of a good apple.

When it came to the more complex concept of a good GP, however, although there was still a

1. Warm-up exercise: what is a "good GP?"
2. The GMC's "good doctor"
3. Introduction to values-based practice
4. Role play: conflicting values and work certification
5. A framework of shared values for *this* practice
6. Conclusions

Workshop Diagram 1. The workshop program.

Get started quickly: write down three words:

(a) To describe a good eating apple.

(b) To describe a good GP.

Do not confer.

Workshop Diagram 2. Warm-up exercise.

Good eating apple	
Group 1	**Group 2**
Tasty	Tasty
Crisp	Crisp
Crunchy	Crunchy
Fresh	Fresh
Tangy	Tangy
Juicy	Juicy
Ripe	Ripe
Clean	Clean
Red	Succulent
Sweet	Reliable
British	
Flawless	
Shiny	

Workshop Diagram 3. Responses to "good eating apple"

Good GP	
Group 1	**Group 2**
Empathetic	Empathetic
Competent	Competent
Knowledgeable	Knowledgeable
Capable problem-solver	Capable problem-solver
Responsible	Trustworthy
Friendly	Affable
Approachable	Caring
Kind	Organized
Considerate	Wise
Attentive	Reliable
Listening	
Committed	
Keen	
Interested	
Curious	
Courageous	

Workshop Diagram 4. Responses to a "good GP."

reasonable level of agreement, there were fewer terms shared between the two groups. Many of the terms used moreover conveyed more complex concepts ("empathetic," for example, as the most frequently used term for good GPs as against "tasty" for good eating apples). Some of the terms led to discussion about what they really meant. Thus, "courageous" was interpreted differently by different members of the group. Several of the doctors noted that they had to have the courage to take decisions under conditions of uncertainty. But one of the Patients' Forum representatives said, "I wouldn't want my GP to be a risk taker!" For many of the values they had assigned a good GP, there were competing interpretations from different perspectives.

So all-in-all, the group came to see that, while the values involved in a concept like "good apple" are relatively simple, the values involved in the concept of a "good GP" are in various ways complex.

Reviewing these "good GP" terms with the group, Dr. Real told them about some work he undertook years back on effective GP education. Of course, the outcome he was interested in was improving the quality of the GP (in order to improve the quality of the patient experience). Like many more experienced researchers before him, he encountered the difficulty of defining for his outcome measure what it is that makes a GP "good." The answer appeared then (and perhaps now) to elude satisfactory succinct research definition. To the

question, "What is a *good* GP?" doctors and their patients tend to respond along the lines of, "I don't know, but I can recognize one if I see one."

By the end of the discussion in this part of the workshop, participants had thus had their "wake-up call" to values. They had understood that values are wider than ethics (notice that "ethical" did not appear on either list of "good GP" terms); and they had seen for themselves that values, even in an apparently well-understood context such as the idea of a "good GP," are complex.

2. The GMC's "good doctor"

"Let's take this idea of a 'good GP' a bit further," Dr. Real now said. "Who else might have ideas about what makes a good GP?" They quickly came up with the GMC, the regulatory authority for doctors in the UK. This led naturally into a second exercise comparing their ideas about a good GP with the GMC's ideas.

For this exercise, Dr. Real gave out copies of the GMC's summary list of the "Duties of a Doctor" shown in Workshop Diagram 5. He again divided the workshop into their two original subgroups, asking them this time to compare and contrast the GMC list with their own lists.

1. Make the care of your patient your first concern

2. Protect and promote the health of patients and the public

3. Provide a good standard of practice and care

- Keep your professional knowledge and skills up to date
- Recognize and work within the limits of your competence
- Work with colleagues in the ways that best serve patients' interests

4. Treat patients as individuals and respect their dignity

- Treat patients politely and considerately
- Respect patients' right to confidentiality

5. Work in partnership with patients

- Listen to patients and respond to their concerns and preferences
- Give patients the information they want or need in a way they can understand
- Respect patients' right to reach decisions with you about their treatment and care
- Support patients in caring for themselves to improve and maintain their health

6. Be honest and open and act with integrity

- Act without delay if you have good reason to believe that you or a colleague may be putting patients at risk
- Never discriminate unfairly against patients or colleagues
- Never abuse your patients' trust in you or the public's trust in the profession.

Workshop Diagram 5. The GMC's definition of a "good GP.".

Good GP	
Group 1 ($n = 17$)	**Group 2 ($n = 13$)**
Empathetic (5)	Empathetic (5)
Competent (3)	Competent (3)
Knowledgeable (3)	Knowledgeable (3)
Capable problem-solver (3)	Capable problem-solver (3)
Responsible (3)	Trustworthy (6)
Friendly (4)	Affable (4)
Approachable (4)	
Kind (4)	Caring (1)
Considerate (5)	Organized (3)
Attentive (5)	Wise
Listening (5)	Reliable
Committed (1)	
Keen	
Interested (5)	
Curious	
Courageous	

Workshop Diagram 6. The workshop's "good GP" suggestions that were not in the GMC's Duties of a Doctor (shown by underlining; numbers in brackets refer to the numbers on the GMC list).

"Caring" and "committed" they said were close to the GMC's "Make the care of your patient your first concern." And then once they had got the idea, they had soon cross-mapped the majority of the items on the two lists.

There were a number of items left on both lists, however, that had not cross-mapped. Dr. Real underlined these, as shown in Workshop Diagrams 6 and 7.

Again, the first response to this was that they now had an even longer list. Yes, the GMC's list covered many of their terms for a good GP, but it extended the requirements for a good doctor to include concerns for colleagues and for the wider public; and the GMC list had missed a clutch of virtues that they as a group had included (their good GP should be "keen, curious, courageous, wise and reliable"). "So we'll all have to be super-docs!" joked one of the senior medical partners.

Picking up on this comment, Dr. Real asked the group, "What do you think about that? Is this a feasible list? Can a doctor show all these qualities? Can a doctor ever be 'good' in the way we've now defined 'good'?"

A longer discussion followed this second exercise. Initially, the groups were surprised at how different their lists were from the GMC's. This was a surprise particularly because a majority of the participants were doctors and hence subject to the GMC's jurisdiction on good practice. Yet the workshop seemed to have come up with rather different ideas from the GMC about what made a good doctor.

So the first outcome of this exercise was to reinforce the message about the complexity of values. But Dr. Real now asked the group to look more closely at the two lists to see if there were any overlaps. They quickly picked out "competent" and "knowledgeable" from their lists as coinciding with the GMC's "Keep your professional knowledge and skills up to date" under their broad category of "Provide a good standard of practice and care."

"Anything else?" Dr. Real pressed them.

Again, there were different views, but the point of Dr. Real's question was soon recognized. The point was

1. Make the care of your patient your first concern

2. Protect and promote the health of patients and the public

3. Provide a good standard of practice and care

- Keep your professional knowledge and skills up to date
- Recognize and work within the limits of your competence
- Work with colleagues in the ways that best serve patients' interests

4. Treat patients as individuals and respect their dignity

- Treat patients politely and considerately
- Respect patients' right to confidentiality

5. Work in partnership with patients

- Listen to patients and respond to their concerns and preferences
- Give patients the information they want or need in a way they can understand
- Respect patients' right to reach decisions with you about their treatment and care
- Support patients in caring for themselves to improve and maintain their health

6. Be honest and open and act with integrity

- Act without delay if you have good reason to believe that you or a colleague may be putting patients at risk
- Never discriminate unfairly against patients or colleagues
- Never abuse your patients' trust in you or the public's trust in the profession.

Workshop Diagram 7. The GMC's Duties of a Doctor not on the workshop's "good GP" list (shown by underlining).

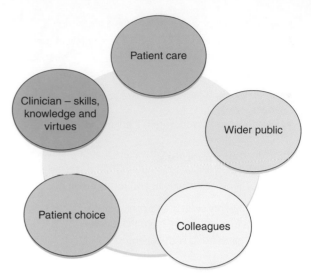

Workshop Diagram 8. The workshop's shared framework of values.

that no one could do all of the things on the list all of the time. This wasn't a matter of being or not being a "super doc." The point was simply that some values on the list were potentially in conflict with other values. The group readily came up with examples from their own experience. One common example involved conflicts between concern for the public and confidentiality. Added to the complexity of values they had taken from the first part of the workshop was now the further challenge that values could also be conflicting.

Here they broke for coffee, which they brought back to drink while Dr. Real gave them a brief introduction to values-based practice.

3. Introduction to values-based practice

This part of the workshop followed essentially the outline of values-based practice given in Chapter 3.

Building on their earlier discussion, the group readily grasped (i) that values-based practice offers a process for dealing with complex and conflicting values, and (ii) that, as such, it is a partner to evidence-based practice. They were surprised by but welcomed Sackett's definition of evidence-based practice as including expertise and values (although they were quick to point out that clinicians' values should be in there as well as patients' values).

Dr. Real then briefly ran through the elements of the process of values-based practice again, building on their earlier exercises in raising awareness of values as a case in point. This prompted a useful discussion about the links between values-based practice and communication skills. They liked the links with person-centered practice and team work. And "dissensus," although initially a less familiar idea, made sense.

"But how does all that work in practice?" the "super doc" partner now asked. Here, Dr. Real gave them the example of the framework of values developed to support balanced values-based decision-making in the use of the Mental Health Act 2007 (see Fig. 3.4).

"We could use a similar approach here," he continued. Then, drawing a number of circles on the flip chart, he asked them to think how the GMC's list could be organized in a similar way. Using a guided discussion approach, they ended up with a picture similar to that shown in Workshop Diagram 8.

Essentially, what they had done was a further mapping exercise in which they had organized all the

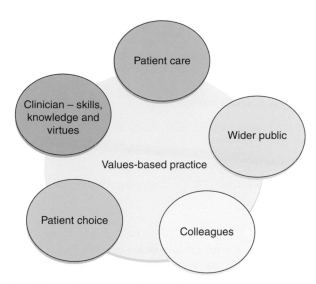

Workshop Diagram 9. Values-based practice and the workshop's shared framework of values.

Group 1: You represent the patient who has:

- Been off work for 4 months already
- Long-standing depression-related and anxiety-related sick notes
- Social issues ++

Group 2: You represent the GP who works with the patient as an ally. Your relationship with the patient is of fundamental importance.

Group 3: You represent the GP who believes in being tough about sick notes.

Workshop Diagram 10. Role play instructions.

diverse elements of their two lists into five main categories covering patient care (the GMC's points 1 and 4), public responsibilities (included in the GMC's points 2 and 6), responsibilities to colleagues (included in the GMC's points 3 and 6), working in partnership with patients (the GMC's point 4) and their competence as clinicians (covered by the GMC's point 3, but also extending to the virtues that they had identified but were absent from the GMC's list).

"So what we have here," Dr. Real explained, "is a framework of values that we as a group all share. And . . ." (adding "Values-based practice" in big letters in the middle of the framework, as in Workshop Diagram 9) ". . . this is where values-based practice comes in to support balanced decision-making within this shared framework of values."

But the "super doc" was not convinced. "So how does it work in practice?" he asked.

"OK, let's try it" replied Dr. Real, thus linking in to the role play.

4. Role play: conflicting values and work certification

Dr. Real then introduced the role play using the scenario he had agreed with Dr. Gulati of conflicting values around the issue of work certification for doctors and patients (although choosing a different condition from Dr. Gulati's case of low back pain). This time he divided the workshop participants into three

groups representing different roles and perspectives, giving each of them the sketchiest of briefs as shown in Workshop Diagram 10.

Each group then had five minutes to imagine their character together and to list the values that influence their character's attitudes to sick notes. The groups then nominated a role player and two role plays were performed in front of the whole group: the first with the patient consulting with the "doctor as ally," and the second with the "doctor as ally" being challenged by the "hard-line doctor" when they met later over a coffee. The rest of the group was tasked with identifying implicit and explicit values at play.

After the role play, Dr. Real asked the group to work in pairs to draw together the values they had identified. He then took feedback, listing them on a flip chart. There was a further brisk discussion during this process with a good deal more disagreement than had emerged at earlier stages in the workshop. We do not have space here to go into the details of this discussion, but we give the list of perspectives that Dr. Real wrote up on the flip chart in Workshop Diagram 11.

"So, who is right?" Dr. Real now challenged the group. Then, before the discussion (it had by now become more of an argument) could re-start, he added, "Let's look at this by going back to our framework of values for a good doctor." And he gave them a final brief task of working in pairs to see how many of their framework values they could identify in the values that had come out of the role play. When he took feedback, he marked up the flip chart of role-play values as shown in Workshop Diagram 12. The message was clear. Judged by their own framework of shared values (which included everything in the GMC list), they were *all* right. They were all expressing

- We have a societal responsibility to maintain the workforce and avoid "skivers" (this particularly from one of the Patients' Forum representatives).
- Off-work certification can only work if it is universally applied fairly.
- It is not a nice part of our job, but if we do it in the right way, helping people instead of just refusing, then in the long-term our patients will benefit (this from Dr. Gulati citing evidence of the benefits of rehabilitation).
- We have a responsibility to support our partners by *all* taking a party line on only issuing sick notes when patients are genuinely incapable of work.
- It is unacceptable for my partners to let me down and leave me exposed as the "tough one" (this from the partner who had role-played the hard-line doctor).
- Refusing sick notes damages our therapeutic relationships and just means patients go "next door" – it is the job of the "benefits doctor" to police the system (this from Dr. Austin).

Workshop Diagram 11. Values drawn out from the role play.

- We have a societal responsibility [Public] to maintain workforce and avoid "skivers" (this particularly from one of the Patients' Forum representatives).
- Off-work certification can only work if it is universally applied fairly [Public and Colleagues].
- It is not a nice part of our job, but if we do it in the right way, helping people instead of just refusing [Partnership], then in the long-term our patients will benefit (this from Dr. Gulati citing evidence of the benefits of rehabilitation [Competences]).
- We have a responsibility to support our partners [Colleagues] by *all* taking a party line on only issuing sick notes when patients are genuinely incapable of work.
- It is unacceptable for my partners [Colleagues] to let me down and leave me exposed as the "tough one" (this from the partner who had role-played the hard-line doctor).
- Refusing sick notes damages our therapeutic relationships [Care] and just means patients go "next door" – it is the job of the "benefits doctor" to police the system (this from Dr. Austin).

Workshop Diagram 12. Values from the role play as shared framework values (shown in blue).

values that are part of what it is to be a good doctor – and the challenge in the values-based practice model of decision-making was to find the right balance between them in individual cases.

5. A framework of shared values for this practice

Summing up, Dr. Real ran over what they had covered writing up brief conclusions on the flip chart as the key points that had come out of each part of the work shop as shown in Workshop Diagram 13.

1. Warm up ("good GP") – values are complex and wider than ethics.
2. Similar to "GMC duties" – but values may also be conflicting.
3. Values-based practice – a process for working with complex and conflicting values (a partner to evidence-based practice) within share frameworks of values.
   And (pointing to the relevant flip chart) we produced our own framework . . .
4. Role play (work certification) – produced complex and conflicting values . . .
   . . . that (now showing them the final flip chart) we mapped onto our own framework of shared values.

Workshop Diagram 13. Conclusion: key points from the workshop.

"So this is where values-based practice comes in to support balanced judgments on individual cases within a shared framework of values. Just how you do this," he finished, turning to the "super doc," "takes us into the whole area of skills development – but that's for another time!"

6. Conclusions to the workshop

But now it was "super doc" who was enthusiastic for more information. In reply to his question, Dr. Real told the group about the wide range of training materials supporting the process of values-based practice that are now available. These included the Royal College of General Practitioners (RCGP) curriculum statement covering values-based practice (Royal College of General Practitioners, 2005) to which Dr. Gulati had referred earlier (see Chapter 2). Drafted primarily by Anne-Marie Slowther at Warwick Medical School, the RCGP statement drew among other resources on a training manual for values-based practice, called *Whose Values?*, which had been developed by Kim Woodbridge and others to support the policy and training developments outlined in Chapter 3 (Woodbridge and Fulford, 2004). The manual and other training resources are included in downloadable forms on the website supporting this series.

Finally, Dr. Real noted a number of related developments internationally. The World Psychiatric Association, in particular, through an Institutional Program on Psychiatry for the Person (Mezzich and Salloum, 2007), has been particularly active in this area with a number of key initiatives, including important innovations in person-centered diagnosis (Mezzich, 2007); and there have been training initiatives in values-based practice in several European countries and in South Africa (Van Staden and Fulford, 2007).

Outcomes from the workshop

As we noted at the start of this chapter, Dr. Gulati, her colleagues and their patients (represented in the PLT workshop by the two members of the Patients' Forum) had to make an investment of time and, as it turned out, self-reflection to develop their shared framework for values-based decision-making. But once made, the investment paid off in many ways. On the specific issue of off-work certification, the practice as a whole had gained a greater understanding of each other's values and the differences of approach between them, although these had become less marked and more balanced between them. This also meant that they found it natural to discuss problem cases and to agree a joined-up approach.

A further outcome from the workshop was that Dr. Gulati and her colleagues now recognized the many areas of their practice that involved complex and conflicting values as well as complex and conflicting evidence. One such area was the recently introduced GP commissioning. They were able to use their shared framework of values in their now established partnership with the Patients' Forum in making shared decisions about local priorities on expenditure. In connection with this, and as a second wider outcome from the workshop, they recognized the need to find out what really were the priorities of the patients and families they served.

These outcomes, together with the work Dr. Gulati and her colleagues did in the workshop itself, thus added a number of additional elements of values-based practice to those that Dr. Gulati had used already in her short-term management of Roy Walker (see Fig. 14.2). We summarize these in Fig. 14.3. Again, the essential point is the added effectiveness of the different elements of values-based practice when they are used together in a fully joined-up way.

Returning to Roy Walker

But what happened to Roy Walker? In our stories in the rest of the book, we have not looked at outcomes, but in this case we have left Dr. Gulati's "master stroke" hanging. As you might expect, Roy Walker found it very hard initially to go along to the PDSA but, supported by the consistent approach from the

Elements of values-based practice	Demonstrated by the practice team
Premise: mutual respect	✓
Skills – awareness	✓
Skills – knowledge	✓
Skills – reasoning	✓
Skills – communication	✓
Person-values-centered	✓
Team values	✓✓
EBP/VBP – Two-feet Principle	✓
EBP/VBP – Squeaky-wheel Principle	✓
EBP/VBP – Science-driven Principle	✓
Dissensus + consensus	✓
Point: balanced decisions	✓
Framework of values	✓✓

Fig. 14.3. Summary of values-based practice demonstrated by Dr. Gulati and her colleagues.

practice as a whole (the physiotherapist gave him much encouragement as well as teaching him his back exercises), he eventually managed it and was pleasantly surprised by the way his offer of help was received. His talent with animals was quickly noted and he soon found that he was a much-valued member of the PDSA team.

With his growing self-esteem and interest in life, he drank less and, being also more active, he lost weight. To this now virtuous cycle was added a positive result from his back exercises. He returned to his old job for a period, but when a paid post came up at the PDSA he took that instead.

Chapter summary

In this chapter, we have followed the story of Dr. Gulati and Roy Walker from where we left them in Part 1 with the aim of showing how the elements of values-based practice set out separately in this book come together in practice. Drawing in part on Dr. Gulati's already well-developed skills for working with values and partly on a PLT workshop on values-based practice, Roy Walker was helped to build on his own hitherto-unrecognized strengths to regain his confidence and sense of self-worth and thereby to avoid becoming a long-term disability statistic.

Not all stories starting with "It's my back, Doctor!" work out so well. Dr. Gulati, you may feel, had an element of good luck. But then luck, as they say, is when opportunity meets preparation.

References

Mezzich, J. E. (2007) Psychiatry for the person: articulating medicine's science and humanism. *World Psychiatry* **6**, 65–67.

Mezzich, J. E. and Salloum, I. M. (2007). Towards innovative international classification and diagnostic systems: ICD-11 and person-centered integrative diagnosis. *Acta Psychiatrica Scandinavica* **116**, 1–5.

Van Staden C. W. and Fulford K. W. M. (2007). Hypotheses, neuroscience and real persons: the theme of the 10th International Conference on Philosophy, Psychiatry and Psychology. *South African Journal of Psychiatry* **13**, 68–71.

Underwood, E. (1998). Crisis: what crisis? *European Spine Journal* 7, 2–5.

Woodbridge, K., and Fulford, K. W. M. (2004). *Whose Values? A Workbook for Values-based Practice in Mental Health Care*. London: The Sainsbury Centre for Mental Health.

Websites

- The *Duties of a Doctor* are given in the General Medical Council's Good Medical Practice at www.gmc-uk.org.
- The Royal College of General Practitioners (2005) Curriculum Statement: Ethics and Values Based Medicine is available at: http://www.rcgp.org.uk/gpcurriculum/pdfs/ethicsAndVBPsf RCGPCouncilDec2005.pdf.

Postscript: the small change of care

The stories in this book have illustrated some of the ways in which the skills and other process elements of values-based practice support balanced decision-making in medicine and health care where complex and conflicting values are in play.

As a response to complexity, values-based practice, as we have emphasized throughout, is a partner to evidence-based practice. Decisions – *all* decisions, whether clinical or otherwise – stand, as we put it in Chapter 1, on *two* feet, a values foot and an evidence foot. The process of evidence-based practice has been developed as a response to the growing complexity of the *evidence* base of clinical decision-making. The process of values-based practice has been developed as a response to the growing complexity of the *values* base of clinical decision-making.

Linking science with people

The complementary relationship between evidence-based practice and values-based practice can be understood in part in terms of the relationship between the sciences and the humanities.

There are overlaps, of course. The founders of evidence-based practice, as we saw from David Sackett's work in Part 1, although focusing on the technical processes required for establishing generalizable conclusions about best scientific evidence, set this in context with the need to link best evidence with clinical experience and patients' values. Values-based practice similarly, although derived primarily from work in analytic and other areas of philosophy, includes knowledge of values (including as we described in Chapter 6, *research*-based knowledge) as one of its four key skills areas; and the process elements of values-based practice include three specific principles (covered in Part 4) directly linking evidence and values.

All the same, there is a broad sense in which, at least in their impact on practice, evidence-based practice and values-based practice can be understood, respectively, as more scientific and more humanistic.

This is why there are no technical complexities in this book (beyond those reflecting scientific clinical issues): there are no "values scanners," as it were, still less a values equivalent of "the number needed to treat." There are, instead, stories from life: examples of best practice in values-based decision-making illustrated by the stories of individual people – clinicians, patients, families and others – working through the complexities presented by the contingencies of the particular practical situations in which they find themselves.

Essential *evidence*-based practice, then, to paraphrase the title of this book, is scientific and general. Essential *values*-based practice is human and individual. This is as it should be. It is in reflecting, respectively, the scientific and human aspects of medicine that evidence-based practice and values-based practice offer complementary approaches to supporting clinical decision-making that, as the subtitle to this book puts it, links science with people.

No villains here

There is, though, one respect in which it may seem that the stories from life in this book have not been entirely stories from *real* life. As one of those who kindly read the manuscript for us put it, "There are no villains here! Even your potential villains, like Roy Walker in the opening chapter, turn out to be decent chaps after all."

This reader went on to add that there are no superheroes either "... so, yes, everything described taken individually could happen. The positives *are* realistic. But where are the negatives? The doctor who is just too lazy to examine a road crash patient's fundi and misses a subdural hemorrhage; the night nurse who writes up her patient's observations in advance to avoid having to go round later; or the manager who takes out his or her frustrations by bullying junior colleagues?" Less dramatic perhaps, we might add, but no less pernicious for that, where are the petty jealousies and putdowns, the hidden agendas, the tribalism, the waste

201

and inefficiencies that are so much a part of the experience of many, no less in healthcare than in any other (always fallible) human endeavor?

"Are not the negatives as much as the positives all part of everyday reality?" our reader concluded. "Where is values-based practice when the fat hits the fan?"

Only one tool in the toolbox

We accept this point. Indeed, we own it. Values-based practice, as we said in the Prologue, is about building on *best* practice. So it is right that the stories in a book setting out the essentials of values-based practice should largely reflect as it were the best of times.

There are, certainly, the worst of times to deal with as well. We've all been there. We've all seen it. We've all, surely, done it. Values-based practice recognizes this. But we have regulatory ethics and law to deal with bad practice. Values-based practice, furthermore, although concerned primarily with building on best practice, includes, as we described in Chapter 3, two distinct mechanisms for excluding practice that is simply *bad*:

- *Definition*: racism and other forms of discrimination are by definition outside the values-based premise of mutual respect: recall here from Chapter 3 the NIMHE Values Framework for policy and service development in mental health (Fig. 3.4).
- *Shared frameworks of values*: other values are excluded from values-based practice because they fall outside the framework of values shared by a given group at a given time (which, as our various examples have indicated, varies from context to context).

Either by definition or through shared frameworks of values then, values-based practice places definite constraints on practice. And when it comes to actually *dealing* with the "villains," we have the other tools of regulation and law to hand. Recent years have indeed seen a proliferation of increasingly powerful regulatory tools – ethical, professional and legal – for dealing with bad practice. Values-based practice, to repeat, is by contrast a tool primarily for building on good practice.

Time to emphasize the positives

We believe there are a number of reasons why it is time to start building on best practice. One reason for this is the danger of regulation turning into *over*-regulation.

"Just one more law and we'll get it right!" a parliamentary legal draftsman of many years' experience commented wryly to one of us recently. He was in a better position than many to have seen at first hand the impossibility of preventing bad practice by regulation alone, however comprehensively drafted.

A second reason for emphasizing the positives is a growing recognition that, however effective regulation may or may not have been in preventing bad practice, it has certainly done little actively to promote good practice. The recent report from the NHS employer's organization, the NHS Confederation, cited in Chapter 3 (NHS Confederation, 2010), drew together the growing evidence for the effectiveness of a positive culture of care, not only in improving the experience of patients and of staff but also in improving clinical outcomes and the cost-effective use of resources. Yet our record in this regard in the NHS is, as the report shows, at best patchy. Indeed, despite the policy priority afforded in recent years to the personalization of services, a recent Commonwealth Fund report cited by the NHS Confederation ranked the UK seventh (out of seven) for person-centered health care.

Many of the key elements of a positive culture of care highlighted in the NHS Confederation report correspond directly with the process elements of values-based practice: a starting point in mutual respect, an awareness of other peoples' values (their wishes, needs, preference and so forth), the importance of really finding out what matters to people rather than just assuming that we know already, a focus on person-centered care, a key role for the extended multidisciplinary team, the importance of combining care with evidence-based provision of services, and the fundamental role of partnership between service users and service providers in every aspect of service provision.

The cost of care

A third reason for believing that it is timely to start emphasizing the positives is the current round of fiscal restraints and budget cuts. This is because values-based practice is about "working smarter, not harder." Getting the values-base as well as the evidence-base of our decision-making right makes our resources (of time, as well as money) go further.

Some up-front investment is needed. But one advantage of the human rather than technical nature of the process of values-based practice is that the investment required to achieve a return in practical efficiency is really quite small. For a "whole-system" impact, as the NHS Confederation report notes, a whole-systems approach is needed: values-based commissioning, in particular, as the subject of a later book in the series, will be important here. High-level and sometimes costly strategies for training and service development have their place.

What the NHS Confederation report also shows, however, and what the stories in this book all illustrate, is that when it comes to the clinical encounter, it is in what might be called the small change of care that values-based practice is most decisively realized.

The cleaner who cared

Our final story (which is based on a real incident and reproduced with permission) illustrates the importance of the small change of care not in a clinical context but in a brief encounter in a hospital corridor between the wife of an elderly dying man and a cleaner.

Mrs. Janice Jones was lost. The hospital in which her 73-year-old husband was dying from cancer of the colon was clean and well organized. The wards were all clearly signposted. But in her preoccupied state, Janice Jones, who was a recently retired head teacher, had found herself wandering down a long corridor clearly in the wrong part of the hospital. The only person she could see to ask for directions was a cleaner who was busy mopping the (already spotless) floor. "You're well out of your way, love," replied the cleaner. "I'll show you ..." And parking her pail and mop, she led Janice Jones right across the hospital leaving her only when she was in sight of the ward she was looking for.

In a more heavily regulated environment, that cleaner would no doubt have been in trouble. But all the essentials of values-based practice were caught in that simple act of care: the key role of skills in the cleaner's perceptive awareness and understanding of Janice Jones' values (her need for support as well as for information); the communication of care (in the cleaner's time freely given); her person-centered priorities (putting people before time-keeping, as it were); and her role as a key provider of care in what we called in Chapter 9 the extended multidisciplinary team.

There was a cost attached to the cleaner ceasing to clean for a few minutes and guiding Janice Jones across the hospital. But it was a small price to pay for laying the foundations for a positive engagement between Janice Jones and the team caring for her husband in his last days.

A bold claim to end this book

We began with our assertion that *the most likely reason why things go wrong in clinician–patient interactions is a failure of values-based practice*, not a failure of evidence-based practice. In light of what you have gleaned about the processes of values-based practice from our clinical illustrations, you may like to test our claim over the coming year.

We end with another assertion. *If you rehearse and practice the elements of values-based practice detailed in this book, you are likely to find your consultations more personally rewarding and your patients are likely to derive more benefit.*

Don't forget you already possess many, if not most, of the skills, and if some (such as dissensus and casuistry) are new to you, you will find them relatively easy to adopt.

Appendix A: VBP summary and definitions of key terms

In this appendix, we summarize the essential features of values-based practice and give brief definitions of some of the key terms used in this book.

NOTE: Terms in bold correspond to terms highlighted in blue in the index, which in turn is supported by an index spreadsheet (on the VBP web site) showing what is covered by each of the highlighted index references.

Values-based practice

Values-based practice is a new approach to working with complex and conflicting values in healthcare that is:

- Complementary to other approaches to working with values such as ethics (medicine's values tool box) in focusing on individual values
- A partner to evidence-based practice in supporting clinical judgment in individual cases.

Values-based practice thus links science with the unique values of the particular people involved (clinicians, patients, carers and others) in a given clinical decision.

Values-based practice builds on a premise of mutual respect to support balanced decision-making through a ten-part process covering clinical skills, professional relationships, links with evidence-based practice and partnership.

Values

Values are anything positively or negatively weighted as a guide to action (for example, needs, wishes and preferences).

Values-based practice is a process that supports healthcare decision-making where complex and conflicting values are in play.

- **Complex values** are values that mean different things to different people (for example, 'best interests')

- **Conflicting values** are values that are in conflict one with another (for example, there are often tensions in healthcare decision-making between 'best interests' and 'freedom of patient choice').

Medicine's values tool box

Values-based practice is complementary to other tools in medicine's values tool box:

- The **values tool box** is the range of disciplines concerned in one way or another with values in health care (examples include **codes of practice**, **medical ethics**, **medical law**, **decision analysis**, **health economics**, **narrative-based medicine** and others, including the psychological and social sciences, medical humanities, history, literature, philosophy, visual arts, and so on).

Values-based practice complements other tools for working with values in focusing particularly on the *unique values of the particular individuals* concerned (*clinicians*, *patients* and *carers*) in a given clinical situation.

Clinical judgement

Values-based practice is a partner to evidence-based practice in supporting the exercise of clinical judgement in individual cases:

- **Clinical judgment** is exercised whenever a clinician uses his or her **clinical expertise** in progressively squaring down on the evidence and values relevant to diagnostic and treatment decisions appropriate to a particular patient in a particular situation
- **Squaring down** is the *process* by which, in exercising clinical judgment, a skilled clinician focuses progressively on the more relevant information (about evidence and values) while

discarding the less relevant information arising from history, examination and investigations.

In exercising clinical judgement, **evidence-based practice** is vital in bringing the clinician's focus onto the most likely diagnostic and treatment possibilities; values-based practice is vital in matching those possibilities with the particular circumstances presented by *this particular patient in this particular situation.*

It is thus through squaring down in the exercise of clinical judgement that values-based practice links science with the unique values of individual people.

The point of values-based practice

The **point of values-based practice** is to support balanced decision-making within frameworks of shared values appropriate to the decision in question:

- **Balanced decision-making** means decision-making that is based on a balance between the (often complex and conflicting) values of those concerned in a given clinical situation
- **Frameworks of shared values** are frameworks of (often complex and conflicting) values that, although shared by those concerned in a given clinical situation, are in tension one with another and hence have to be balanced according to the particular circumstances presented by that situation.

The premise of values-based practice

The **premise of values-based practice** is the 'democratic' premise of mutual respect for differences of values.

Mutual respect for differences of values avoids moral relativism ('anything goes') by marking out excluded values and by shifting the emphasis in decision-making from pre-set 'right outcomes' to good process:

- **Excluded values** are values (like racism) that are incompatible with the premise of mutual respect and hence (however widely shared) are by definition excluded from values-based decision-making
- **Good process** in values-based practice is decision-making that is guided by one or more of ten key process elements of values-based practice (see below).

The 10-part process of values-based practice

The **process of values-based practice** includes ten key elements covering four key clinical skills, two aspects of professional relationships, three close links with evidence-based practice and a dissensual basis for partnership in decision-making.

Clinical skills

The four key **clinical skills** for values-based practice are: awareness, reasoning, knowledge and communication skills.

1. **Awareness of values** includes awareness of the **diversity of individual values**, awareness of clinicians' **own values** as well as the values of others, and awareness of **positive values** (StAR values, i.e. strengths, aspirations and resources) as well as negative values (such as needs and difficulties).

2. **Reasoning about values** in values-based practice is aimed at **expanding our values horizons** rather than (directly) deciding what is right. Reasoning thus directed may include any of the established methods of ethical reasoning (such as **principles reasoning**, **case-based reasoning** (or **casuistry**), **utilitarianism**, **deontology** and **virtue ethics**).

3. **Knowledge of values** as derived from research and clinical experience has the important **limitation** that it can never 'trump' the actual values of a particular individual. Nonetheless, as in any other area of medical knowledge, knowledge of values includes both **tacit** (or **craft**) **knowledge** and **explicit knowledge**; and it includes the skills for **knowledge retrieval** from electronic databases (including the use of values-specific sources (such as **Healthtalkonline** and the **VaST** search manual).

4. **Communication skills** include skills for **eliciting values** (including **strengths**, as in **ICE-StAR**) and skills of **conflict resolution**.

Professional relationships

The two aspects of **professional relationships** important for values-based practice are person-values-centered practice and extended multidisciplinary team work.

5. **Person-values-centered practice** is practice that focuses on the values of the patient while at the same time being aware of and reflecting the values of other people involved (clinicians, managers, family, carers, etc.): this is important in tackling two particular problems of person-centered care,

problems of mutual understanding and **problems of conflicting values**.

6. **Extended multidisciplinary team work** is practice that draws effectively not only on the diversity of skills represented by different team members but also on the **diversity of team values**: this is important both in identifying the values in play in a given situation and in coming to balanced decisions about what to do.

Science and values-based practice

Values-based practice has three key **links with science** defined by three principles: the Two-feet Principle, the Squeaky-wheel Principle and the Science-driven Principle.

7. The **Two-feet Principle** is that *all* decisions, whether overtly value-laden or not, are based on the two feet of values and evidence: clinically, this translates into the reminder "*Think facts, think values!*"

8. The **Squeaky-wheel Principle** is that we tend to notice values only when (like the squeaky wheel) they cause trouble: clinically, this translates into the reminder "*Think values, think facts!*"

9. The **Science-driven Principle** is that advances in medical science and technology in opening up new choices (hence diversity of values) drive the need equally for values-based practice and for evidence-based practice: clinically, this translates

into the reminder that, above all, in high-tech medicine it is vital to "*Think both facts and values!*"

Partnership

As the tenth element of the process of values-based practice, **partnership in decision-making** depends on both consensus and dissensus:

- **Consensus** involves differences of values being resolved (as in the development of shared frameworks of values)
- **Dissensus** involves differences of values remaining in play to be balanced sometimes one way and sometimes in other ways according to the particular circumstances presented by different situations.

Learning and teaching

As a primarily skills-based process, doing values-based practice for real depends critically on the availability of training resources.

In this connection, Appendix B gives a VBP Teaching Framework that includes learning outcomes and suggested methods of assessment for each of the key elements of values-based practice; and this VBP Summary can be used in conjunction with the terms highlighted in blue in the index and with the index spreadsheet on the VBP website to track aspects of values-based practice as they are mapped across different chapters of the book. (See also Prologue, Ways of using this book, pp. xvi–xvii.)

Appendix B: Values-based practice teaching framework

An essential understanding of values-based practice comprises:

1. The point of values-based practice. Values-based practice, rather than giving us answers as such, aims to support **balanced decision-making within frameworks of shared values** appropriate to the situation in question.
2. The premise of values-based practice. The basis for balanced decision-making in values-based practice is the 'democratic' premise of **mutual respect for differences of values**.

3. The process of values-based practice. Again, like a political democracy, the values democracy of values-based practice supports **decision-making through good process rather than prescribing pre-set right outcomes**. There are **ten key elements of the process** of values-based practice covering clinical skills, professional relationships and the inter-relationship of science (evidence-based practice) and values-based practice, as well as dissensus in partnership decision-making.

Element	Title and Content Descriptor	Knowledge, Skills and Attitudes/ behaviours	Possible Assessment Methods
1	**Awareness of values:** self-aware of one's own values **and** aware of others' values. **Central premise = respect for differences of values**	**K** What are values? **A** Self awareness **KS** Eliciting Ideas, Concerns and Expectations (ICE) **KS** Eliciting Strengths, Aspirations and Resources (StAR) **K** Legal and human rights frameworks **A** Respect for difference	EMQ Significant event analysis; reflective portfolio; talk-aloud protocol (can be OSCE station) OSCE OSCE Written questions 'White space' examples OCE Station 'Healthtalkonline' examples'
2	**Reasoning about values:** **T**he importance of clinical ethics and professional codes Why different processes are needed in complex situations and if values conflict	**K** Professional codes (e.g. Good Medical Practice) **K** 'Four principles' and other ethics precepts **K S** Principles reasoning **K S** Case-based reasoning (casuistry) **K S** Decision analysis **A** Clinical judgment	MCQ MCQ and short-answer questions OSCE station OSCE station OSCE station, two different methods of DA Mini-CEX

Element	Title and Content Descriptor	Knowledge, Skills and Attitudes/behaviours	Possible Assessment Methods
3	**Knowledge about values:** where and how to search for evidence about values	**S** Critical analysis **K** Why is values evidence more difficult to access than biomedical scientific evidence? **K S** Conventional searching techniques (Google Scholar and Medline) **K S** VaST searching	OSCE station or short-answer question Short-answer question On-line computer OSCE station On-line computer OSCE station
4	**Communication skills:** extending the basic clinical communication skills to skills for eliciting values	**S** Asking the appropriate values questions – progressing from ICE to ICE-StAR **S A** Identifying value agendas **S** Conflict resolution **K** Adaptive work, non-confrontational communication and clinical leadership	OSCE OSCE OSCE (video scenario) Mini-CEX Reflective portfolio
5	**Person-values-centred practice**	**K** Many varieties of person-centred medicine **S** Overcoming problems of mutual understanding **S** Overcoming problems of conflicting values **S** Case-based reasoning and person-centred medicine **SA** Applying clinical guidelines in a person-centered way	Short-answer question Scenario-based OSCE Scenario-based OSCE Written or OSCE DOPS, Mini-CEX or OSCE station based on a NICE guideline (UK)
6	**Extended multidisciplinary teamwork**	**K** Shared sets of values K Differences of values (importance for balanced decision-making) **K** Protocols and toolkits : the advantages and disadvantages for teams **S** Balanced decision-making and risk-sharing	Safeguarding scenario OSCE Written question Written question OSCE 360-degree feedback
7	**The Two-feet Principle**: clinical decisions based on evidence and values	**K** Understanding that failure to elicit values is more often responsible for consultation failure than ignorance about science and treatment options **S** Applying best available evidence to the individual (based on knowledge of their values)	OSCE: locating relevant sectors on Dowie's diagram Mini-CEX and DoPS OSCE
8	**The Squeaky-wheel Principle:** where to focus attention on values	**S** Maintain a focus on the appropriate clinical evidence when immersed in value-laden situations **A S** Applied cultural awareness	Mini-Cex DoPS, OSCE and reflective portfolio Mini-Cex DoPS, OSCE and reflective portfolio
9	**The Science-driven Principle**	**K** Advances in medical science and technology drive development of evidence-based and values-based practice	Written questions

Element	Title and Content Descriptor	Knowledge, Skills and Attitudes/behaviours	Possible Assessment Methods
10	**Partnership in decision-making**	**K** Consensus and dissensus **S** Applied clinical leadership in dissensus	Written questions OSCE
Universal	**A shared framework for values-based practice**	**K** Basis for balanced decision-making in individual cases	Can only be tested in group exercise

Assessment of the global understanding of values-based practice and the extent to which it has been incorporated into practice relies on the ability to test interrelated elements:

- V-BP elements which are based on clinical skills
- V-BP elements which are based on professional relationships
- V-BP elements which are based on the interrelationship of evidence and values
- The V-BP elements of partnership in decision making

Additionally, clinicians should demonstrate that they have understood the basic premise of values-based practice and the point about shared frameworks for values-based practice.

Index

Entries in blue correspond to terms defined in the Summary, and the page references are included in the Index Spreadsheet available on the website. Bold terms correspond to key terms and corresponding rows in the spreadsheet, while bold numbers indicate a main treatment of a given topic.